David Irving has written a masterpiece of investigation into the mysteries of why people continue to eat a diet that damages their long-term health. This is a must-read for all health-care and public policy professionals, and especially for all students in those fields. Better yet, it is a must-read for anyone who eats.

George Eisman, MA, MSc., RD., Registered Dietician, Coalition for Cancer Prevention

An incisive analysis of current key public health concerns, deserving a must-read recommendation.

Dr. Samuel S. Epstein, author of *The Politics of Cancer, Cancer-Gate: How to Win the Losing Cancer War,* and *What's in Your Milk?* Professor Emeritus at the University of Illinois School of Public Health.

David Irving reveals the science which can eliminate our common chronic killing diseases. His blistering exposé of the politics, institutions, corporations, and governments which are geared to thwart this life-saving message is a powerful read.

Caldwell B. Esselstyn, Jr., MD, author of *Prevent and Reverse Heart Disease.*

Reading and following the message in The Protein Myth *could be the best health insurance policy you could buy for you and your family. This common sense approach to health management will be the best investment you could ever make in your future.*

Howard Lyman, author of *Mad Cowboy: Plain Truth From the Cattle Rancher Who Won't Eat Meat.*

The Protein Myth *dispels misinformation that is making more than a billion people sick and destroying planet Earth. This book will also be a big step to stopping the hazardous high animal food, low-carb craze. Those seeking the truth will find this book a worthwhile read.*
John McDougall, MD, Founder of the McDougall Program.

This book is LONG overdue. For decades, those of us who've made our diet humane and healthy have had to answer the insatiable question, 'but how do you get enough protein?' The simple answer lies within the covers of this book — along with a shocking and gut-provoking exposé of the dangers inherent in the ancient tradition of consuming animal flesh. From human health to animal cruelty to environmental safety to world peace, The Protein Myth challenges us to reconsider our diets and our ethics — both of which are crucial to creating a better world for ourselves and generations to come.
Laura Moretti, Founder & Editor of *The Animals Voice*.

The Protein Myth *is a powerful indictment of the healthcare establishment for ignoring the evidence that could save the lives of millions of people. At the same time, it's a vivid portrayal of how our treatment of animals is ruining the health of the nation and stealing the public's wealth.* The Protein Myth *shows that compassion toward other species is not merely an act of kindness. It is what is required to restore our health and move us toward a world without slavery, genocide or war.*
John Robbins, author of *The New Good Life: Living Better in an Age of Less, The Food Revolution,* and *Diet for a New America.*

The Protein Myth *thoroughly debunks most everything we've been told about food, and does a great job summarizing the latest research, as well as following the money trail that brings such high profits to a few while causing sickness and suffering to so many. This is a great book to help liberate yourself from the medical delusions that harm us, and cause so much animal suffering.*
Will Tuttle, Ph.D., author of # 1 Amazon best-seller, *The World Peace Diet.*

The
Protein
Myth

Significantly Reducing the Risk of Cancer,
Heart Disease, Stroke, and Diabetes
While Saving the Animals and Building
a Better World

The
Protein
Myth

Significantly Reducing the Risk of Cancer,
Heart Disease, Stroke, and Diabetes
While Saving the Animals and Building
a Better World

David Gerow Irving

BOOKS

Winchester, UK
Washington, USA

First published by O-Books, 2011
O-Books is an imprint of John Hunt Publishing Ltd., Laurel House, Station Approach,
Alresford, Hants, SO24 9JH, UK
office1@o-books.net
www.o-books.com

For distributor details and how to order please visit the 'Ordering' section on our website.

Text copyright: David Gerow Irving 2010

ISBN: 978 1 84694 673 8

A CIP catalogue record for this book is available from the British Library.

Design: Stuart Davies

Printed in the UK by CPI Antony Rowe
Printed in the USA by Offset Paperback Mfrs, Inc

CONTENTS

How We Got to Where We Are

Suffer the Little Children

The Road to a Solution

Dedication

To Barbara Priest
whose many years of friendship
inspired this book.

Acknowledgements

To Tysonia Read
with love and appreciation for
always being there whenever needed.

With special thanks to Darrel Irving for his outstanding
critique and insightful reading of the manuscript
and for his wholehearted support and encouragement.

With grateful appreciation to Julie Beckham
and Riccardo Ferreira
for helping to show the way.

To my very special cat friends Goldie Boy, Looney, and
Lewie-Lew Thank you for your amazing companionship.

To all my friends with deepest appreciation.

Correspondence e-mails can be addressed to:
dgsworkshop@earthlink.net

In Remembrance

Laurence Gerow Irving (1900-2002) and
Adeline Thomas Irving (1899-1997)
With much love and gratitude for the influence
of these good people

Ann Irving
1926-2007
Prima donna of aria and song
Leading lyric soprano with the Lyric Opera of Kansas City
Cio-Cio-San (Madama Butterfly), Gilda (Rigoletto),
Lauretta (Gianni Schicchi), Marguerite (Faust),
Mimi (La Boheme), Violetta (La Traviata)

Ann Scofield
1944-1998
Actress, director, therapist, teacher, and
visionary founder of Montreal's Transformative Theater —
workshops for empowering women based on improvisation,
movement, written scripts, storytelling, pantomime, and ritual

Martin Silver
1933-2009
Flutist, Antiquarian, Head Music Librarian
The University of California, Santa Barbara
President, Association for Recorded Sound Collections
Radio show host KCSB-FM: New Releases
from the Arts Library
Representative for employee rights on the
board of Local 2141, AFT

One of the truly good guys in life.
He stood up for what he believed in
whether it was excellence in music performance
or social justice for all people.

Animal Research

Any mention of animal research in this book should in no way be construed as an approval of the practice by the author. In his estimation, it is time to turn the page on the history of animal research and enter a new phase where cures for human disease are sought not by a dependency on defenseless, unconsenting animals, but founded on a growing appreciation of the magnificent diversity of the planet that surrounds us and a deeper comprehension of the profound interrelatedness of all forms of life.

* * *

The man of science, the naturalist, too often loses sight of the essential oneness of all living beings in seeking to classify them in kingdoms, orders, families, genera, species, etc., taking note of the kind and arrangement of limbs, teeth, toes, scales, hair, feathers, etc., measured and set forth in meters, centimeters, and millimeters, while the eye of the Poet, the Seer, never closes on the kinship of all God's creatures, and his heart ever beats in sympathy with great and small alike as "earth-born companions and fellow mortals" equally dependent on Heaven's eternal love.

John Muir

Prelude to Health

In January of 2005 a monumental event happened in the field of healthcare when one of America's most eminent scientists presented compelling evidence to the public that the cause and the means for the prevention of cardiovascular disease, stroke, many forms of cancer, diabetes, and other chronic diseases had been found. Some of these diseases could even be reversed.

The scientist was T. Colin Campbell, and the format in which he presented his evidence was his book *The China Study*. The *New York Times* called it the "Grand Prix of Epidemiology." The book is a report on the author's 20 plus years of research on rural and semi-rural China connecting the various links between nutrition, health, and disease.

Campbell is not the first to study these kinds of relationships. Scientists have been making the connection between nutrition and disease for decades (even centuries), often with little recognition for their efforts. But the Campbell project, arranged by Cornell University, Oxford University, and the Chinese Academy of Preventive Medicine, is the largest and most comprehensive study ever undertaken to analyze the correlation of disease to diet and lifestyle.[1] Its conclusions carry considerable weight and stand prominently as an authority that is not easily dismissed.

The China Study is thorough in its scholarship, human in its perceptions, and penetrating in its analysis. The media described the work as a "landmark study." The Saturday Evening Post said it "should shake up medical and nutrition researchers everywhere."[2]

In June of 2008 Dr. Campbell taped a two-part interview

conducted by Dennis McQuistion for FRTV (Foundation for Responsible Television), a Dallas-based foundation that specializes in presenting programs about "business, social, economic and public policy concerns" that challenge prevailing attitudes.[1] The program was picked up by PBS for broadcast by some of its stations in the ensuing months.

The interview was the first encounter with Campbell for many of the viewers who would tune in to watch the show. What they saw was a scientist who said that not only had his work uncovered overwhelming evidence of the cause of breast cancer and how to greatly reduce the risk of getting it, but that the discovery also applied to many additional forms of cancer as well as to heart disease and heart attacks, stroke, diabetes, and various other chronic diseases.

It would seem that by the time the McQuistion interview was aired, news of this magnitude would already have been broadcast on the major media outlets and displayed in bold headlines in magazines and newspapers all across the country in a way that no one could miss. After all, *The China Study* had been published three years earlier to excellent reviews. But even today with more than 350,000 copies in print and though the book continues to make an impact, thanks to programs like the McQuistion interview and other efforts on the book's behalf, most people have still never heard about Campbell's discoveries. And when they do hear about them it is usually by accident.

The reason is that the healthcare establishment and most of the media have ignored the results of Campbell's work. Why this has happened is a mystery that needs to be unraveled. With so many people suffering and dying from heart disease, heart attacks, stroke, diabetes, osteoporosis, Alzheimer's disease, multiple sclerosis, breast cancer, prostate cancer, colorectal cancer, and other forms of cancer, it seems tragically unfortunate that people have not been informed about the kind of information presented in *The China Study* which could greatly reduce the risk of getting these diseases.

No one can predict, of course, what people will do with any kind of knowledge once they have it, whether they will use it or whether they will pay no attention at all. But one fact remains perfectly clear. There is no plausible reason why the evidence contained in *The China Study* and in other studies of a similar nature should not be out circulating in the public forum and throughout the medical community. People are dying of the killer diseases daily in vast numbers. Yet the means for preventing and even reversing many of these diseases is available backed by solid, scientific evidence that is irrefutable. There is no magic to it, no quackery, no super exotic formula to follow, no special vitamin supplements to take, no drugs, and no surgery.

Why are government healthcare agencies, our major nonprofit health organizations, doctors, and medical professionals not telling the public about this breakthrough? People are just not being offered the information. In the chapters that follow we will examine some of the reasons why this message is having so much difficulty in getting through.

Peeling back the layers of the healthcare establishment to get to the root of matters like these is an eye-opening experience. Often one just finds human nature at work, indifference, prejudice, and resistance to change. But sometimes what lies just below the surface is far from innocent.

As the cases examined in this book bear out, when it comes to nutrition and diet, the medical establishment is all too often a group-think enterprise. Repetition of doctrine and acceptance of institutional authority has ingrained certain theories in the healthcare system so deeply that they dominate the industry. Medical professionals rely upon these concepts for information that they communicate to the public. When theories are inaccurate, however, as is the case for some of the most notable ones, they can have life-threatening consequences.

3

The same can be said about healthcare reports that are supposed to be based upon the most expert research to date, but are, in fact, defective. A famous study done at Harvard University, the Nurses' Health Study, funded by the National Institutes of Health (NIH), turns out to have been conducted on a flawed premise in regard to diet and in the process has misled members of the public, the scientific and academic community, and the media, resulting in far-ranging consequences that continue to make a negative impact on the public health. Other studies like the equally famous Women's Health Initiative Dietary Modification Trial funded by the National Heart, Lung, and Blood Institute (NHLBLI), have done the same.

Investigating the healthcare system turns up many surprises — like opulent fundraising balls for a major cancer organization that end up promoting products that cause cancer. We will attend one of these balls and see for ourselves.

Also, we will examine alternative cancer therapies that for decades the healthcare establishment has been reluctant to test to find out if they are effective or ineffective because of a prevailing "I'm right, you're wrong" mentality. As a result no one knows whether these therapies are any good or not and to what extent they may help, even though many sick and desperate people continue to turn to them as a last resort.

It is equally intriguing to learn how science has sometimes pursued a certain direction for decades, even centuries, based on hypotheses that are never tested until someone finally stands up and says that something does not seem quite right. Only then is the scientific method sent out to test the original hypothesis. Of course, the reason scientists allow this to happen is because there is something in it for themselves that they do not want to give up. What that something is becomes clear upon examination.

The degree to which the thirst for corporate profit and conflicts of interest have hindered finding a cure for the killer diseases also raises important questions that deserve careful scrutiny. Seeing the extent to which ethics and profit are divorced in the pursuit of profit and how this standard has created the massive problems with which the entire world is now confronted is mind-boggling. In this realm corporations and special interests steal the dreams of school children and stuff them with junk food, fill a beguiled public with drugs, misuse the lands of impoverished nations, and torture and abuse innocent animals in research laboratories and on factory farms.

Standing in this land is like being inside an asylum where the keepers have convinced the entire world that insanity is sanity, but where their actions reveal that they are the ones who are insane. This is especially evident on factory farms, in university and medical center animal research laboratories, and in school cafeterias.

Years before T. Colin Campbell wrote *The China Study*, his work and that of other researchers was available to the science and healthcare community through many papers published in peer scientific and academic reviews, yet it was mostly ignored. How many women might have been spared getting breast cancer if they had been aware of these findings? How many men might have escaped prostate cancer? How many people might not have suffered cardiac arrest and stroke? How many amputations for diabetes might never have been performed?

These are not frivolous questions. Knowing that tobacco causes lung cancer and heart disease has provided ample inspiration for many people to stop smoking, erasing the risk of getting the diseases caused by tobacco. Knowing the causes of cancer, heart disease, heart attacks, stroke, and diabetes and how to greatly reduce the risk of getting them can have the same result.

A growing number of scientists, healthcare professionals, and concerned individuals are forging a new path paved by changing concepts of the causes of disease that lead toward greater health for ourselves, our families and loved ones, our society, the country, and the world. This is a journey offering many rewards, none greater than a growing respect for our neighbors at the far corners of the earth and increased understanding of our unity with all forms of life that cohabit our planet.

Part I

The Road to Better Health

How Our Diet Endangers Our Health

Chapter I

The Killer Diseases

Is There a Cure?

We live with the uncomfortable realization that at any moment a phone call can come telling us that one of the major killer diseases has struck someone close to us, our mother or father, our husband or wife, a brother or a sister, a relative, a close friend, a co-worker or an associate, all too often, a child.

The inescapable fact is that Americans of all ages face an obstacle course of health risks over which they are required to run as they simultaneously seek fulfillment in their personal lives. As the years pass by, we can only hope we are able to achieve our personal objectives without disease striking first. Most of us have friends who have fallen along the way. The death toll for the most catastrophic diseases is tragically high.

The American Cancer Society informs us that 565,650 people died of cancer in the year 2008.[1] This represents approximately one quarter of all deaths in the country.

The figures for cardiovascular disease are even more dramatic. According to the American Heart Association, preliminary data shows that of the 2,425,900 deaths in 2006, 829,072 resulted from cardiovascular disease, about 1 in every 2.9 deaths.[2] That's 34.2%. Some 2400 Americans die of cardiovascular disease every day. One death every 37 seconds. It doesn't get any better. Approximately 785,000 people will have their first heart attack this year and 470,000 more will have a recurrent one.

Like the Energizer Bunny, the disasters keep going and going. One in seventeen Americans died of stroke (cerebrovascular disease) last year, the third highest cause of death in the country where about one stroke occurs every 40 seconds. A 2009 report indicates 610,000 people experienced their first stroke in 2008 and another 185,000 had at least their second.[3]

The incidence of another dreaded disease, diabetes, lurks not far behind. The American Diabetes Association tells us that diabetes was the 7th leading cause of death in 2006 with 72,507 reported cases, though death by diabetes goes considerably unreported so that the figure is probably much higher. In 2004, about 71,000 lower-limb amputations were performed on people with diabetes. It is estimated that 23.6 million people, 7.8% of the population, have this disease which is the leading cause of blindness in adults aged 24 to 70 and the leading cause of kidney failure.[4] Many other complications can result from diabetes, especially if uncontrolled, like severe periodontal disease, complications with pregnancy in which excessively large babies are born, and biochemical imbalances that can lead to life-threatening conditions that induce coma.[5]

The landscape portrayed above is not a pretty one. Behind each breath we take lives a nagging disquiet that one of these killer diseases might someday invade our own bodies. If we are fortunate during our lifetimes not to belong to the third of Americans who will fall prey to heart disease, the quarter who will get cancer, the one in seventeen who will suffer a stroke, or the eight percent of the population who will get diabetes, we are still victimized by a kind of nervous apprehension that hovers over our lives with the threat that one of these killer diseases may have already made its way into our system where it is silently at work undermining our health. Then one day a visit to the doctor reveals the bad news we would do anything to avoid hearing. You've got cancer. You've got heart disease. You're bordering on a stroke. Diabetes will force you to have your toes amputated, and who knows how much more will have to be cut away after that, bit by bit.

Some Americans like to think they are number one in everything good when compared to other countries. But the United States also ranks high in things not so good like cancer, heart disease, stroke, diabetes, and other diseases. America ranks only 46th in life expectancy worldwide and our healthcare costs are astronomical.[6] In 1980, $250 billion went to healthcare.[7] By 2006 the figure had risen to two trillion. By the year 2113, it is estimated that healthcare will cost four trillion dollars. In terms of disease and economics, America is in the midst of a health crisis that the nation seems unable to shake. It lumbers ahead like a dinosaur on the way to extinction.

But what if we suddenly learned that all of this could be avoided? What if we didn't have to go through life wondering if we were some kind of ticking time bomb just waiting to go off? What if we could practically eliminate the risk of cancer, heart disease, stroke, and diabetes from our lives entirely? What if we could even greatly reduce the risk of Alzheimer's disease, osteoporosis, macular degeneration, and multiple sclerosis?

This is not only possible, but the path to freedom from these killer diseases that plague our society and our lives has already been discovered, and it is open to everyone free of charge.

But how could that be? If that were true, why haven't we heard of it before? Why have we been permitted to wander in the dark groping for the light when the light switch was there fixed to the wall just waiting to be turned on? Is someone concealing the truth? Those are good questions. Questions this book will try to answer.

In the meantime there is good news. The possibility of significantly reducing the chance of getting one of the major killer diseases really has been discovered and that path has been and continues to be chartered by some of the nation's leading scientists. We will profile one of these scientists in chapter 3 and make reference to his work in other portions of this book. The discovery he and other scientists have made in this area is not hype, it is not fakery, and it is not one more phony diet invented to bring its inventor untold riches. It is rather a journey that leads away from disease and toward greater health that can benefit ourselves, our families and loved ones, our society, the country, the international community, and the planet. But before we meet this scientist and learn a little about what he and his colleagues have discovered, a little background will help.

Chapter 2

The Evolution of the Role of Nutrition in the Treatment of Disease

Government healthcare agencies and nonprofit health organizations like the National Institutes of Health, the National Academy of Sciences, the United States Department of Agriculture, the American Cancer Society, the American Medical Association, the American Heart Association, and other healthcare organizations have known about the nutritional link to chronic disease since at least the 1960s when cardiologists were studying nutrition and making their voices heard about the connection between diet and disease.

The American Heart Association offered diet recommendations to reduce heart disease in the 1970s, and Senator George McGovern's Senate Select Committee on Nutrition and Human Needs issued a major report in reference to heart disease and stroke in 1977.[1,2]

Today, more than thirty years later, much has been learned about diet and nutrition that is well known by the medical establishment that could prevent the occurrence of many diseases. Yet this information has often not been communicated to the public in ways that could make an impact in disease prevention. In fact, news about nutrition is frequently presented to the public in a puzzling and even questionable manner.

The National Cattlemen's Beef Association, the National Dairy Council, and other food lobbyists are only too happy to keep it this way, for if people were fully aware of just how dangerous some of the foods they eat are, the meat and dairy industries might find their profits dwindling rapidly. Meanwhile, because nutritional advice is often contradictory, the public is bewildered, caught in a mass of confusion about what to believe and what not to believe about a healthy diet. For example, one of the premier government healthcare agencies, the Food and Nutrition Board (FNB) of the Institute of Medicine of the National Academy of Sciences, set the upper level for protein intake in its 2002 annual report at 35% (as a percentage of calories). That was 25% higher than the amount recommended the previous 50 years.

No explanation accompanied the new FNB recommendation. It was especially mysterious because of the little known fact that only a 5% to 6% intake of protein is really needed. (This will be more fully explored in chapter 17.) Another rarely disclosed fact is that protein intake within a 10% to 20% range (which is what most people consume) is "associated with a broad array of health risks, especially when most of the protein is from animal sources" which, among other problems, raises blood cholesterol levels.[3] The 35% figure recommended by the FNB was, therefore, excessive in the extreme. Why had the agency suddenly issued this inflated figure for protein consumption that had the potential for damaging the public health?

One possible explanation was that some members of the FNB panel were thought to have been sympathizers with the Atkins Diet (an "extreme" diet based on high protein consumption). Another reason for consideration was that the chair of the panel left the committee "shortly before its completion for a senior executive position in a very large food company," the kind that would benefit from a high protein recommendation. Other facts that emerged were that some panel members either were not aware the recommendation had been made and had not participated in the decision, or knew almost nothing about nutrition.[4,5] It seems likely that a mixture of these factors, lack of knowledge, biases, poor management, and conflicts of interest, may all have been involved in making the FNB recommendation to up protein intake to 35%.

Conflicts of interest and biases all too often do play a role in the health advice that gets transmitted to the public, sometimes taking control so completely that the public is entirely misled. This creates a sense of ambivalence for the public which has grown suspicious about the wisdom of relying upon the healthcare organizations. (See chapter 8 and chapters 14 and 15 for a closer examination of some of these biases and conflicts of interest.)

A major feature in the debate about diet and disease is the reluctance of doctors to give nutrition its due. Many physicians are predisposed against nutrition from the onset of their careers. This is encouraged by the medical profession itself as demonstrated by the following. In 1961, nearly 50 years ago, "the American Medical Association Council on Foods and Nutrition reported that nutrition in the U.S. medical schools received inadequate recognition, support and attention." Little had changed by 1985 when the National Research Council disclosed that doctors received only about two credits worth of nutrition training in their entire medical school careers.[6] The same conditions still prevail today with "the medical status quo [continuing to rely] heavily on medication and surgery at the exclusion of nutrition and lifestyle."[7] Doctors just do not believe that nutrition is important and seldom mention it to their patients.

Prejudice and indifference toward nutrition within the medical profession has influenced and divided the healthcare industry. On the side that has the upper hand, doctors and scientists commit to healthcare treatment and research through drugs and surgery. This has created an enormous money-attracting industry with skyrocketing costs for finding new drugs and the development of surgical procedures at the expense of sick people who have to suffer through them and pay exorbitantly for the treatment. However, another side has made its presence felt. Here treatment is reflected in the search for the underlying cause of disease from environmental and other external factors including nutrition. In recent years this side has placed a major emphasis on the investigation of food and its role in promoting and reducing disease.

Conflicts between the two sides is part of the reason why the healthcare establishment is unable to supply the public with a unified approach to better health upon which the public can rely. At the present time drugs and surgery have the upper hand, but nutrition is gaining ground.

The quest to find the causes of various diseases dates far into the past. Egyptian healers were discussing tumors as early as 1500 BCE.[8] A few centuries later a physician came along who named the disease. This was Hippocrates (460-377 BCE). He thought cancer was an "imbalance of bodily 'humors' caused by an excess of black bile that resulted from improper diet and exercise and the vagaries of climate, age, and season."[9],[10] Following Hippocrates, the physician Galen (129 – 199 CE) also thought a strict dietary regimen was necessary to restore the body's "humors" in the elimination of cancer and believed certain nutrients like walnuts should be avoided.

Since Galen many other theories have been investigated, but the role of nutrition in disease formation frequently emerges as one of the prime suspects.

In the 16th and 17th centuries physicians sought to broaden the search and suggested that cancer might result from alchemical arsenic, bumps and bruises, arterial blockages, or emotional stress. In 1676, Richard Wiseman, a prominent English surgeon, wrote that diet could promote cancer, especially the consumption of meat and alcohol.[11] (It would take another three centuries for this idea to really gain a firm foothold, but today all the major healthcare organizations recognize the connection of meat and alcohol to cancer and disease to some degree.)

By the 18th century physicians were taking note of environmental factors in instigating disease by linking substances like lead and mercury to the poisoning of potters and gilders (crafts people who applied overlays of gold or gilt onto various objects). These physicians continued to keep a watchful eye open for the causes of cancer and connected soot with the high occurrence of cancer in chimney sweeps.[12] In the 19th century statistical research showed that cancer incidence was higher in Paris than in the suburbs (an early epidemiological study).[13] The search for causes and cures sometimes bordered on the exotic. For example, in 1910 President William Howard Taft urged Congress to spend $50,000 to determine if drinking water from trout-fed streams was a major cause of cancer.[14] Congress turned him down.

During the latter half of the 20th century, concerns about radon gas in basements, electromagnetic fields from high-voltage wires, dental X-rays, hair dye, radiation from television sets, and asbestos in buildings captured the headlines and the imagination as being possible, and in some cases, probable causes of cancer.[15] People also worried whether nutrients like barbecued meats, peanut butter, spinach, and bruised broccoli contained natural carcinogens. They wondered if low-level ionizing radiation from flying in airplanes increased cancer risk. Did chlorinated water cause bladder and rectal cancer? Did drinking beer and alcoholic beverages pose a threat? Were the chances of getting breast cancer raised by having an abortion? What about breast feeding? Did that lower the risk of breast cancer? These kinds of questions and their resolution or lack of one have been raised in recent years only to fade from the headlines, at least momentarily, though they linger in memory while many concerns remain unresolved.

Meanwhile, new questions continue to emerge. Does red meat and pesticides in sushi and salmon put people at risk for non-Hodgkin's lymphoma? Do computers emit radiation that could contribute to cancer? Do cell phones pose a risk?

The role of pollutants, carcinogens, chemicals, and pesticides in the development of cancer continues as a topic of debate. Generally, their risk potential is dependent upon their relation to each individual — smoking, for example. Causes are sometimes group-specific, as in the case of workers who develop lung cancer from working with arsenic and uranium. At other times a large segment of the public is affected, like an overall Japanese susceptibility to stomach cancer related to the Japanese diet.[16]

Nutrition poked its head into the discussion circle and started insisting on a place at the table in 1977 with the McGovern report mentioned above. This was followed in 1982 by a National Academy of Sciences report on *Diet, Nutrition, and Cancer.* (Both of these reports will be referred to in more detail in coming chapters.)

Since then diet and nutrition has become a major component of healthcare and has established itself as a fixture in the debate on finding a cure for the most notorious diseases. It is especially appealing because individuals have some control over the nutrients that affect their health, which often cannot be said about environmental factors.

A collection of government healthcare agencies, nonprofit health organizations, university medical centers, hospitals, and medical practitioners and administrators make up that portion of the U.S. medical establishment concerned with eliminating debilitating diseases from our lives. These are government agencies like the National Institutes of Health including the National Cancer Institute and the National Heart, Lung, and Blood Institute; the National Academy of Sciences and the Institute of Medicine (including the Food and Nutrition Board); the United States Department of Agriculture; and the Food and Drug Administration. They also include nonprofit healthcare organizations like the American Cancer Society, the American Heart Association, the American Diabetes Association, and the American Medical Association. And they include hospitals, medical centers, and university and private research facilities, plus an army of physicians, nurses, medical practitioners, medical writers, and administrative personnel, all functioning in a variety of medical settings.[17]

The purpose of this healthcare establishment is to find, treat, cure, and prevent disease and to keep the public informed. But individuals and groups who supervise the healthcare organizations sometimes become entrenched in organizational protocols, and a kind of group-think takes over making progress in achieving national health-care goals difficult to achieve. When that happens the public suffers and information that could save people much anxiety and misery either gets buried (sometimes intentionally) or somehow falls through the cracks. Not many people are aware, for example, that "impressive evidence now exists to show that advanced heart disease, relatively advanced cancers of certain types, diabetes and a few other degenerative diseases can be reversed by diet."[18] These are the words of Dr. T. Colin Campbell in his landmark study on nutrition, *The China Study*, which he wrote with his son Thomas.

The Campbells and a handful of other pioneering scientists and researchers have put their cards on the table that demonstrate to the healthcare establishment and the public in terms that cannot be scientifically refuted that the cause of the major killer diseases has been uncovered. To date, the healthcare profession has been ignoring this information because it steps on the toes of established interests that, for reasons we shall explore, are resistant to change.

If people want to continue along the path of healthcare that for many ends in unnecessary drugs, surgery, and, all too often, death, that is one choice that is available. But if people want to take a new path that offers relief from the failed policies of a healthcare system that, after decades of trial and error, has yet to find a cure for the major killer diseases, that should also be a choice that is theirs to make.

Chapter 3

Introducing Dr. Campbell

The Discovery of a Dark Secret

At the beginning of his career, T. Colin Campbell, the Jacob Gould Schurman Professor Emeritus of Nutritional Biochemistry at Cornell University, could never have imagined that nutrition played any role in the cause or prevention of disease. Nor could he have foreseen that one day he would compile the results of a 40 year career investigating the subject in a book he would title *The China Study*.

"I started at the opposite end of the spectrum," Campbell says, "as a meat-loving dairy farmer in my personal life and an "establishment" scientist in my professional life. I even used to lament the views of vegetarians as I taught nutritional biochemistry to pre-med students."[1]

T. Colin Campbell grew up on a Virginia dairy farm where he learned to work the fields, drive a team of horses, and herd cattle. Like many Virginia farm boys, he hunted, fished, and developed a strong sense of independence. His mother raised the family from produce that grew in the garden, and livestock that fed in the barnyard and grazed in the pastures.

Early in life Campbell learned that cow's milk built strong, healthy bones and teeth. He had no reason to question his diet or to think that dairy products could be linked to "prostate cancer, diabetes, osteoporosis, multiple sclerosis or other autoimmune diseases, or to worry about how casein, the main protein in dairy foods, has been shown to experimentally promote cancer and increase blood cholesterol and atherosclerotic plaque."[2] Like almost everyone else in every other generation of Americans, he gave little thought to the food he ate so long as it followed general societal norms.

Campbell was the first in his family to go to college. He studied pre-veterinary medicine at Penn State University and afterwards attended veterinary school at the University of Georgia. Then Cornell University offered him a scholarship to do graduate research in animal nutrition. Eventually he gained considerable recognition working at the Massachusetts Institute of Technology where he helped discover dioxin, part of the herbicide in Agent Orange, and "arguably the most toxic chemical ever found."[3]

When Campbell left MIT he took a faculty position at Virginia Tech and "began coordinating technical assistance for a nationwide project in the Philippines working with malnourished children." Part of the project was to discover the cause of an "unusually high prevalence of liver cancer, usually an adult disease, in Filipino children." The suspected villain was one of the most potent carcinogens known, "aflatoxin," a corn and peanuts mold toxin.[4]

For ten years the objective of the Philippines project was to ensure adequate nutrition for the Filipino children specifically by getting them to consume as much protein as possible since it was commonly thought that malnutrition in children was caused by a lack of protein, particularly animal protein. During the project, however, Campbell discovered what he calls "a dark secret." The secret was that "children who ate the highest-protein diets were the ones most likely to get cancer. They were the children of the wealthiest families."[5]

This was Campbell's first discovery on his journey of scientific ground-breaking in the field of nutrition. It was a journey that would teach him that cancer and other diseases could be prevented and reversed by diet.

Campbell tells us that after discovering the negative effects too much protein had on Filipino children, he next noticed a research report from India that had studied two groups of rats. He relates that:

> ...in one group, [the Indian researchers] administered the cancer-causing aflatoxin [discussed above in relation to Filipino children], then fed [the rats] a diet that was composed of 20% protein, a level near what many of us consume in the West. In the other group, they administered the same amount of aflatoxin, but then fed [them] a diet that was only composed of 5% protein. Incredibly, every single animal that consumed the 20% protein diet had evidence of liver cancer, and every single animal that consumed a 5% protein diet avoided liver cancer. It was a 100 to 0 score, leaving no doubt that nutrition trumped chemical carcinogens, even very potent carcinogens, in controlling cancer.[6]

The information that Campbell was learning went against everything he had been taught and was the defining moment in his career. He tells us that "it was heretical to say that protein wasn't healthy, let alone say it promoted cancer....Questioning protein and animal-based foods in general ran the risk of my being labeled a heretic, even if it passed the test of 'good science.'"

The discovery prompted Campbell "to start an in-depth laboratory program that would investigate the role of nutrition, especially protein, in the development of cancer."[7] He conducted his own tests with aflatoxin. What Campbell learned was "shocking." He found that:

> ...low-protein diets inhibited the initiation of cancer by aflatoxin, regardless of how much of this carcinogen was administered to these animals....Low protein diets also dramatically blocked subsequent cancer growth....In fact,

dietary protein proved to be so powerful in its effect that we could turn on and turn off cancer growth simply by changing the level consumed...casein, which makes up 87% of cow's milk protein, promoted all stages of the cancer process...the safe proteins were from plants, including wheat and soy.[8]

Campbell tells how the picture that emerged began to "challenge and then to shatter some of [his] most cherished assumptions."

One of the problems with animal studies, however, besides being objectionable to an increasingly large segment of the public, is that tests on animals cannot be considered reliable unless "the appropriate epidemiological study has been done and its results are conclusive beyond doubt — which is rare," according to Professor Samuel S. Epstein, Professor Emeritus of Occupational and Environmental Medicine at the School of Public Health at the University of Illinois Medical Center at Chicago.[9]

Campbell was also aware that his hypothesis needed to be corroborated and correlated accurately with epidemiological studies. By a stroke of luck, Dr. Junshi Chen, one of the first Chinese scholars to visit the United States following the opening of relations between China and the United States in late 1978, was sent to Dr. Campbell's lab at Cornell University.

In the 1970's Chou EnLai, the Premier of China, was dying of cancer and had initiated a monumental survey of death rates of twelve different kinds of cancer in 2400 Chinese counties involving 880 million citizens.[10] This represented 96% of the entire population of China. It resulted in a color-coded atlas showing where cancer rates were high and where they were almost non-existent all across China.[11]

As they became better acquainted, Chen and Campbell discovered their mutual interest in investigating the causes of disease based on nutrition, and the color-coded atlas provided the perfect underpinning for such an undertaking. The two scholars began to frame a plan that would lead to what turned out to be the largest epidemiological study ever done. They assembled a team that consisted of Dr. Chen, who was the deputy director of the most important government diet and health research laboratory in China, Dr. Junayao Li, one of the authors of the color-coded Cancer Atlas Survey inaugurated by Chou EnLai and a top scientist in China's Academy of Medical Sciences in the Ministry of Health, Richard Peto of Oxford University, one of the premier epidemiologists in the world (he has since been knighted and has received several awards for cancer research), and Dr. Campbell himself.[12]

Campbell says that he likes to practice the type of science that originated 2400 years ago by the Father of Medicine, Hippocrates, who said, 'There are, in effect, two things: to know and to believe one knows. To know is science. To believe one knows." is ignorance."[13] That is the kind of foundation upon which *The China Study* is based. It "is largely empirical, obtained through observation and measurement. It is not illusory, hypothetical or anecdotal; it is from legitimate research findings."[14]

Campbell illustrates the procedures he followed:

My colleagues and I were cautious in framing our hypotheses, rigorous in our methodology and conservative in interpreting our findings. I chose to do this research at a very basic science level, studying the biochemical details of cancer formation....By carefully following the rules of good science, I was able to study a provocative topic without provoking knee-jerk responses that arise with radical ideas....Then our results were reviewed...for publication in many of the best scientific journals.

The China project surveyed a vast range of diseases and diet and lifestyle factors in rural China. The following describes some of the results.

A plant-based diet high in carbohydrates and fiber protects against and dramatically lowers the risk of the major killer diseases. Campbell refers to the diseases caused by the consumption of animal protein and fats as "diseases of affluence" because these are the diseases which people living in affluent countries are prone to get and die from. They are heart disease [and stroke], cancer (colon, lung, breast, brain, stomach, liver, esophageal, leukemia), and diabetes.[15] According to statistics taken from the American Cancer Society, in an affluent country like America where animal protein and fat consumption is high, males have a significantly high chance of getting cancer (47%), and females are not far behind (38%).[16]

Poorer societies fall victim to what Campbell terms "diseases of poverty," not because of diet, but because of other factors like the environment, prenatal care, malnutrition, and their healthcare system. These diseases are pneumonia, intestinal obstruction, peptic ulcer, digestive disease, pulmonary tuberculosis, parasitic disease, rheumatic heart disease, metabolic and endocrine disease other than diabetes, diseases of pregnancy, and many others.[17]

People living in poorer countries consume little animal protein and live largely on a plant-based diet. But when these countries manage to climb the economic scale of achievement to enter the ranks of the affluent nations, they soon become subject to the diseases of affluent nations, and their citizens die accordingly.[18] That is because their diets change from one that is based on plants to one that is based on animals.

It defies the imagination that our healthcare organizations and medical researchers have not eagerly welcomed these discoveries about animal protein that could save so many lives. On the contrary, they resist learning about them, and, in some cases, as we shall see, do their best to discredit the research. Yet scientists have consistently made and continue to make the same kinds of observations.

In 1981, world-renowned epidemiologist Sir Richard Doll, working with Richard Peto, completed studies showing that approximately 30 percent of cancer is diet related, second only to smoking as a principal cause.[19] (Peto would later become a member of Campbell's China team.)

A University of Oxford Vegetarian Study conducted between 1980 and 1984 comparing 6000 vegetarians and 5000 non-vegetarians with cross-sectional vegan analysis revealed that vegans had lower LDL (bad) cholesterol levels with intermediate values for the vegetarians. [The diet of vegetarians may include some animal products. Vegans consume no animal products.] The non-meat eaters also had a lower mortality rate for heart disease and cancer, with a higher death rate from heart disease associated with total animal fat, saturated animal fat, and dietary cholesterol.[20] A fourteen year study completed in 1988 of 34,000 Seventh-Day Adventists in California against other Californians showed that the people who avoided meat, fish, and poultry had a far lower incidence of prostate, ovarian, and colon cancer than meat-eaters.[21] An 11 year study done in Germany that was finished in 1992 reported that 1,904 vegetarians and persons leading a healthy life style had less cancer than half of the population, with less ischemic heart disease for strict vegetarians who avoided meat.[22] (Ischemic refers to a blockage, stoppage, or constriction of a blood vessel leading to decreased blood flow to bodily tissue or an organ.) In addition, the Physicians Committee for Responsible Medicine, in assessing a 1994 study in the United Kingdom, showed that "cancer rates for vegetarians are 25 to 50 percent below population averages, even after controlling for smoking, body mass index, and socioeconomic status."[23]

The trend is unmistakable. A study in the British Medical

Journal made in 1998 noted that about half of lung, bowel, breast, and prostate cancer deaths in the United Kingdom were virtually absent in much of the developing world, and that migrants from the developing world began to develop these diseases once they moved from low risk to high risk areas.[24] The study concluded that these cancers should be largely preventable.

The link between animal protein and disease has been reported by a number of other sources as well, and the evidence continues to mount. A 2006 study at Harvard involving 135,000 people revealed that those who ate grilled skinless chicken had a 52 percent higher chance of developing bladder cancer than those who did not.[25] Concerning breast cancer, a 2007 study of more than 35,000 women published in the British Journal of Medicine found that women who ate the most meat were more likely to develop the disease.[26] And, in the same journal, an earlier study found that "up to 80% of bowel and breast cancer may be preventable by dietary change."[27] Pancreatic cancer has also now been identified with the consumption of animal protein. In the Journal of the National Cancer Institute, researchers recently reported that people with the most animal fat in their diets had a higher risk for developing this killer disease. According to the study, researchers "observed positive associations between pancreatic cancer and intakes of total, saturated and monosaturated fat overall, particularly from red meat and dairy food sources." The researchers "did not observe any consistent association with polyunsaturated or fat from plant food sources."[28]

As significant as these kind of studies appear to be, such evidence seems to mean little to the American Cancer Society which states that it "it is not possible to conclude at this time [2006]...that a vegetarian diet has any special benefits for the prevention of cancer."[29]

This, in general, describes the attitude of mainstream

healthcare thinking. When this position is examined closely, though, as it will be in this book, it cannot withstand careful scrutiny. It becomes further untenable in light of breakthroughs in disease prevention involving nutrition that the public has begun to pick up on and recognize as having real applicability to their personal lives. This includes the work of Dr. Caldwell B. Esselstyn, Jr., and Dr. Dean Ornish, whose work will be examined more closely in chapter 10. These physicians have proved conclusively that heart disease can be arrested and reversed through nutrition by means of a plant-based diet. Nutritional disease prevention and reversal therapy like this has also been successfully carried out for prostate cancer (Dr. Ornish), and diabetes. (See chapter 10.)

In the United States and Western societies, where most people die from diseases of affluence, they are already free from the tyranny of diseases of poverty. But they also have the opportunity to escape the tyranny of the diseases of affluence. As the facts now undeniably show, all they have to do is to stop consuming a high-fat, animal-based protein diet and change to one that is plant-based.

Chapter 4

Got Cancer?

The American Cancer Society

The American Cancer Society in the largest nonprofit health organization in America. Its job is to encourage early cancer screening and diagnosis, maintain research and education programs, supply the public with the latest information and most up-to-date and effective recommendations for cancer treatment, and engage in nation-wide fundraising efforts.

Founded in 1913 as the American Society for the Control of Cancer, the organization changed its name to the American Cancer Society in 1946. It grew from a small group of concerned medical practitioners and laypersons into an organization that at one point had a House of Delegates with 194-members and a National Board of Directors with 116-members. Presently, it is governed by a National Assembly with 78 delegates drawn from 13 Divisions and a National Board of Directors consisting of 43 Directors. Up to 12 past officer delegates may also be called upon for votes in the National Assembly along with some non-voting honorary life members. Leadership of the ACS includes doctors and scientists in conjunction with executive officers and directors of banks, insurance companies, advertising firms, and pharmaceutical corporations.[1]

Today the American Cancer Society gets high marks from many sources for its work in fighting against tobacco use. That is one of the society's highest priorities, although this has not always been true. Prior to 1962 the ACS would admit that only a possible link existed between smoking and lung cancer and even worked with tobacco companies in trying to build a safer cigarette (as opposed to working to ban tobacco altogether like many citizen's groups and other organizations were doing). But in 1962 the Royal College of Physicians in England shook the healthcare establishment and the public by announcing that "cigarette smoking is a cause of lung cancer and bronchitis, and probably contributes to the development of coronary heart disease and various other less common diseases."[2] The ACS followed suit, switching from its previous stance of tobacco tolerance to one in which it denounced smoking as "a major cause of lung cancer." Two years later the United States Surgeon General joined in, declaring that smoking was responsible for a 70 percent increase in the mortality rate over non-smokers, that smoking was responsible for chronic bronchitis with a correlation to emphysema and heart disease, that smokers had a nine to ten times increased risk of developing lung cancer, with heavy smokers having a 20 percent risk, and that the risk rose according to the duration of smoking and decreased with the cessation of smoking.[3]

The combined force of these censures made a major impact in the war against tobacco, the Surgeon General's report being the final straw. Within three months of the announcement smoking had declined by 20 percent nationwide. Panicked, the tobacco industry began a campaign of obfuscation and deceit aimed at preventing any limitations from being placed on tobacco, including advertising aimed at children.

Tobacconists were often aided in their survival efforts by government agencies like the USDA, which for over a century has been openly offering tobacco allotments (price support and production controls) to tobacco farmers. Critics say this is nothing but a subsidy for the tobacco industry. Private corporations like the American Medical Association (AMA), anxious not to lose lucrative tobacco advertising contracts, also supported tobacco.[4] But mostly the tobacco industry was put on the defensive. It managed to sustain itself by raising doubts about the accuracy of anti-tobacco cancer reports and by demanding absolute proof for any claims targeting tobacco.[5] Doubts can be voiced about anything, no matter how absurd they are, and this was the strategy the tobacco companies relied upon for survival. The opposition to tobacco was caught off guard by the extent to which the tobacco companies would go to try to discredit the truth. Even as recently as 1994 the heads of the major tobacco companies swore before a congressional subcommittee that tobacco might not be a cause of cancer after all and that nicotine was not addictive.[6]

After initially denouncing tobacco the ACS had a change of heart and soon backed away, according to some critics, including Lester Breslow, who in those days was Dean of the UCLA School of Public Health and President of the American Public Health Association.[7] In speaking about the early 1970s Breslow said "the ACS directly delayed many things that could have helped a lot of people back then. They kept reports on the hazards of smoking locked up a lot longer than they should have. They delayed getting the Pap smear in use. They had a lot to be embarrassed about, and they weren't the only ones."[8]

Part of the problem was due to conflicting loyalties. For example, until he resigned his post in 1993, ACS lobbyist for Pennsylvania, Eugene F. Knopf, was working behind the scenes in support of tobacco and tried to get the ACS to back a Pennsylvania law that prevented localities from limiting smoking in public places. His loyalties surfaced when he announced his resignation from the ACS, stating that "the reason for my withdrawal is that I am being retained by the American Tobacco Institute." As a registered lobbyist for tobacco, Knopf was paid $85,000 a year up until 1996.[9]

Forty-seven years after the Surgeon General's 1964 report, smoking has decreased in the United States, but not enough to prevent 20 percent of the adult population from continuing the deadly addiction which still accounts for 443,000 deaths annually.

As for the ACS, many believe the agency has succeeded in weeding out internal conflicts of interest along with officials who were wedded to tobacco companies and has evolved into an organization committed to an aggressive policy that fully addresses the tobacco menace.[10] Today the ACS carefully monitors tobacco expansion and keeps the public alerted to the facts about tobacco such as that smoking accounts for more deaths than alcohol, car accidents, suicide, AIDS, homicides, and illegal drugs all put together.[11]

The ACS also keeps track of smoking in the developing world where the tobacco industry has sought to compensate for its revenue losses in the Western world by gradually and steadily carving out new customer bases. This has resulted in more and more deaths from lung cancer. Trying to keep pace, world health organizations are now calling on the United States to help ratify an international tobacco control treaty in an effort to reign in tobacco proliferation.[12]

The ACS hopes to do its part. John Seffrin, the CEO of the ACS, said that "if we take action, we can keep the numbers from going where they would otherwise go."[13]

Tobacco use has grown rapidly with all too little opposition in Asia, and Seffrin notes that forty percent of the world's smokers now live in China and Japan. In China, home to 350 million smokers, people who smoke already outnumber the entire population of the United States. One program the ACS plans to inaugurate is a smoking cessation counseling service in India, where 250 million smokers live.

Tobacco is succeeding beyond its wildest expectations. Five million people now die from smoking-related illnesses worldwide with the number growing every year.[14]

Global efforts in which the ACS is involved, like the counseling service in India, plus domestic programs at home that include state tobacco control programs, national smoke-out days, and smoking cessation hotlines, lead the casual observer to conclude that the ACS position on tobacco today is far different than in the past. A general perception prevails that CEO Seffrin and the ACS are knights in shining armor that deserve laurels and wreaths for their aggressive stand against tobacco.

Yet criticisms and doubts remain. One reason is that the ACS has been unable to shake off its past history of coziness with the tobacco companies. Professor Samuel Epstein (briefly introduced in chapter 3), an outspoken critic of the ACS, wrote in an article titled "American Cancer Society: The World's Wealthiest Non-Profit Institution," that the ACS spends most of its money on overhead, salaries and fringe benefits, but little on cancer prevention and education. In an interview with Amy Goodman on PBS's *Democracy Now* in the year 2000, Epstein accused the agency of spending only $1,000,000 for tobacco related programs out of a total budget of $700,000,000 and said that ACS salaries were "bloated."[15] As a consultant to the U.S. Senate Committee on Public Works and recipient of the 2005 Albert Schweitzer Golden Grand Medal "for Humanitarianism, and International Contributions to Cancer Prevention," Epstein's panning of the ACS is not easily brushed aside. Items that emerge such as that according to a December 2008 report by the American Institute of Philanthropy, CEO Seffrin's salary was $953,132, indicate that Epstein's allegations are not without merit.[16] Further, Epstein's criticisms directly contradict the ACS claim it has staked out over the past few years that it is a major player in the fight against tobacco and lung cancer.

Is the ACS commitment to fighting tobacco and lung cancer real or is it hype? And if the agency is getting more credit than it deserves, then how involved is it in fighting other forms of cancer?

Today, there is no need for stripping tobacco of protectionist organizations. Nonprofit healthcare organizations no longer dare hold hands with the industry. Everyone knows that tobacco causes lung cancer, cardiovascular disease, emphysema, chronic bronchitis, and many other health problems.

But what about the latest enemies destroying the public's health that we have been focusing on, meat and dairy foods. Only a few progressive doctors and scientists have dared to challenge and speak out publicly against these products, along with a small body of concerned citizens and private organizations. Because it is a major player in the debate about cancer, it is important to determine what kind of a role the American Cancer Society plays in this endeavor, whether it is contributing to the cause or whether it is once again siding with the enemy by limiting its opposition and supporting the parent industries responsible for this plague like it did with tobacco.

It was back in 2005 that T. Colin Campbell's *The China Study* first showed conclusively that there was a definitive link between animal protein and cancer and other diseases. Not only is his study incontestable, he has published many other articles on the subject dating back more than a decade. It would hardly be possible for the American Cancer Society, or for that matter, the other healthcare organizations, not to be aware of Campbell's work and that of other researchers doing similar studies. Just as studies linking tobacco with cancer were known to the healthcare establishment years before the 1964 Surgeon General confirmed the indisputable connection, studies today have also revealed the unmistakable link between animal protein and cancer. So how has the ACS responded to this evidence?

One of the surest ways to answer this question is by examining the nutrition recommendations the ACS makes in regard to some of the most notorious cancers like breast cancer, colorectal cancer, and prostate cancer. The ACS issued specific cancer prevention guidelines in 2006 in *Ca*, the society's official journal, titled *Reducing the Risk of Cancer with Healthy Food Choices and Physical Activity*. These are guidelines that the ACS publishes every five years which it describes as being "consistent with guidelines from the American Heart Association and the American Diabetes Association for the prevention of coronary heart disease and diabetes, as well as for general health promotion, as defined by the Department of Health and Human Services' 2005 *Dietary Guidelines for Americans.*"[17]

The following is the advice that the ACS offers in this publication for reducing the risk of getting breast cancer.

Although reduction of fat intake to very low levels may reduce breast cancer risk, results from the recent intervention trial found that lowering fat intake to 29% of calories had only a very small effect on risk among postmenopausal women. At the present time, the best nutritional advice to reduce the risk of breast cancer is to engage in moderate to vigorous physical activity 45 to 60 minutes on 5 or more days per week, minimize lifetime weight gain through the combination of caloric restriction and regular physical activity, and avoid or limit intake of alcoholic beverages. [18]

According to these guidelines, the only advice the ACS can offer to women for reducing the risk of getting breast cancer is to try not to gain too much weight by doing moderate or vigorous physical activity 45 to 60 minutes daily at least 5 days a week, to restrict caloric intake, and to not drink too much alcohol, if at all. Reducing fat intake to very low levels may also reduce breast cancer risk, but this can only have a very small effect and that is for postmenopausal women.

Is this some kind of bad joke? This is all that millions of research dollars and years of investigative scientific research has produced to inform women what to do to reduce the risk of getting breast cancer? If this is where we stand, we have advanced little from the days over 200 years ago when medical practitioners like George Bell (an English surgeon (1788)) speculated that "breast cancer might be caused by a 'languid circulation' occasioned by an arterial blockage, by a sudden or intense cold, or by anger, fear or anxiety acting to impede the circulation, especially in 'the delicate frame of the female sex.'"[19]

Some might contend that the ACS advice is all that can be expected considering that no cure for breast cancer has yet been found. They would point out that the ACS goes to great lengths to report the known facts and all mainstream research findings about all forms of cancer, including breast cancer, in some detail. And they would be correct. But compare the above recommendations with the ones offered in the Campbell study:

Eating diets higher in animal-based foods...expand [a woman's] reproductive life by about nine to ten years[20]....The risk of breast cancer increases when a woman has early age of menarche (first menstruation), late age of menopause, high levels of female hormones in the blood, and high cholesterol. A diet high in animal foods and refined carbohydrates lowers the age of menarche, raises the age of menopause, increases female hormone levels, and increases blood cholesterol levels....There is overwhelming evidence that estrogen levels are a critical determinant of breast cancer risk. Estrogen directly participates in the cancer process. It also tends to indicate the presence of other female hormones that play a role in breast cancer risk. Increased levels of estrogen and related hormones are a result of the consumption of typical Western diets, high in fat and animal protein and low in dietary fiber....This suggests that the risk of breast cancer is preventable if we eat foods that will keep estrogen levels under control. The sad truth is that most women simply are not aware of this evidence.[21]

The ACS *Ca* journal's cancer prevention guidelines for breast cancer makes no reference to the connection of raised levels of estrogen to nutrition, or how a low-fat diet that eliminates animal protein can reduce estrogen levels, and, consequently, breast cancer risk.

If the American Cancer Society wants to be reliable and credible, it must report the known fact that the consumption of animal protein is a major factor in breast cancer risk just as smoking is in lung cancer risk. Breast cancer will be diagnosed in 25 million women over the next 25 years.[22] Women need to know that nutrition can be used to lower estrogen levels in order to limit their risk of becoming one of those statistics. And they need to know that the "consumption of typical Western diets, high in fat and animal protein and low in dietary fiber" results in increased levels of estrogen and related hormones.

How the ACS guidelines approach another deadly cancer, colorectal cancer, offers further insight into the efficacy of the ACS guidelines for reducing cancer risk.

Colorectal cancer is the fourth most common cancer in the world and the second most common in the United States. Six to seven percent of Americans will get this disease during their lifetimes.[23]

Studies done three decades ago indicated that increased meat consumption was associated with far higher rates of colon cancer. A famous project called *The Seven Countries Study* showed that an increase of fiber by ten grams daily lowered the long-term risk of colon cancer by 33%.[24] Ten grams is equal to about a cup of fruit, beans, or peas, a pretty fair price for some major insurance against colorectal cancer. Other studies showed that those who ate the most fiber had a 43% lower risk of colon cancer than those who consumed the least fiber.[25] Similarly, those who ate the most vegetables had a 52% lower risk than those who ate the least vegetables.

T. Colin Campbell puts it this way.

What is clear is that diets naturally high in fiber and low in animal based foods can prevent colorectal cancer....*The data clearly shows that a whole foods, plant-based diet can dramatically lower colorectal cancer rates. We don't need to know which fiber is responsible, what mechanism is involved or even how much of the effect is independently due to fiber.*[26] [Emphasis by T. Colin Campbell]

But consider what the ACS guidelines recommend nutritionally as a means for reducing the risk of getting colon cancer. After assessing the various factors involved, the agency concludes that:

Diets high in vegetables and fruits have been associated with decreased risk, and diets high in processed and/or red meat have been associated with increased risk of colon cancer....The best nutritional advice to reduce the risk of colon cancer is to increase the intensity and duration of physical activity; limit intake of red and processed meat; consume recommended levels of calcium; eat more vegetables and fruits; avoid obesity; and avoid excess alcohol consumption (e.g., no more than one drink/day in women, two drinks/day in men).[27]

Nutritionally, this recommendation suggests only that "limiting" the intake of red and processed meat and "eating more" vegetables and fruits and recommended levels of calcium are associated with decreased risk for colon cancer. The very important role played by fiber, which comes from plant foods, not animal foods, in reducing the risk of colon cancer is not even mentioned. That is because the ACS does not recognize fiber as playing a major role in reducing cancer risk.

In another section discussing whole grains, the report reads: "data for an association between fiber and cancer risk are limited." There the ACS does, at least, recognize fiber as a risk factor in diabetes, cardiovascular disease, and diverticulitis prevention, in fact, enthusiastically. But it is not about to prescribe fiber as a means for lowering cancer risk since its investigation shows only a weak association with cancer. Therefore, the ACS does not even mention fiber in connection with colon cancer. Anyone relying on the ACS recommendation for colon cancer would never learn about the connection between fiber and reduced risk for colon cancer.

An American Cancer Society review of a January 11, 2005 report titled "Eating Lots of Red Meat Linked to Cancer: Risk Less than Posed by Obesity" that was published in the *Journal of the American Medical Association*, discusses the results of a long-term study of nearly 149,000 adults between the ages of 50 and 74 in relation to colon cancer.[28] It tells us that "eating large amounts of red or processed meat over a long period of time can raise colorectal cancer risk."[29] The co-author of the report, Michael Thun, MD, MS, chief of epidemiology and surveillance research at the ACS, assured, however, that "this is not a condemnation of red meat, but it is part of a growing body of evidence that red meat shouldn't be the mainstay of your diet."

But why should red meat [defined in the report as beef, lamb, or pork] not be condemned if it is a source of colorectal cancer? The report stated that men who ate three or more ounces of red meat a day (a hamburger is about four ounces) and women who ate two ounces or more daily (half a hamburger) were 30% to 40% more likely to develop cancer in the lower colon than people who ate red meat only two times a week. People were also 50% more likely to develop colon cancer who ate processed meats (hot dogs, bacon, bologna, salami, etc.) and 20% more likely to develop rectal cancer, compared to people who ate meat the least.

Obviously, then, this data reveals that consuming a little less than one hamburger a day, or the equivalent in red meat, puts a man at risk of developing colon cancer at least 30% to 40% more than people who eat red meat twice a week. At the same time, women need to eat only two-thirds that much to be put at similar risk. Certainly the report is startling in that it seems to indicate that virtually everyone who eats meat is at some risk of developing colon cancer and at considerably greater risk than people who consume no meat at all.

From this study it is apparent that the American Cancer Society is aware that people who eat meat are at risk for developing colon cancer. The organization will not have met its obligations to the public until it announces unequivocally, "If you eat meat you are at risk of getting colon cancer." This is demonstrated by the agency's own data. [See also chapter 6 on the report by the Second Expert Panel of the American Institute of Cancer Research which found that red meat is a probable cause of colorectal cancer.]

The title of this chapter, "Got Cancer? The American Cancer Society," is a take-off on the dairy industry's "Got Milk" ad campaign that was popular a few years ago. This campaign has featured fictional characters like Batman, Shrek, and Yoda, and celebrities like Christie Brinkley, Martha Stewart, and Alex Rodriquez wearing a milk moustache. First created in 1993, the ad was voted the best commercial of all time in a USA Today poll done in 2002.

People for the Ethical Treatment of Animals (PETA) parodied the ad in the year 2000 by placing its own ad in the media showing former mayor of New York City, Rudy Giuliani, who had been diagnosed with prostate cancer and was undergoing radiation treatment at the time, wearing a milk moustache under the heading "Got Prostate Cancer?" The point was to advertise the dangers of milk as a risk factor in prostate cancer. Mayor Giuliani, along with the dairy industry and many others, did not see the humor. Giuliani threatened to sue PETA, and PETA apologized and removed the ad, saying it was intended to be provocative, not hurtful. But prostate cancer is the most common cancer in men in the United States.[30] As many as half of men over 70 years of age are estimated to have latent prostate cancer, and the PETA ad did succeed in raising a question in many people's minds. Does milk increase the possibility of getting prostate cancer?

If one follows the guidelines for reducing the risk of prostate cancer provided by the ACS in its journal *Ca*, the answer to that question is "not significantly." This is what the ACS guidelines conclude:

> Several studies suggest that diets high in certain vegetables (including tomatoes/tomato products, cruciferous vegetables, soy, beans, or other legumes) or fish are associated with decreased risk....Several studies have observed that greater consumption of red meat or dairy products may be associated with increased risk of prostate cancer....At the present time, the best advice to reduce the risk of prostate cancer is to eat five or more servings of a wide variety of vegetables and fruits each day, limit intake of red meats and dairy products, and maintain an active lifestyle and healthy weight.[31]

These guidelines tell us that "Several studies have observed that greater consumption of red meat or dairy products may be associated with increased risk of prostate cancer" and conclude that "the best advice to reduce the risk of prostate cancer is to...limit intake of red meats and dairy products." This counsel is mild at best. At worst, it is playing Russian roulette. Many studies have shown conclusively that dairy products put men at high risk for developing prostate cancer. A 1998 review of the published literature said the following:

> In ecologic data, correlations exist between per capita

meat and dairy consumption and prostate cancer mortality rates [one study cited]. In case control and perspective studies, the major contributors of animal protein, meats, dairy products and eggs have frequently been associated with a higher risk of prostate cancer...[23 studies cited]. Of note, numerous studies have found an association primarily in older men [six studies cited] though not all [one study cited]....The consistent associations with dairy products could result from, at least, in part, their calcium and phosphorous content.[32]

A 2001 Harvard University review was even more explicit.

...twelve of...fourteen case-control studies and seven of...nine cohort studies [have] observed a positive association for some measure of dairy products and prostate cancer; this is one of the most consistent dietary predictors for prostate cancer in the published literature. In these studies, men with the highest dairy intakes had approximately double the risk of total prostate cancer, and up to a fourfold increase in risk of metastatic or fatal prostate cancer relative to low consumers.[33]

The ACS *Ca* journal agrees, at least to a certain extent, that dairy products are a risk factor when it says "dairy products may be associated with increased risk of prostate cancer." But after making this admission, then all it does in following up is to suggest that men should "limit intake of red meats and dairy products" to reduce prostate cancer risk.

What needs to be determined conclusively is whether the ACS is offering advice that really will help men avoid prostate cancer, or if it is making suggestions that might even contribute toward getting the disease by refusing to sufficiently condemn red meat and dairy products proportionate to their risk in getting prostate cancer.

The ACS is going in all kinds of different directions at once. For example, while offering the advice to limit diary products, it also recommends milk and dairy foods as a good source of calcium but ignores the evidence that high calcium intake has been linked to osteoporosis (as will be discussed in chapter 5). And though recommending the consumption of dairy products for calcium, the *Ca* journal acknowledges that calcium is a risk factor for prostate cancer as follows. In the journal it states "...because of a potential increase in risk of prostate cancer associated with calcium intake, it would be *prudent* [author's emphasis] to limit calcium intake in men to less than 1500 mg/day until further studies are conducted."[34]

As noted, these recommendations contradict each other.

Concerning the ACS advice to limit calcium to 1500 mg/day, it should be pointed out that an 8-ounze glass of milk is equal to about 300 mg of calcium. Two slices of firm cheese equal the same, and two ounces of yogurt equal 100 mg.[35] To limit oneself to 1500 mg/day of calcium does not really seem like much of a sacrifice. One could consume five glasses of milk, ten slices of cheese, or almost four cups of yogurt containing eight ounces each (or any combination of these) to reach 1500 mg/day of calcium. In fact, the American Institute for Cancer Research reports that the current federal guidelines for calcium intake is between 1000 and 1200 mg per day.[36] By these standards, the ACS advice to limit calcium intake to 1500 mg per day does not even constitute a reduction. Considering the known danger of diary products in prostate cancer risk, of which the ACS has taken note, to recommend *prudently* limiting calcium intake to lower prostate cancer risk is like advising smokers to *prudently* limit smoking in order to reduce lung cancer risk. It would be far more *prudent* to recommend cutting out all dairy products entirely.

The above examples illustrate the reluctance of the ACS to

acknowledge the cancer risk inherent in consuming meat and dairy products. At the same time, the text in the ACS *Ca* cancer guidelines reveals convincingly that the agency is fully aware of the risks to cancer meat and dairy products pose. For example, the *Ca* guidelines state:

> Many epidemiologic studies have examined the association between cancer and the consumption of red meats...and processed meats...Meat contains several constituents that could increase the risk of cancer. Mutagens and carcinogens (heterocyclic amines and polycyclic aromatic hydrocarbons) are produced by cooking meat at high temperatures and/or by charcoal grilling. The iron content (heme) in red meat may generate free radicals in the colon that damage DNA. Substances used to process meat (nitrates/nitrites and salt) contribute to the formation of nitrosamines that can damage DNA. It is also possible that the fat content in meat contributes to risk. For example, foods that are high in fat increase the concentration of secondary bile acids and other compounds in the stool that could be carcinogens or promoters of carcinogenesis.[37]

This passage describes meat as a dangerous product in no uncertain terms noting that the iron content in "red meat may generate free radicals in the colon that damage DNA" and "...foods that are high in fat increase the concentration of secondary *bile acids* and other compounds in the stool that could be carcinogens or promoters of carcinogenesis." [Author's emphasis.]

The ACS guidelines cited above state that "foods that are high in fat increase the concentration of secondary bile acids and other compounds in the stool that could be carcinogens or promoters of carcinogenesis." But in the discussion under the heading "Fat" in the same report, the guidelines state that "there is little evidence that the total amount of fat consumed increases cancer risk." The inconsistency could hardly be more visible. On the one hand high-fat foods increase bile acids that could promote cancer, but on the other hand there is little evidence that fat increases cancer risk. This represents yet more contradictory advice the ACS is offering to the public. Small wonder that the public is confused.

Dr. Leo Galland, a New York University trained physician who did his training at Bellevue Hospital in New York City and who takes an integrative approach to medicine, has also written about the dangers of bile acids and says that "this is the Western degenerative disease pattern which results from diets high in fat and meat and low in fiber. These enzymes may then metabolize *bile acids* to tumor promoters and deconjugate excreted estrogens, raising the plasma estrogen level." [Author's emphasis.] He goes on to say: "Epidemiologic data implicates this type of dysbiosis [bacterial imbalance in the gut] in the pathogenesis of colon cancer and breast cancer. It is usually corrected by decreasing dietary fat and flesh, increasing fiber consumption and consuming probiotic preparations."[38]

[Dr. Galland's book, *Power Healing*, is endorsed by Dr. Dean Ornish, referred to earlier, who is celebrated for his landmark research proving that heart disease can be arrested and reversed through nutrition.][39,40]

Both the ACS and Dr. Galland say that they are relying on epidemiologic evidence. But when it comes to counseling the public on how to avoid getting cancer, the ACS avoids the kind of epidemiological evidence that Dr. Campbell has assembled, even though his study is the most "comprehensive study of diet, lifestyle and disease ever done with humans in the history of biomedical research."[41] Campbell's study affirms categorically that meat and dairy products promote cancer. The American Cancer Society apparently does not want to admit this and so cites several epidemiological studies that show, for instance, in the case of colon cancer, that while meat may be responsible for "an increased risk of cancers of the colon and/or rectum" this is not important enough to warrant more than a caution for the public to *limit* red meat intake. In fact, as observed earlier, the ACS chief of epidemiology, Michael Thun, goes out of his way to pacify and reassure the public that his findings in regard to colorectal cancer were "not a condemnation of red meat."

We have now seen evidence that the ACS is aware of just how dangerous red meat and processed meats are to increased cancer risk. When it comes to actually advising people what to do to avoid this risk, however, the agency takes a step backwards and advises only to *limit* the consumption of these foods.

"Tobacco is a cause of lung cancer" gets the ACS stamp of condemnation. "Animal protein is a cause of cancer" gets the label of "uncertainty" and "may cause" or "may or may not," but still gets the ACS stamp of approval so long as meat and dairy consumption is limited to lean cuts and smaller portions, and low-fat and nonfat dairy products.

Some might contend that to expect more is to expect too much considering the complexities of modern life and the problems in deterring disease. But the facts are now known with certainty that consuming animal protein, both meat and dairy products, puts people at high risk for developing breast cancer, colon cancer, and prostate cancer. This is strongly suggested even by the ACS reports described in this chapter. That is noteworthy and surely deserves to be lit up in red, white, and blue lights so that no one can miss it.

When the American Cancer Society's recommendations for reducing cancer risk are put under the microscope, as has been done in this chapter, it becomes clear that the agency is ambivalent about the dangers posed by meat and dairy products just as it was with tobacco when it first came under attack. (This ambivalence will be more thoroughly addressed in chapter 11.)

The question that must be asked and answered is why the ACS would not want the American people to know that animal products pose a significant risk in promoting cancer when the facts clearly reveal that they do. If the American Cancer Society, the largest and most prominent of all the health organizations, adopts this kind of policy, are other healthcare organizations doing the same, and if so, why?

The answers to these questions will become increasingly clear as the narrative proceeds.

Chapter 5

Milk and Dairy Products

Do They Prevent or Cause Osteoporosis?
Can Eliminating Animal Products From the Diet Help Prevent Alzheimer's Disease, Diabetes, Macular Degeneration, Multiple Sclerosis, Kidney Stones, and Arthritis?

Mainstream organizations like the American Cancer Society, the American Heart Association, and the Mayo Clinic all recommend milk and dairy foods for calcium. Their views reflect those of the dairy industry which universally advertises that dairy products are necessary because they are the best sources for calcium which builds strong bones and teeth in children and prevents osteoporosis in adults.[1]

The ACS list of recommended foods for a well-stocked refrigerator includes reduced-fat or fat-free milk, reduced-fat sour cream, reduced-fat yogurt, and reduced-fat cream cheese, plus a variety of other reduced-fat cheeses: cheddar, mozzarella, Swiss, Monterey Jack, cottage cheese, and Parmesan — all high calcium dairy products.[2,3]

What needs to be determined is whether high doses of calcium from dairy products really are necessary for good bone health, or whether the healthcare organizations are just falling in line behind the dairy industry and helping to promote a product that factually is dangerous to our health. Opponents of dairy products claim that their calcium content does not increase bone strength, but is a cause of osteoporosis. So who is right and who is wrong about calcium intake?

A good starting place is a report in CyberParent which states that according to a Michigan study of 1600 women published in the American Journal of Clinical Nutrition, those [women] who had been vegetarians for at least 20 years lost only 18 percent of bone mineral density by the time they were eighty years of age compared to a 35 percent loss for women consuming a typical American diet. That is nearly double the loss.[4]

Another challenge to dairy industry claims comes from retired Harvard Professor of Nutrition Mark Hegsted, who was a principal architect of the nation's dietary guidelines produced in 1980 by the USDA and the Department of Health and Human Services. He points out in the American Journal of Clinical Nutrition that "osteoporotic fractures are, like coronary artery disease, largely a disease of Western societies." He notes that "the international epidemiologic data show an association between [animal] protein consumption and osteoporotic fractures," and that "the aciduria caused by such diets promotes urinary calcium loss."[5] [See directly below for more on urinary calcium loss.] He also remarks that "we know that populations around the world that use few dairy products and have relatively low calcium intakes develop reasonably well and are obviously not falling apart from fractures. On the other hand, fracture rates are obviously high in the countries that consume the Western-type diet." Hegsted further comments that there is "now considerable data indicating that high intakes of fruit and vegetables protect against fractures." He observes, however, that "high-calcium diets have been promoted by the dairy industry, the nutrition establishment, and much of the medical profession for 80 years or more. The dairy interests have a large stake in this and cannot be expected to be unbiased."

In regard to urinary calcium loss, Professor Hegsted describes it as a process in which high calcium intake causes a decrease in the calcium that is absorbed by the body by excreting the excess in the urine. This inefficient process of calcium absorption damages the ability "to effectively use dietary calcium or even to conserve calcium in the bones later in life," putting the bones at increased risk for osteoporosis.[6] Conversely, with a lower calcium intake, the body takes the calcium it needs and is not burdened by having to sort out and excrete the unnecessary calcium excess.

Hegsted is not alone in making these kinds of observations. T. Colin Campbell concurs that the cause of this excessive calcium excretion is animal protein.[7] It increases metabolic acid which draws calcium from the bones, resulting in an increase in the amount of calcium in the urine. He points out that a study found that after six months people on the high animal protein, low-carbohydrate Atkins Diet excreted 50% more calcium in their urine. Campbell further reports that this process of calcium excretion has been known for 80 years but is widely ignored.

Dr. Dean Ornish states the same. "The real cause of osteo-porosis in this country is not insufficient calcium intake, it's excessive excretion of calcium in the urine....Vegetarians, in contrast, excrete much less calcium, and this is why they have very low rates of osteoporosis even though their dietary intake of calcium is lower than those on a meat-eating diet."[8]

For decades the dairy industry has successfully convinced Western societies that dairy products are necessary for strong bones just because dairy products contain a high calcium content. But this view has come under increasing suspicion, as indicated by sources like those cited above.

A report put out by the Compassion in World Farming Trust is also largely negative about dairy products. It points out that the World Health Organization (WHO) and the Food and Agriculture Organization of the United Nations (FAO) recommend eating more fruits and vegetables rather than consuming milk for good bone health. The report also sees "no correlation between increased calcium intake and a decreased risk of bone fractures" and further quotes Professor Walter

Willett, discussed later in connection with the Harvard Nurses' Health Study, in stating that "drinking three (eight ounce) glasses a day [this is the amount of milk commonly recommended] would be equivalent to eating twelve strips of bacon or a Big Mac and an order of fries."[9] The report further contends that the saturated fat in every ounce of cheese is equal to that contained in a glass of milk, or, according to Willet's calculation, about four strips of bacon. It further states that skimmed [2%] milk contains about half the amount of fat contained in whole milk (equal to two strips of bacon).

In addition, the report notes that three quarters of adults in the world are lactose intolerant while some evidence also shows that milk, contrary to increasing bone strength, may raise the risk of bone fractures. It suggests that the calcium people absorb from dairy products may be used up in neutralizing the acid created by the animal protein contained in the dairy products. [10] Finally, the report comments that calcium is thought to be assimilated better when magnesium is present but points out that magnesium is largely absent in dairy foods. It argues that calcium is "most beneficially assimilated" not by consuming dairy products but by eating broccoli, kale, and other green, leafy vegetables.[11]

These views by respected sources all seem to support charges that far from increasing bone strength, dairy products may cause bone density loss. But the healthcare establishment has kept silent about the possible link between dairy products to increased risk of bone fractures and osteoporosis. It could scarcely be unaware of the evidence. If dairy products increase osteoporosis because their consumption triggers a process in which an overload of calcium caused by the high calcium content in dairy products has to be excreted — thus leading to calcium deficiencies — then this needs to be reported to the pubic, not ignored in order to protect the dairy industry. And even if the proponents of dairy products want to insist that the evidence is inconclusive, this information still needs to be communicated to the public so that people can decide for themselves which side to believe.

Besides osteoporosis, other research connects Alzheimer's disease, macular degeneration, multiple sclerosis, kidney stones, arthritis, and diabetes directly to the consumption of animal protein either in the form of flesh or dairy products.

One study compared Alzheimer's disease rates in eleven countries and found that people with a higher fat intake and lower cereal and grain intake had higher incidences of Alzheimer's.[12] Another study of 5,000 people showed that a higher intake of fat and cholesterol tended to increase the incidence of Alzheimer's specifically and dementia generally.[13] (Cholesterol ingestion occurs through animal products only. There is no other dietary source.)

Still another study showed that Alzheimer's risk was greater for those whose blood folic acid was in the lowest one-third range and blood homocysteine was in the highest one-third range.[14] Folic acid comes exclusively from plant foods like green and leafy vegetables. Homocysteine comes from animal products. Hence a diet low in plant foods and high in animal products can put people at greater risk for Alzheimer's disease than a diet high in plant foods and low in animal products. It follows logically that a diet with no animal products would reduce the risk even further.

Another study done at Columbia University of 2148 elderly people showed that "individuals who consume a diet rich in nuts, fish, poultry, vegetables, fruits, and olive oil-based salad dressings but low in high-fat dairy products, red meats, organ meats, and butter have a reduced risk for Alzheimer's disease."[15]

The message seems clear enough to post red flags all around animal products warning of the distinct possibility that they can be high-rate risk factors for Alzheimer's disease. The public needs the healthcare organizations to broadcast this information to the nation so that people can make use of it.

In regard to macular degeneration, studies have shown that consuming carotenoids can reduce the incidence of the disease by as much as 88%. That is because people who have more carotenoids in the blood are two-thirds less likely to develop the condition. Carotenoids are antioxidants found in the colored parts of fruits and vegetables. Green leafy vegetables (like broccoli, spinach, and collard greens), carrots, and citrus fruits (like grapefruit, lemons, limes, kumquats, oranges, and tangelos) are especially good sources. These antioxidants can repress the free radicals that can destroy the tissue around the macula and the macula itself (the "biochemical intersection in the eye — where the energy of the light coming in is transformed into a nerve signal") and can lead to macular degeneration.[16]

Western diet has also been strongly implicated in multiple sclerosis. Dr. Roy Swank (1909 – 2008), who was head of the Division of Neurology of the University of Oregon Medical School (Oregon Health & Science University) for 22 years, conducted a well-known long-term trial on 144 multiple sclerosis patients at the Montreal Neurological Institute and found that a low-saturated fat diet greatly reduced the progression of the disease even for people with initially advanced conditions.[17] Of the group in the early stages of the disease, only 5% of the patients consuming the low saturated fat diet died after thirty years and remained only mildly disabled. Of those who consumed the high-saturated fat diet, 80% died in the same time frame.

New epidemiological studies also show that cow's milk is strongly linked to multiple sclerosis and Type 1 diabetes.[18]

With diabetes there are two kinds to contend with, Type 1 and Type 2. The difference is that in Type 1 the insulin-producing cells of the pancreas have been destroyed whereas in Type 2 the pancreas produces insulin but it is "rendered ineffective, and the blood sugar is not metabolized properly."[19]

Evidence strongly links Type 1 diabetes, which is presently incurable, to dairy products. In addition, "the ability of cow's milk protein to initiate Type 1 diabetes is well documented."[20]

One theory suggests the process could commence when infants are bottle fed cow's milk which is inadequately digested so that fragments of the cow's milk protein makes its way into the baby's intestines where it gets absorbed into the blood. There the immune system, thinking the fragments are invaders, goes on the attack destroying both the "cow's milk" invaders and the pancreatic cells This happens because the "invaders" and the pancreatic cells responsible for producing insulin resemble each other. In the process "the child's ability to produce insulin" is eliminated, thus rendering the baby a Type 1 diabetic for life.[21]

Even though no cure for Type 1 diabetes is known, researchers are still working to find effective treatments. James Anderson, M.D., an endocrinologist specializing in diabetes, and a Professor of Medicine and Clinical Nutrition at the University of Kentucky, gave 25 Type 1 diabetics an experimental vegetarian diet for three weeks after which they were able to lower their insulin medication by an average of 40% and their cholesterol levels plummeted 30%, a dramatic drop for this incurable disease.[22] Dr. Joel Fuhrman, who will be referred to in chapter 21, reports fundamentally the same results in his book *Eat to Live and Eat for Health* with the difference that he was able to lower medication by about 50%.

When Anderson tried the same experiment on 25 Type 2 diabetics, 24 were able to discontinue insulin medication entirely. One of these diabetics had a 21 year history of diabetes. In another study involving 14 patients, Anderson was able to reduce their cholesterol on average from 206 mg/dL to 141 mg/dL in only two weeks.[23] Dr. Fuhrman also had extremely positive results in controlling Type 2 diabetes with a diet consisting of fruits, vegetables, nuts, and seeds.

Because heart disease and stroke are a serious problem for diabetics, a cholesterol reduction below 150 is particularly impressive and important considering that a 150 mg/dL cholesterol count is the heart attack safe level, according to the Framingham Heart Study, an ongoing study of the causes of cardiovascular disease begun in Framingham, Massachusetts in 1948.

[The Framingham Heart Study is one of the most widely cited of all heart disease studies from which much of the common knowledge about heart disease is derived. Heart attack safe cholesterol levels in connection with the Framingham Project will be discussed further in chapter 9.]

In another 22 week randomized clinical trial for individuals with Type 2 diabetes, Dr. Neal Barnard and an investigative team of the Physicians Committee for Responsible Medicine (PCRM), compared a low-fat vegan diet to an American Diabetes Association (ADA) low-fat plant-based diet in which no proscriptions were made on animal products. Results showed that 43% of vegan dieters compared to 26% of ADA dieters were able to reduce diabetes medications. Both diets yielded favorable results, but the non-animal diet was more effective than the diet permitting animal products.[24]

Dr. Barnard, an adjunct associate professor at George Washington School of Medicine in Washington, D.C. and the head of the Physicians Committee for Responsible Medicine, described the process of diabetes and how to control it during an interview about his book, *The Reverse Diabetes Diet*:

When someone has diabetes, insulin (the hormone produced in the pancreas) has a difficult time moving sugar out of the bloodstream and into that person's cells. That's because tiny amounts of fat in the person's cells prevent the insulin from "opening" the cell membrane, or what can essentially be thought of as a lock. Instead, these bits of fat which build up when a person eats a high-fat diet clog up the cell and the insulin can't do its job. With the low-fat vegan diet, however, individuals can essentially alter what goes on in their cells. By eliminating most fat from their diet, that person is basically cleaning up his or her cells, which allows the insulin to move the glucose into the cells where it belongs.[25]

In a study of Japanese American men, those who developed Type 2 diabetes consumed the most animal-based foods. Another study of 1300 people in the San Luis Valley in Colorado found that "high-fat, low-carbohydrate diets are associated with the onset of" Type 2 diabetes.

In Iowa, researchers studied 36,000 diabetes-free women over six years during which 1,100 of the women developed the disease. Those least likely to get it consumed the most whole grains and fiber which means they were getting plenty of plant-based foods (since fiber is found only in plant-based foods). At the Pritikin Center, 34 diabetic patients out of 40 were able to discontinue all insulin medication after 26 days on a low-fat, plant-based diet with exercise.[26]

From the above brief review, it should be apparent that a plant-based diet can help in controlling Type 1 and Type 2 diabetes, even having the capacity to eliminate the Type 2 form entirely, so long as the right kind of diet is maintained.

When it comes to kidney stones, Professor W.G. Robertson of the Medical Research Council in Leeds, England, and one of the world's foremost experts on diet and kidney stones, said:

Urolithiasis [kidney stone formation] is a worldwide problem which appears to be aggravated by the high dairy-produce highly energy-rich and low-fibre diets consumed in most industrialized countries....Evidence points, in particular, to a high-meat protein intake as being the dominant factor.[27]

The antioxidant properties of plant-based foods are also beneficial in the fight against the free radicals that, according to recent research, may be responsible for the formation of kidney stones.[28]

Arthritis is a condition that afflicts 33% of Americans and half of those over the age of 65. It is an inflammation of the joint and can be caused by injury (traumatic arthritis), bacterial infection of a joint (suppurative arthritis), and the accumulation of uric acid crystals (gouty arthritis). The more common types are those with no known cause: inflammatory arthritis (rheumatoid arthritis), and degenerative arthritis (osteoarthritis).[29]

A white paper study put out by Johns Hopkins Hospital suggests that those who suffer from rheumatoid arthritis may be protected from heart disease and stroke associated with the condition through a vegan diet. The study asked a group of 38 people suffering from rheumatoid arthritis to follow a diet that eliminated meat, dairy products (including eggs), and glutens (grains like wheat, oats, rye, and barley) for one year. A control group of 28 people with rheumatoid arthritis consumed their normal diet. At the end of the trial, the vegans had lost nine pounds compared to two pounds lost by the control group, and had lower total cholesterol and LDL (bad) cholesterol. They also had higher levels of anti-PC IgA, an antibody associated with lower rates of atherosclerosis, and lower levels of CRP (C-reactive protein), a marker associated with insulin resistance and excess weight.[30]

Dr. John McDougall also reports that a vegan diet "has been found to change the fecal microbial flora in rheumatoid arthritis patients, and these changes in the fecal flora are associated with improvement in the arthritis activity."[31] One of the pioneers in the study of how diet relates to disease and a highly respected nutritionist, McDougall got his start in the field of nutrition when he lived on a sugar plantation in Hawaii. There he noticed that first, second, third, and fourth generation Filipinos, Japanese, Chinese, and Koreans who ate a meatless, dairyless diet "avoided heart disease, diabetes, breast cancer, prostate cancer, and arthritis, by and large, and that they also lived to work and function fully into their eighties and sometimes nineties on a diet primarily of rice and vegetables."[32] He also noticed that succeeding generations became fatter and sicker as they followed Westernized diets. The observation caused McDougall to revise what he had been taught about nutrition. He subsequently developed his own nutrition program for treating arthritis consisting of a starch-based diet with the addition of fruits, and vegetables (low-fat and devoid of all animal products). (See chapter 17 for McDougall's evaluation of starch in relation to protein.)

Osteoarthritis is comparatively rare in African and Asian countries which rely on a plant-based diet. In the United States osteoarthritis appears in the x-rays of the hands of 70% of people over the age of 65. According to McDougall, the Western diet can lead to osteoarthritis by damaging the joints through excessive weight, malnourishment (depriving the joints of needed nutrients to withstand wear and tear), poor circulation (resulting from fat floating around in the bloodstream after eating), as well as inflammation-promoting components in the diet, particularly the proteins in dairy foods.[33] Eliminating dairy and meat products can reduce the risk of developing osteoarthritis.

Several physicians, including McDougall, have also reported significant benefits in treating osteoarthritis through daily supplements of glucosamine. Glucosamine is an amino sugar the body produces and distributes to the cartilage, adding thickness and increasing its cushioning effect. One supplement is manufactured commercially from shellfish powder, though the long-term effects of consuming shellfish powder are unknown. Glucosamine is often combined with chondroitin, a supplement made from cow cartilage which many people object to because it is an animal product. (The same objections apply to shellfish.) Dr. McDougall has expressed concern about chondroitin because it may contain infectious microbes like those found in mad cow disease.[33] For people who wish to avoid animal products and take chondroitin, some companies, like Cargill, have developed a vegetable glucosamine supplement made from corn.

Clinical trials on glucosomine have produced varying results.

The old model for disease is an unhealthy life style that ends in surgery or drugs. The drugs frequently have to be taken for life, and surgery often has to be repeated because the diseases causing the problem are not cured. Many of these diseases are now being linked directly to animal protein, and with that discovery, new parameters for cures are being explored.

Several dynamics can be involved in disease creation, including as discussed earlier, environmental factors. But nutrition is one element that individuals can control. With more research and clinical trials like the ones conducted by the Physicians Committee for Responsible Medicine, the Anderson diabetes' study, the Swank multiple sclerosis study, and the Johns Hopkins white paper referred to above, more and better treatments are certain to evolve.

The new concept for reducing the risk of disease is simple and it costs next to nothing. Just say no to animal products (meat, poutlry, fowl, and fish). That is all that is required, and that is the new model for a healthy life style. It leads toward good health, not in the direction of the surgery room or a trip to the pharmacist to pick up the week's bundle of prescription drugs loaded with potentially life-shortening side effects.

Chapter 6

The Uniformity of the Healthcare Organizations

Did the Second Expert Report of the American Institute for Cancer Research Get It Wrong? The Need for a National Debate

Government healthcare agencies, nonprofit health organizations, hospitals, and medical facilities have arrived at a near consensus about what kind of diet they believe works best to promote good health and keep the killer diseases at bay. It narrows down to: 1) eating low-fat foods, low saturated fat foods, and low cholesterol foods; 2) consuming monounsaturated fats like olive oil, canola oil, oatmeal, avocados, nuts and seeds; and polyunsaturated fats like safflower oil, soybean oil, corn oil, sunflower oil, and cottonseed oil, as well as bananas, nuts, and seeds; 3) reducing saturated fats and trans fats (hydrogenated foods); 4) consuming whole grain products; 5) consuming plenty of fruits and vegetables; 6) switching from whole milk and dairy foods to low-fat dairy products; 7) limiting red meats and processed meats; 8) limiting sugar and high-sugar products like candy and pastries; 9) limiting refined and processed foods like white flour foods; 10) limiting salt; and 11) limiting alcohol intake.[1] In addition, they recommend plenty of exercise.

This is the basic model the healthcare establishment turns to in making dietary recommendations to the public. It is derived from the USDA and Department of Health and Human Services *Dietary Guidelines for Americans* issued every five years along with the USDA five foods pyramid. The pyramid recommends

1) whole grains; 2) vegetables; 3) fruits; 4) low-fat or fat-free milk; and 5) low-fat or lean meat, poultry, fish, eggs, beans, peas, nuts, and seeds.

Many healthcare organizations and hospitals like the American Medical Association, the National Cancer Institute, the Johns Hopkins Hospital, and the Massachusetts General Hospital of Boston follow the USDA recommendations directly or provide links to the USDA guidelines from their websites.[2] The Mayo Clinic acknowledges closely following the USDA guidelines in setting up unified dietary guidelines, but also offers several alternative diets for consideration which, nevertheless, are similar.[3] Other organizations like the American Heart Association and the American Cancer Society create their own guidelines that also resemble the basic structure of the USDA guidelines.[4,5] In addition, the National Heart, Lung, and Blood Institute has developed a diet for lowering blood pressure called the Dash Diet.[6] It, too, follows the same basic principles.

In 2007, after a rigorous five-year investigation, the American Institute for Cancer Research (AICR) in conjunction with the World Cancer Research Fund (WCRF) completed its Second Expert Report. Titled *Food, Nutrition, Physical Activity, and the Prevention of Cancer: a Global Perspective*, the report added its nutrition guidelines to the mix. According to the panel of experts who prepared the report, the plan was structured on "the total body of scientific evidence on the relationship of diet, physical activity and weight management to cancer risk" and made specific recommendations for avoiding the risk of cancer as follows:[7]

Be as lean as possible without becoming underweight; be physically active for at least 30 minutes every day; avoid sugary drinks; limit consumption of energy-dense foods (particularly processed foods high in added sugar, or low in fiber, or high in fat); eat more of a variety of vegetables, fruits, whole grains and legumes such as beans; limit consumption of red meats (such as beef, pork and lamb) and avoid processed meats; if consumed at all, limit alcoholic drinks to 2 for men and 1 for women a day; limit consumption of salty foods and foods processed with salt; don't use supplements to protect against cancer.

This program also contains most of the elements featured in the other plans. While the panel chose to offer no advice in regard to dairy products, the Spring 2009 AICR newsletter advises that good protein sources include "...low-fat and nonfat dairy products..."[8] Dairy products are also recommended at other places on the AICR website.

Except for a few minor differences, the above brief survey of nutritional guidelines reveals that the major healthcare organizations are more or less in agreement about what kind of diet works best for optimal health and warding off disease. It boils down basically to a diet of lean meats, beans, peas, nuts and seeds; low-fat dairy products; plenty of fruits, vegetables, and whole wheat grains; and limited intake of salt, sugar, and alcohol. Getting lots of exercise is also recommended.

Still, none of these organizations have taken the next vital step in disease prevention, which is to declare that animal-based foods, including dairy products, are the definitive nutritional cause of the killer diseases, and that the best way to significantly reduce their risk is to remove animal protein from the diet. Until the healthcare organizations are willing to make this or a similar announcement to the world, they are limiting the impact they can make in helping people achieve the best possible health attainable, and they are continuing to make recommendations that can be harmful to the health and well-being of the public.

The AICR's panel of experts assert that they reviewed and analyzed "the total body of scientific evidence on the relationship of diet, physical activity and weight management to cancer risk" in completing the 2007 Second Expert Report just described. This means that they would have evaluated the work done by T. Colin Campbell in his monumental epidemiologic study on China, especially considering that Dr. Campbell was the co-chair for the First AICR Expert Report on nutrition completed in 1997. Apparently, though, this second influential panel did not think Dr. Campbell's findings merited inclusion in their nutritional guidelines since they do not even come close to suggesting the possibility of eliminating animal-based products from their diet guidelines. In fact, a review of the Second Expert Report offers no indication that the panel even considered T. Colin Campbell's work at all in its particulars when it comes to the dangers of consuming animal protein.

This differs noticeably from the respect accorded to Dr. Campbell by the President of the AICR, Marilyn Gentry, who praised his work in the testimonials section of *The China Study*, stating that "today, AICR advocates a predominantly plant-based diet for lower cancer risk because of the great work Dr Campbell and just a few other visionaries began twenty-five years ago."

These words would have been written prior to the publication of *The China Study* which occurred in 2005. At that time the AICR was still under the influence of its First Expert Report of 1997 which suggested not only to limit red meat to less than 3 ounces a day, but added the caution "if eaten at all."[9] But today, as indicated on the AICR website, the organization expresses a different perspective as follows:

Most adults can easily meet their protein needs with a balanced diet that includes five to six ounces a day of lean poultry, fish or meat and three servings of dairy products (or alternatives) in addition to the protein from plant based foods. Those who prefer to omit or minimize meat or dairy products need to include multiple servings of vegetarian sources of protein like beans, nuts, seeds and perhaps some eggs.

This is unmistakable advocacy for making animal protein the first choice for meeting protein needs and plant protein the second, plus this recommendation even advises consuming from 5 to 6 ounces of animal protein daily, double the amount recommended by the 1997 panel. The AICR also posts many recipes for meals on its website that include turkey, chicken, fish, and cheese. One recipe reads "many health professionals recommend eating at least one meatless meal each week."[10] A statement of this nature hardly indicates an exceptional concern about limiting meat consumption or advocating a "predominantly plant-based diet." Has the AICR shifted its position?

The AICR Second Expert Report completed in 2007 recommended limiting red meats, like all the healthcare organizations previously referred to have done, but it also concluded that "...many foods of animal origin are nourishing and healthy if consumed in modest amounts." [See the AICR Second Expert Report Summary.] And it stated this even while reporting in practically the same breath that "people who eat various forms of vegetarian diets are at low risk of some diseases including some cancers, although it is not easy to separate out these benefits of the diets from other aspects of their ways of life, such as not smoking, drinking little if any alcohol, and so forth."

Coming from a panel of experts, the implied authority with which the first statement is made without any supporting evidence and for the second statement, the lack of any serious attempt to drill down to try to determine how a group of people [vegetarians] have found a way to avoid cancer and other diseases, suggests a narrowness of point of view that is troubling. The first statement, by reporting to the public that the consumption of animal foods is nourishing and healthy, even in moderation, could encourage people to eat meat which could result in very negative health consequences for some but more probably many people. The second statement implies that the disease prevention aspects of a vegetarian diet need not be taken too seriously because life style factors may be the true reason for the benefits of a vegetarian diet. Both statements have no scientific basis.

The panel justifies recommending the consumption of meat on the supposition that "an integrated approach to the evidence also shows that many foods of animal origin are nourishing." Since the panel does not indicate what this integrated approach is or upon what evidence this statement is made, it might be assumed that they mean, as stated further, that meat can be "a valuable source of nutrients, in particular protein, iron, zinc, and vitamin B12."

As noted in this book, and backed by solid scientific evidence, animal protein, including meat, can also be a source of cancer and other diseases no matter how many wonderful nutrients it may contain. [For reasons why a diet consisting of as much as 18 ounces of red meet weekly, which is what the AICR Second Expert panel recommends, is not only inadvisable but dangerous in relation to heart disease, see chapter 9. Also, as noted above, the AICR itself recommends from 5 to 6 ounces of animal protein daily [plus three servings of dairy products], or 35 to 42 ounces weekly, which is far more dangerous.]

It might also be noted that in the panel's review of the findings of other outside expert reports in regard to preventing chronic disease and cancer, the panel took 44 of these reports concerning the moderate consumption of meat, fish, and eggs into consideration but evaluated none which were concerned with eliminating meat, fish, and eggs entirely from the diet. This seems much more like a one-sided than an "integrated" approach and suggests a bias against evaluating non-meat (vegan) diets.

In regard to the second statement about vegetarians, apparently the panel did not reflect long on the possibility that the reason vegetarians and vegans get far less cancer than the general population is exactly because they are vegetarians or vegans and therefore do not eat animal protein. This is not the first cohort study that has leaned toward discrediting the benefits of a non-meat diet by suggesting that other non-nutritional factors might account for the benefits of a non-meat diet without investigating exactly what those non-nutritional factors might be or what impact they might or might not make. Since cohort (large group) studies are available that specifically target the absence of animal consumption as the source of the health benefits a vegetarian or vegan diet provides, it is surprising that the AICR panel of experts would minimize the value of a vegan diet while recommending the consumption of meat when it is a known cause of cancer. The panel even acknowledges that red and processed meats are convincing and probable causes of some cancers, like colorectal cancer, as we shall see momentarily.

On the surface, at least, it appears that the Second AICR panel did not place much faith in studies that reject the consumption of meat. It is important, therefore, to take a brief look at the methodology the panel members employed in order to try to determine how they made the decision to recommend the moderate consumption of meat as a healthy, nourishing product to the public.

Essentially the Second AICR panel followed a comparison protocol whereby they compared different kinds of studies to determine causal relationships of different factors to the incidence of particular kinds of cancer, for example, dairy products to prostate cancer. To find a "probable causal relationship," which stood at the apex of the matrices they designed as cancer indicators, they set as a standard the requirement to find evidence from at least two independent cohort studies and at least five case control studies (in which people with a specific type of cancer are compared to people without cancer) plus lesser factors.

In following this protocol, the Second Expert Report arrived at some conclusions that coincided with and in some cases even strengthened the findings of the First AICR Expert Report conducted in 1997, such as that red and processed meats are convincingly a cause of colorectal cancer. However, their conclusions also contrasted sharply with the first panel in finding, for example, that there was little evidence based on current research to show that diets high in fats and oils were the cause of any kind of cancer. This accounts, perhaps, for why the Second panel so easily recommended the moderate consumption of meat as a healthy product, in spite of its finding that red meat is convincingly a cause of colorectal cancer.

Obviously, this conclusion differs substantially from those made by Dr. Campbell and other researchers according to which animal fat is a major promoter of several forms of cancer, including breast cancer, the risk of which can be vastly reduced by eliminating the source of estrogen producing nutrients, namely the same source that produces colorectal cancer, animal protein. The problem with a comparison protocol, such as the one upon which the Second Expert Report panel relied in which cohort studies are the most important determinant of a probability, is that cohort studies can themselves be significantly mistaken. The AICR panel relied especially on cohort studies made from the mid 1990s forward and said that these studies tended to weaken the evidence supporting fats and oils as a cause of cancer.

It should be noted, therefore, that in *The China Study*, T. Colin Campbell reported that *every single epidemiological study done* has been *seriously flawed* and that together they have been a disaster for discovering the causal link between nutrition and disease. One of those he singled out above all others for employing faulty methodology was the Nurses' Health Study which turns out to be one of the large cohort studies the panel for the AICR Second Expert Report relied upon in arriving at their conclusions. If Dr. Campbell's analysis is correct, then the panel's conclusion specifying that it is healthy to consume red meat moderately and even processed meat to a more limited extent must be regarded with suspicion since it relied in part on the Nurses' Health Study which Dr. Campbell asserts is flawed. (His reasons for this contention are set out in chapter 8 where the Nurses' Health Study and two other well-known cohort studies are examined.) In fact, as shown, he asserted that every single epidemiological study (in relation to fat as a cause of cancer) was flawed. If he is right, then the Second AICR report is also flawed.

A comparison study, which is what the AICR Second Expert Report essentially is, may be extremely comprehensive and it may contain endless amounts of data cross-checked in many elaborate ways. Still it can only summarize the most notable and likely to be true events and try to mold them into some kind of conclusion, the process of which cannot avoid a certain amount of subjectivity on the part of the researchers. Does a methodology like this meet standards high enough to justify making a serious nutrition recommendation to the public that it is healthy to consume red meat in moderation, especially when alternative authoritative sources claim the evidence being relied upon is flawed? Remember, the Campbell China study is the largest epidemiological study ever undertaken anywhere by anyone. Beyond *The China Study*, however, other studies, some of which have been referred to in this book, also strongly indicate that animal protein is a definitive cause of cancer.

The AICR Second Expert Report stated that it had reviewed "the total body of scientific evidence" in arriving at its dietary conclusions. Well, if it reviewed Dr. Campbell's important discovery exhaustively but still disagreed, it does not help the public to keep silent about the reasons for the disagreement. The AICR panel did, after all, ignore Dr. Campbell's findings that the cause of many cancers is the consumption of animal protein when it advised that it is healthy to eat meat in moderation. A precise and unequivocal explanation is, consequently, warranted.

People make life and death decisions based on nutrition advice put out by our healthcare organizations. If there is disagreement and conflict about what the guidelines conclude, this needs to become a matter of public debate. Dr. Campbell, Dr. Esselstyn, Dr. Ornish, as well as Dr. John McDougall have all put their evidence on the table stating unequivocally that the cause of the killer diseases is the consumption of animal protein. It is unjust to the public for the member organizations of the healthcare community to ignore this assertion when they do their own research, or to just cover it over with their own conclusions, which is what the AICR report would accomplish if it is accepted. Fortunately, and to its credit, the AICR has undertaken a Continuous Update Project to keep the evidence related to the Second Expert Report updated and current. It is possible, then, for the Update Project to take this issue under advisement and review impartially whether or not the recommendation to consume meat in moderation and the statement that meat is healthy and nourishing should be excluded from the report and, as well, the unscientific suggestions made in regard to vegetarians (vegans). Hopefully, it will do this.

The entire healthcare establishment has been ignoring or downplaying arguably the most significant breakthrough about nutrition ever made, that the consumption of animal protein is the major cause of the killer diseases. Experts in the field like Dr. Campbell, Dr. Esselstyn, Dr. McDougall, and Dr. Ornish have made this discovery available to the healthcare industry not only through books but through well-researched papers that have been published in scientific and academic journals for many years.

An article on Dr. Campbell's work, for example, appeared in

the Fall 1994 edition of the Cornell University Human Ecology Journal. It took note of Campbell's report that "rising plasma cholesterol levels in China were associated with a greater prevalence of stomach, liver, colon, lung, breast, and blood cancers," and that "even small intakes of animal products...were associated with elevated concentrations of plasma cholesterol and increased prevalence of these cancers."[11] This describes animal protein as a cancer-promoting substance and along with all the similar evidence should cause considerable reflection at the AICR about the advisability of including a recommendation in its Second Expert Report that describes meat as a healthy product if eaten in moderation.

The healthcare establishment seems unwilling to accept the message that animal protein is a major cause of the killer diseases, in spite of compelling evidence that supports the assertion, and is also unwilling to debate the issue. But it is no longer a matter of what the healthcare organizations want. The country needs and deserves a good old fashioned debate pitting the forces of those who state unequivocally that animal protein is a source of the killer diseases against those who refuse to take any kind of stand on the subject except to ignore it, or, as in the case of the panel for the AICR Second Expert Report, make their own brand of nutrition recommendations to the public without evaluating the opposing view. That just discredits the opposition without a hearing and tends to bury it.

Both sides need to be brought to the debate table on this important life and death issue for a full public airing of the facts. If the United States healthcare establishment is afraid to participate in this debate, it is letting down not only the American people, but all the people of the world.

Chapter 7

Grading the Healthcare Organizations

Is It Time for Women to Start Putting Up a Fight Against the Healthcare Establishment?

We have grown up with the sense that our healthcare organizations are designed to protect us. We have taken for granted that their job is to assemble knowledge, conduct research, and keep us up-to-date with the most accurate and current healthcare information available. We have been confident that the officers of these organizations are objective reporters without a hint of special interests or interagency rivalry attached to the work they perform. But today with growing suspicions that our personal health is being seriously compromised by the failure of our healthcare organizations to reveal the facts, questions are beginning to mount.

Contributing to the confusion is the incorrect information that gets communicated to the public by the healthcare system based on dogmatic parroting of doctrinaire ideals. The most transparent example is especially visible in the manner in which the healthcare system scripts dairy products as necessary components of good health when the scientific evidence reports just the opposite. (See chapters 5 and 23.) In addition, sometimes wrong information haphazardly assessed gets communicated that can have serious negative repercussions.

For example, the American College of Physicians (ACP) issued health guidelines in 1996 stating that there was not enough evidence to recommend that people over 65 should test for high cholesterol, based in part on an analysis of data from numerous sources including the famed Framingham Heart

Study. But Dr. William Castelli, who had been director of the Framingham study for 16 years, read the ACP report and strongly disagreed with the ACP analysis. In an open letter to doctors to be used by patients over the age of 65 to get their personal physicians to take their cholesterol concerns seriously, Castelli sharply criticized the ACP guidelines, pointing out its faults, and said that "lowering blood cholesterol lowers heart-attack risk in older people, just as it does in younger people." He protested that "if we do not concern ourselves with cholesterol in people over age 65, we will allow more than half of those people destined to get a heart attack in this country to go on and get that heart attack."[1]

It does seems self-evident that many people over the age of 65 could easily be at risk for heart disease and should do what is possible to limit the risk if they are able and if they are so inclined, including having their cholesterol tested.

The information that healthcare organizations are providing to people can have dangerous consequences for the public health as illustrated in the above instance and in other cases as well, for example, the advice that they do or do not make available concerning breast cancer. It has already been shown that the American Cancer Society ignores reporting that diet can reduce estrogen levels that in turn can reduce breast cancer risk. (See chapter 4.) But the ACS is not the only major cancer organization to do so.

Navigating to the web link for breast cancer on the website of the National Cancer Institute, one of the most notable of the 27 institutes of the National Institutes of Health, the web browser finds that the NCI does report that drugs like Tamoxifen, Raloxifene, Aromatase inhibitors, and a type of vitamin A called Fenretinide, all of which can have serious side effects, are able to reduce breast cancer risk.[2] The web page also discusses prophylactic mastectomy and oophorectomy in which women choose to have both breasts or both ovaries removed when there is no sign of cancer as a method of lowering breast cancer risk.

The NCI openly converses about radical procedures like prophylactic mastectomy and oophorectomy for reducing breast cancer risk and has no hesitation in providing the information that prophylactic oophorectomy "decreases the amount of estrogen made by the body and lowers the risk of breast cancer." Obviously, then, the NCI knows that estrogen levels are directly related to breast cancer. It would be difficult not to know considering that the majority of breast cancers are treated by suppressing the production of estrogen in the body, whether by drugs or more drastic procedures. That is because these cancers depend upon estrogen to grow. Yet, like the American Cancer Society, the NCI makes no mention of nutrition as a means for reducing estrogen levels in order to reduce breast cancer risk. In fact, about diet and breast cancer, the NCI says this:

> Diet is being studied as a risk factor for breast cancer. It is not proven that a diet low in fat or high in fruits and vegetables will prevent breast cancer. For more information on diet and health, see the Fruits and Veggies website.[3]

While it is commendable that the NCI is studying diet "as a risk factor for breast cancer," it is not satisfactory to just shuttle cancer inquirers about this serious matter off to visit an attractive Fruits and Veggies website with which the NCI has partnered, pretty though it may be. The question that must be asked is why the NCI has not considered the "overwhelming" evidence that already exists showing that the right kind of diet can lower estrogen levels in women and therefore can reduce the risk of breast cancer, especially since the NCI acknowledges that a decrease in estrogen made by the body "lowers the risk of breast cancer."

As we saw in chapter 4, the evidence tells us that "a diet high in animal foods and refined carbohydrates lowers the age of menarche, raises the age of menopause, increases female hormone levels [including estrogen], and increases blood cholesterol levels," so says T. Colin Campbell. Moreover, he says "there is *overwhelming* evidence that estrogen levels are a critical determinant of breast cancer risk."[4] [Author's emphasis.] The NCI acknowledges that "being exposed to estrogen over a long time may increase the risk of breast cancer."[5]

Since the NCI says that "it is not proven that a diet low in fat or high in fruits and vegetables will prevent breast cancer," and since an eminent researcher like Dr. T. Colin Campbell, one of the top scientists in the world, says that the proof unambiguously and overwhelmingly exists that "increased levels of estrogen and related hormones" [are] "a critical determinant of breast cancer risk" resulting from "the consumption of typical Western diets, high in fat and animal protein and low in dietary fiber," and further that "a plant-based diet will lower estrogen levels and reduce breast cancer risk," the stage is set for a serious disagreement if not an out and out confrontation over the facts.

Many men are tired of seeing their wives, daughters, sisters, mothers, grandmothers, girl friends, friends, and associates getting breast cancer and would like to see a public airing of this dispute about estrogen. Certainly, many women would like to see the disagreements brought out into the open. That is because the advice women follow about breast cancer that is put out by organizations like the NCI and the ACS can spell the difference between life and death. This is one big issue that needs to be broadcast across America so that the women of the entire country can hear it and make up their own minds.

The question that must be fought over and answered is quite simply this. Can a plant-based diet lower estrogen levels and consequently lower breast cancer risk to a considerable extent? It is not sufficient to ignore the question and shunt visitors off to visit a veggies website when so much is at stake. Women deserve an answer to this question by the National Cancer Institute and the American Cancer Society. Way back in 1996 the January/February issue of the Nutrition Action Health Letter reported that Regina Ziegler, a nutritional epidemiologist at the National Cancer Institute, said "we have consistent evidence that an affluent, Western diet is associated with higher risk [of breast cancer]."[6] That was fifteen years ago.

It is more than apparent that by Western diet Ziegler was referring to a low carbohydrate, high animal protein diet. How many women have developed breast cancer in the last fifteen years and died of the disease without the benefit of this knowledge of which the NCI was fully aware? So what is the answer, NCI and ACS? Can estrogen levels be lowered with plant-based foods and by eliminating animal products from the diet thus significantly reducing the risk of breast cancer? Is the answer Yes or is it No? In-betweens do not suffice.

The National Cancer Institute says that its "struggle to fully understand and ultimately defeat malignant disease requires the constant and timely sharing of information among cancer researchers, health professionals, patients and their families, and the general public, as well as the continuous training of new cadres of investigators." It also boasts that "through the years, the NCI has been a leader in exploiting new communications technologies to share cancer information."[7] If this is true, then the NCI must account for why it has not shared information like that uncovered by Dr. Campbell's 30 plus years of research on cancer that among other discoveries, directly links an animal-based diet to high estrogen levels that promotes breast cancer, and a plant-based diet to low estrogen levels that, in consequence, reduces the risk of breast cancer. Our healthcare agencies like the NCI need to stop resisting new discoveries that are backed with solid, scientific evidence just because they have policy differences, because they personally disapprove, because of institutional prejudices, because they are envious, because they are so buried in their own research they can hardly keep track of what their own policies are, or, because it does not meet their financial objectives.

As we have discussed, in 1996 Regina Ziegler, a nutritional epidemiologist at the NCI said "we have consistent evidence that an affluent, Western diet is associated with higher risk [of breast cancer]." Why then, in 2010 does the agency say: "It is not proven that a diet low in fat or high in fruits and vegetables [the opposite of the Western diet] will prevent breast cancer."

It is curious that just like the American Institute for Cancer Research, as discussed in chapter 6, the National Cancer Institute seems to have taken a step backwards when it comes to admitting the connection between animal protein and disease. It almost seems like whenever these organizations get closer to making significant progress in reducing the risk of cancer — which, incidentally, if achieved, could spell a reduced need of funding for cancer research — it becomes time to take a step backwards. The possibility should not be overlooked either, that this step backwards is a further consequence of flawed epidemiological research like that produced by the Nurses' Health Study discussed in chapter 6 and to be further addressed in chapter 8.

Today it seems the only way women can get truly accurate information about breast cancer risk is to accidentally stumble across it in a book like *The China Study*, or from independent sources not employed by mainstream healthcare organizations. Dr. Dean Ornish, referred to earlier because of his landmark research on heart disease prevention and reversal, who was also appointed to the 1992 National Institutes of Health Planning Panel to Assess Unconventional Medical Practices, is one of those independent sources. He wrote the following.

...a diet high in animal fats increases both the production and the biological activity of estrogens. Non-vegetarian women have about 50 percent higher blood estrogen levels than vegetarians. High levels of estrogens, in turn, promote the growth of many breast tumors.[8]

So Dr. Campbell is not the only healthcare expert sounding the alarm about the connection between diets high in animal fats to estrogen levels and breast cancer. Add also the name of Dr. John McDougall plus a growing number of other sources struggling to communicate this information to the public. These include websites offering nutrition advice like Health-Science.com and eHow.com; medical professionals like Robert Kradjian, MD (author of *Save Yourself from Breast Cancer*), and William Sears, M.D. with Martha Sears, RN (askdrsears.com); and independent researchers like Dr. Lesley M. Butler at Colorado State University. This represents only a few of the people working to get out the message that a low-fat diet can significantly reduce estrogen levels which will reduce breast cancer risk.

The problem with relying on independent sources to transmit "new" cancer information like this to the public is that it can take years and years for it to circulate, and many people will never hear about it. Certainly it is not likely that their personal physicians will tell them the news because, just like our healthcare organizations, most medical professionals do not get overly enthusiastic about information that does not emanate from mainstream establishment sources. As noted by Dr. Ornish, "breast cancer ...afflicts one in nine American women. [But] if you ask American physicians what women can do to prevent breast cancer, they usually reply, 'Get a mammogram every year after age 40.' Yet mammograms do not *prevent* cancer, they *detect* cancer."[9] [Emphasis, Ornish]

The effects of the failure of our healthcare system to communicate the most up-to-date scientific evidence to the public about disease and its prevention should be a matter of deep concern for everyone. In reference to their failure to communicate the facts about nutrition and estrogen in relation to breast cancer, women, especially, have every right to feel profoundly aggrieved.

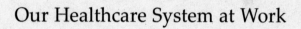
Our Healthcare System at Work

Chapter 8

The Influence of Cultural Biases on Science

Flawed Research: the Women's Health Initiative, the Nurses' Health Study, and the Women's Health Trial

When anyone tries to suggest changes to the medical establishment concerning its nutrition policies related to consuming meat and dairy products they are certain to encounter a host of biases. This was evident when the committee working on the 1982 *Diet, Nutrition, and Cancer* report for the National Academy of Sciences recommended reducing fat intake from 40% to 30% of calories with the proviso that the data could justify an even lower reduction. One of the committee members, the director of the United States Department of Agriculture, responded that if the committee recommended going below 30% consumers would have to "reduce animal food intake and that would be the death of the report."[1]

Because of concerns like this some researchers try not to panic people by telling them something about nutrition they would prefer not to hear. In the process these researchers abandon the rigors of good science and give in to the cultural biases of their times. The result is that facts get concealed and the public gets misled.

Only a very small percentage of the budget of the National Institutes of Health goes for research in nutrition.[2] So when an Institute of the NIH funds a nutrition study it is a key event. The chief healthcare organizations and interested members of the medical community and the public perk up their ears, open their eyes, and listen and watch.

This is what happened in 1993 when the National Heart, Lung, and Blood Institute of the NIH funded the Women's Health Initiative Dietary Modification Trial (which was one of three components comprising a Women's Health Initiative trial) created for the purpose of testing the effects of a low-fat diet in the prevention of breast cancer, colon cancer, and heart disease. The trial involved 49,000 women aged 50 to 79 of which 19,541 were randomly assigned to follow a low-fat diet. The cost to taxpayers was 415 million dollars.[3]

On February 8, 2006 the researchers released the results of the trial to the public. As reported by the Journal of the American Medical Association, the study showed that there was no significant benefit to a low-fat diet in reducing the risk of breast cancer, colorectal cancer, or heart disease.[4],[5],[6]

The results also caused the Harvard School of Public Health to issue a report that practically rated a low-fat diet in reducing the risk for cardiovascular disease as having little importance:

This [WHI Dietary Modification] eight-year trial, which included almost 49,000 women, found virtually identical rates of heart attack, stroke, and other forms of cardiovascular disease in women who followed a low-fat diet and in those women who didn't.[7]

The Harvard critique also stated that "the low-fat, high-starch diet that was the focus of dietary advice during the 1990s — as reflected by the USDA food guide pyramid — is dying out. A growing body of evidence has been pointing to its inadequacy for weight loss or prevention of heart disease and several cancers."[8]

These reviews were devastating blows to the people who had been advocating a low-fat diet for the prevention of cancer and heart disease that got its start with the National Academy of Sciences report on *Diet, Nutrition, and Cancer* in 1982. Years and years of hard work showing the link between dietary fat and disease was in danger of being undone.

The Dietary Modification Trial of the Women's Health Initiative (WHI), however, was deeply flawed from the beginning. Because the food industry has created many low-fat and nonfat products (meats, cheeses, yogurts, milk, cereals, crackers, dressings, cookies, etc.), it is easy enough to reduce fat intake and still maintain high levels of cholesterol and animal protein in the diet.[9] Dr. McDougall, the health nutritionist we met in previous chapters, reported that "the women in the WHI trial "continued to eat nearly the same amounts of fiber, protein, red meat, chicken, fish, and grains [as they normally did.]"[10]

Dr. McDougall personally spoke to the architects of the WHI study, Ernst Wynder (now deceased) and Rowan Chlebowski, on McDougall's syndicated radio show during the trial.[11] There and on many other occasions he challenged Wynder and Chlebowski to teach the women participating in the trial to use a very low-fat, plant-based diet, but Wynder and Chlebowski were not interested. They proceeded with a low-fat diet that included meat and dairy products. This was curious because prior to the WHI study Wynder had himself "published extensively on the benefits of a very low-fat (10% of calories), almost vegetarian, Japanese diet for prevention and treatment of breast cancer."[12] [The usual recommended level of fat intake today is 30%.][13] As we have seen, nevertheless, when he and his colleague Chlebowski conducted the WHI study they relied on a moderate, low-fat diet that was so temperate in scope that the women in the study assigned to the low-fat diet lost only one pound in eight years. Their blood levels of cholesterol, triglycerides, and blood pressure changed little. Obviously, something was way off. People who switch from a "normal" diet to a low-fat, plant-based diet can expect to lose far more than one pound in eight years with a meaningful change in their cholesterol, triglycerides, and blood pressure levels.

But the WHI Dietary Modification trial had little to do with being a low-fat, plant-based diet. Because Wynder and Chlebowski permitted the women to engage in their customary consumption of animal protein, any hypotheses related to reducing fat by reducing animal fat, and by consuming plant-based foods naturally low in fat in order to lower the risk for colon cancer, heart disease, and breast cancer, were not even tested. Because of these faults the public has been misled to believe that a "low-fat diet" is ineffective in reducing the risk of breast cancer, colon cancer, and heart disease. McDougall believes that "people worldwide have been, and are still being, betrayed by investigators who spend taxpayer's dollars on useless dietary research."[13]

Other notable studies of recent years that have minimized the importance of a low-fat diet in the prevention of chronic disease based upon flawed research are the famous billion dollar Nurses' Health Study and the Women's Health Trial (different from the Women's Health Initiative).

The Nurses' Health Study funded by the NIH is a Harvard initiative begun in 1976 that enrolled 120,000 nurses across the country to "investigate the relationship between various diseases and oral contraceptives, post-menopausal hormones, cigarettes and other factors." Data has been "collected for over two decades" from the study that is "widely known as the longest-running, premier study on women's health." It has "spawned three-satellite studies, all together costing $4 to 5 million per year."[14]

Professor Walter Willett of the Harvard School of Public Health decided to use the study to test the hypothesis that fat causes breast cancer which he accomplished by adding a dietary questionnaire to the study. It seemed like a good strategy since the study was already set up. As in the Women's Health Initiative, however, when the women reduced their fat intake, they could do so by using low-fat and nonfat animal products so that they were still ingesting animal protein.

In *The China Study*, reduced fat intake correlated to reduced animal protein intake with a consequent reduction in the incidence of cancer and vice versa. In the Nurses' Health Study, however, as stated, the women reduced their fat intake not by reducing animal protein, but by consuming low-fat or nonfat animal-based foods. Low-fat diets of this kind can contain "more than double the amount of protein of [a] high-fat meal," most of it coming from animal products. A"low-fat meal [like this also] contains almost twice as much cholesterol" as a plant-based meal.[15]

This is the same manner in which people are being fooled every day. They think that because they are consuming low-fat foods that their diet is healthy. In reality, they may be consuming a diet high in animal protein and high in cholesterol. A diet like this can lead to cancer and heart disease.

In the Nurses' Health Study between 78% to 86% of the protein the nurses consumed came from animal-based foods. Their average protein intake in terms of calories was around 19% as compared to the national average which is about 15% – 16%. The nurses therefore consumed even more animal protein than most people and consumed very few foods that were plant-based.[16] It was not possible to correctly measure the breast cancer risk associated with a "low-fat diet" by means of this study because the study did not measure the effects of animal protein and it did not measure the effects of a plant-based diet. Nevertheless, the Nurses' Health Study has led people to believe that there is no significant correlation between fat and breast cancer.

Flawed research like Professor Willet conducted with the Nurses' Health Study chips away at sound discoveries and makes damaging claims that can lead people to arrive at faulty conclusions like that breast cancer is unrelated to diet.

The Women's Health Trial, a 1991 – 1996 study to determine

if women could decrease the incidence of cancer through a low-fat diet, was sponsored by the National Cancer Institute.[17] Like the Nurses' Health Study and the Women's Health Initiative, it also did not ask the participating women to reduce their fat intake by reducing their consumption of animal-based foods. Instead, the women reduced their fat intake by using low-fat, nonfat animal products and less fat in cooking. As in the other studies, the participants could actually eat more animal products while consuming less fat through low-fat foods. This was once again a study that ignored the effects of animal-based and plant-based foods in relation to health and disease.

T. Colin Campbell said "we might as well conclude that diet is completely unrelated to cancer."[18] He believes the Nurses' Health Study "has virtually nullified many of the advances that have been made over the past fifty years without actually posing a scientifically reliable challenge to earlier findings regarding diet and cancer." Campbell says further that "hardly any study has done more damage to the nutritional landscape than the Nurses' Health Study, and it should serve as a warning for the rest of science for what not to do."[19] He notes that some "people within the scientific community are already beginning to say that diet may have no effect on cancer."

That some people have been influenced to change their point of view can be observed by taking a look at what the Harvard School of Public Health had to say about Willett's conclusions. It reported that in the Nurses' Health Study:

...no link was seen between the overall percentage of calories from fat and any important health outcome, including cancer, heart disease, and weight gain.[20]

We have also discussed in chapter 6 how the Nurses' Health Study may have influenced the AICR Second Expert Report to draw the false conclusion that fat is not a cause of cancer.

Unfortunately, the faulty conclusions have not stopped. An article by the popular nutritionist Dr. Andrew Weil published in the July 2, 2010 Huffington Post debunked the dangers of saturated fats, and suggested that they might even be good for us compared to processed carbohydrates and sugars. Weil backed up his contention with a study published by Dr. Ronald Krauss in the March 2010 American Journal of Clinical Nutrition which proposed that there is "no difference in the risk of heart disease or stroke between people with the lowest and highest intakes of saturated fat." This is similar to the conclusions drawn by the Harvard School of Public Health and the Health Professional's Follow-up Study just mentioned. The Krauss study, however, consisted of a comparison of several epidemiological studies involving 348,000 participants. Weil viewed the Krauss study as a "significant exoneration" of saturated fat as a factor in heart disease. The problem for both Dr. Weil and Dr. Krauss, is that of the 348,000 participants upon which the Krauss study relied, almost half were taken from the Nurses' Health Study, which, as we have seen, also sees little importance between a high-fat and a low-fat diet as a cause of disease. Because we have just taken a look behind the scenes, however, we know that this study is flawed. And this does not preclude other studies upon which Dr. Krauss relied from being equally flawed, especially since, as reported below, Dr. Campbell has asserted that virtually every other epidemiological study of this nature is seriously flawed for the same reasons. Consequently, the Krauss study must be regarded as suspect and, as should now be apparent, does not really deserve scientific validation. However that may be, it does not prevent hypotheses like Krauss and Weill have proposed from making their way out into the public forum where they exert an influence not only on the public, but on scientists and medical personnel who are not aware of the flaws underlying the research.[21]

When Dr. Campbell ran into Professor Willett on several

occasions, he pointed out to Willett that the Nurses' Health Study did not include plant-based foods naturally low in fat. Willet consistently replied, "You may be right, Colin, but people don't want to go there."[22]

But what people want should not be a controlling factor in conducting scientific research.

John McDougall, in referring to the Women's Health Initiative, makes the same point. In talking about the relationships of doctors with their patients, McDougall discusses the role cultural biases play in doctor/patient interactions:

My nearly 40 years of experience, working with hundreds of influential doctors and scientists, leads me to believe they have a very low opinion of patients and the public in general. They believe we are too stupid and uninterested in our own welfare to make meaningful changes in our diet — specifically to follow a plant-food based diet. When I suggest such powerful dietary changes, they respond with, 'That's unreasonable; no one will follow a vegetarian diet.' Even if they were correct, you and I still deserve to know the truth, so that this option for preventing illnesses and premature death is open to us. [23]

Dr. Campbell says virtually the same:

Scientists should not be ignoring ideas just because we perceive that the public does not want to hear them. Too often during my career, I have heard comments that seem to be more of an attempt to please the public than to engage in an open, honest debate, wherever it may take us. This is wrong. The role of science in society is to observe, to ask questions, to form and test hypotheses and to interpret the findings without bias — not to kowtow to people's perceived desires. Consumers have the ultimate choice of whether to integrate our findings into their lifestyles, but we owe it to them to give them the best information possible with which to make that decision and not decide for them. It is they who paid for this research and it is only they who have the right to decide what to do with it.[24]

The examples referred to in this chapter illustrate how some medical professionals and healthcare organizations are not acting in accordance with an unbiased perspective in conducting scientific inquiries and arriving at conclusions about the effects of animal protein on the public health. In fact, Campbell insists that practically all of the other human epidemiological studies "published to date have been seriously shortchanged in their investigations of diet and disease associations....Because of these very serious flaws, these studies have been a virtual disaster for discovering the really significant effects of diet on these diseases."[25]

As long as researchers give in to popular culture and design their research accordingly, the public will pay the consequences. In order to build an informed and accurate consensus of the best diets available to assist the population in living the healthiest possible life, it is vital that healthcare researchers keep the doors of inquiry open for new discoveries uninfluenced by cultural biases. If they do not, their research can only produce results that impact the public health in harmful ways and start a chain reaction that is difficult to overcome. Once the genie escapes, it can take decades, even centuries to get it back in the lamp.

Chapter 9

The Story Behind Cholesterol and Statins

Is the Information Distributed by the Healthcare Establishment Causing People to Have Heart Attacks?

In recent years the medical profession has been relying on people's cholesterol count as the major factor in estimating risk for heart attacks and cardiovascular disease. Though this method has been coming under some criticism, healthcare organizations also follow this procedure and use cholesterol guidelines that are more or less standard throughout the healthcare industry. These are put out by an expert panel of the National Heart, Lung, and Blood Institute (an Institute of the NIH) which passes them down to the National Cholesterol Education Program (NCEP) for distribution. The NCEP, whose main job is to raise public awareness about the dangers of high cholesterol, is responsible for communicating the cholesterol guidelines to the medical institutions and the public.

The NCEP cholesterol guidelines advise that a total cholesterol count of 200 mg/dL and below is desirable with a count of 200 – 239 mg/dL being borderline high. (mg/dL = milligrams of glucose per decileter of blood) A cholesterol count above 240 mg/dL is considered high.[1] The American Medical Association follows this standard and also warns that any count above 240 mg/dL means that people are at twice the risk of having a heart attack as someone within the borderline high range of 200 – 239 mg/dL.[2] Other major healthcare organizations concerned with cholesterol levels like the American Heart Association employ the same guidelines as do hospitals like the Massachusetts

General Hospital, the New York-Presbyterian Hospital/ Columbia University Medical Center, the Mayo Clinic, Johns Hopkins, etc.[3] These are also the guidelines that get passed along to physicians for use in their private practice all across the country.

About the best thing that might be said about a threshold safety level of 200 mg/dL for preventing heart disease and heart attacks is that it is an improvement over the guidelines of previous decades. For years "it was the conventional wisdom that blood levels of cholesterol up to 300 mg/dL were perfectly normal."[4] But what the medical establishment is unwilling to say these days is that "35% of heart attacks strike Americans who have cholesterol levels between 150 and 200 mg/dL."[5] In other words, a total cholesterol count of 200 mg/dL is not really a heart attack safe level at all.

This is what T. Colin Campbell tells us. He is not the only one and no one in the medical establishment is denying it. Campbell writes that some of the most "innocent [and unsuspecting] victims [of heart attacks] are health-conscious Americans who follow [the recommendations of the medical experts], keeping their total cholesterol around 180 or 190 mg/dL, only to be rewarded with a heart attack leading to premature death."

Dr. Caldwell B. Esselstyn, to be focused upon more closely in chapter 10, also points out that one out of every four persons who has a heart attack has a blood cholesterol level between 180 and 210 mg/dL and that a third of those in the Framingham Heart Study who had heart disease had total cholesterol levels between 150 and 200 mg/dL.[6]

As mentioned earlier, the Framingham Heart Study is an ongoing study of the causes of cardiovascular disease begun in Framingham, Massachusetts in 1948. The heart-safe cholesterol level according to the Framingham Heart Study is 150 mg/dL. In fact, Dr. William Castelli, known as the originator of the terms "good cholesterol" and "bad cholesterol," tells us that they never "had a heart attack in Framingham in 35 years in anyone who had a total cholesterol count under 150."[7] As indicated earlier, Castelli was the Director of the Framingham Heart Study for 16 years. (He was a laboratory blood technician there for an additional 14 years before becoming Director.) Esselstyn further warns that the safety threshold chosen by the government and our healthcare organizations of 200 mg/dL "virtually guarantees — if everyone actually met their stated goal — that every year more than 1.2 million Americans will suffer heart attacks and that millions more will watch the inevitable progression of their coronary artery disease."

According to this standard, all government and nonprofit healthcare organizations, and also all physicians (private and institutional) who recommend a cholesterol threshold level of 200 mg/dL as a safety level for heart disease are giving out information that puts millions of Americans at greater risk for heart attacks and cardiovascular disease. While some physicians may not be aware of the Framingham Heart Study figures, it is difficult to believe that the healthcare organizations are not familiar with them, which means that they are knowingly ignoring this evidence. Why they would do this may appear enigmatic, but one very good reason will be suggested after first examining some of the factors that can precipitate and prevent heart disease.

[It should be noted that from 5 to 10 percent of people who have heart disease are genetically predisposed to get the disease. This group includes approximately 85% of people under the age of 65 who have heart attacks. Medications can help lower their cholesterol and save their lives if they are identified with this genetic predisposition in time.][8]

Atherosclerosis (commonly referred to as hardening of the arteries) is one of the primary causes of cardiovascular disease and happens when high blood pressure, smoking, or LDL cholesterol (the bad cholesterol) damages the endothelium, the cellular lining of blood vessels, carrying blood to the heart, according to Richard Stein, of the American Heart Association.[9] At that point, plaque, which is a "jumble of lipids, or cholesterol, cells, and debris," builds up creating a "bump on the artery wall." Over the years the plaque grows and can result in a narrowing of the arteries and diminished blood flow. "The worst-case scenario" happens when plaques "suddenly rupture, allowing blood to clot inside an artery. In the brain, this causes a stroke; in the heart, a heart attack."

(LDL (low density lipoprotein) is called the "bad" cholesterol because LDL particles being transported in the blood stream from the liver that are not diffused into the cells can be carried into the artery wall where they can start the formation of plaque. HDL (high density lipoprotein), which is also circulating in the blood, is called the "good" cholesterol because it carries excess LDL back to the liver for storage or disposal, thus reducing plaque buildup.)

As indicated by many sources, including Merck Pharmaceuticals (now Merck/Schering Plough), the leading sources for cholesterol that can cause atherosclerosis are meat, eggs, and dairy products which are high in saturated fat and cholesterol.[10] Saturated fat, which comes mostly from animal foods, including meat, poultry, fowl, and fish, is the main villain because it stimulates the liver to produce more cholesterol. (A few non-animal foods are also high in saturated fats like coconut and palm oil, and hydrogenated oils like shortening and margarine.)

It is important to bring the issue of strokes into the discussion at this point because the dangers of cholesterol apply equally to stroke. According to Teresa Fung, a researcher who studies stroke at the Harvard School of Public Health, "in essence, an ischemic stroke is much like a heart attack that occurs in your brain and can result from atherosclerosis."[11]

Ischemic strokes account for 83% of all strokes. The

remaining 17 percent are defined as hemorrhagic strokes and are caused by hemorrhaging.[12] Hemorrhagic stroke may be congenital, but most strokes are caused by high blood pressure which can also be related to diet. Plaque debris flaking off from the aorta that then travels to the brain is another event that can precipitate a stroke.[13]

High blood pressure is the single-most important risk factor for stroke, according to the American Heart Association. As previously noted, on average, vegetarians have lower blood pressure than consumers of meat. In a study published in the American Journal of Clinical Nutrition, researchers found that only 2 percent of vegetarians suffered from high blood pressure compared to 26 percent of people who eat meat.[14] Other studies by scientists at the Harvard Medical School have found that "[s]trict vegetarians, who eat little if any animal products, have lower blood pressures than the general population after adjustment for the effects of age, sex, and body weight."[15]

Because vegetarians have lower blood pressure in comparison to meat-eaters, they reduce their chances of suffering a stroke or developing cardiovascular problems associated with high blood pressure. And, they also are not so inclined to get hardened and clogged arteries (atherosclerosis) that are precursors to stroke and heart attacks.[16] Researchers who followed 72,000 women for 14 years also found that the women who adhered to diets rich in fruits, vegetables, and grains were less likely to suffer a stroke compared to those who ate a meat-based diet.[17] Additionally, the Framingham Heart Study found that every three additional servings of fruits and vegetables per day reduced the risk of stroke by 22%.[18] A dab of spinach, a dab of peaches, a dab of carrots. Add them together, and that's all it takes to put one great safety measure against stroke on people's side.

In an attempt to get their cholesterol levels down, eighteen million Americans take cholesterol-lowering statins like Lipitor or Crestor at a cost of $33 billion annually.[19] But the effectiveness of these drugs has been brought into question (see also chapter 15), and it appears that people have been fooled into thinking that statins provide an umbrella of protection that does not really exist.

In 2008, Merck/Schering Plough released the results of a clinical trial for Zetia, a non-statin cholesterol lowering drug prescribed to about one million people. The trial combined Zetia with simvastatin (a statin) and compared it to simvastatin used alone. Dr. Steven E. Nissen, chairman of cardiology at the Cleveland Clinic, called the results of the trial "shocking."[20]

While Zetia did lower cholesterol levels, the study failed to show that any measurable medical benefits resulted. Dr. John Abramson, a clinical instructor at the Harvard Medical School, and the author of *Overdosed America*, answered the question of whether or not cholesterol lowering drugs do any good as follows:

...statins show a clear benefit for one group — people under 65 who have already had a heart attack or who have diabetes. But, there are no studies to show that these drugs will protect older patients over 65 — or younger patients who are not already suffering from diabetes or established heart disease, from having a fatal heart attack. Nevertheless, 8 or 9 million patients who fall into this category continue to take the drugs, which means that they are exposed to the risks that come with taking statins — which can include severe muscle pain, memory loss, and sexual dysfunction.[21]

Equally disturbing is that eight percent of patients whose cholesterol is being successfully reduced with statins will have a serious coronary problem like a heart attack or angina.[22] And for those under 65 who have diabetes or who have had a heart attack, while statins lowered their cholesterol levels, many researchers believe that this will not help them avoid a second one.

One line of thought maintains that eighteen million Americans are taking statins because the American Heart Association and the College of Cardiology have pushed the concept of cholesterol-lowering drugs so hard that everyone accepts it.[23] So many people were having heart attacks that the idea evolved of trying to give cholesterol lowering drugs to anyone who was at risk for developing cardiovascular disease. A few researchers even "half jokingly" suggested that statins be put in the water supply.[24]

But there is good reason for concern about relying too heavily upon statins as a cure-all for heart disease. A 2007 report from the Canadian Women's Health Network, "Evidence for Caution: Women and Statin Use," called what was happening in medicine the "'cholesterolization' of cardiovascular disease — that is, emphasis on a single risk factor."[25] The report contended that "cholesterol has come to represent a virtual disease state in itself, rather than one risk factor among many, and has distracted from grappling with other risk factors that are strong indicators of cardiovascular disease and cardiovascular risk."

Some researchers even question the role of high cholesterol as a causative agent in heart disease. It has been observed, for example, that Spaniards have an LDL cholesterol level about the same as Americans, but only half the rate of heart disease.[26] The Swiss have even higher levels, but also have less heart disease, and Australian aborigines have a low cholesterol, but a high rate of heart disease. Examples like these are puzzling and suggest that other factors contributing to heart disease may deserve more attention than they are getting, factors like those studied in the Framingham Heart Study such as lack of physical activity, obesity, stress, smoking, and alcoholism.[27]

Of prime importance in this debate is the fact that no one in the Framingham Heart Study with a cholesterol count below 150 mg/dL has ever had a heart attack. This would seem to indicate categorically that people with a cholesterol level above 150 mg/dL may be in a range in which they are at risk for cardiovascular disease.

The most important element of all, however, in assessing how best to reduce the risk for cardiovascular and cerebrovascular disease, is the connection of animal protein to higher blood cholesterol levels. That is because the elimination of animal protein from the diet eliminates the high blood cholesterol for which animal protein is responsible thus eliminating the need for statins or other cholesterol lowering medications to reduce it. Unfortunately, this factor has not even made its way into the mainstream medical discourse where saturated fats and cholesterol intake are adversely associated with coronary heart disease, but not animal protein. Dr. Campbell points out that few doctors "will say that animal protein has anything to do with blood cholesterol levels."[28]

The American Medical Association seems to agree that animal protein is not an important factor as a cause of heart disease. It advises that we meet our protein requirements with a combination of dairy products, meat, poultry, and fish. For dairy products, three or more servings daily are recommended (four servings if you are 51 or older). To this add no more than two servings daily of meat or fish (especially oily fish), totaling 6 ounces.[29]

The Mayo Clinic is in almost perfect stride with similar recommendations for dairy (two to three servings of low-fat or nonfat milk, yogurt or cheese) and meat (two to three 2 or 3 ounce servings of lean meats, poultry, fish, dried beans, eggs or nuts).[30] Johns Hopkins Hospital also recommends two or more servings of preferably low-fat dairy foods and no more than six ounces of meat, poultry, or seafood. [31] And we have already seen in chapter 6 that the American Institute for Cancer Research recommends 5 to 6 ounces of red meat daily along with three servings of low-fat dairy products.

Lean meats, low-fat and nonfat dairy products, and poultry and fish: these are the main sources from which the public should satisfy protein needs, according to the healthcare establishment. But the connection between animal protein and dairy products with high saturated fats, high blood pressure, and high blood cholesterol, which, as discussed above, are the main causes of atherosclerosis and heart disease — even according to a mainstream source like Merck/Schering Plough — should not be so easily dismissed. This should, in fact, be a major cause for concern. It should also not be forgotten that those who want to live with a heart-safe cholesterol level need to reduce their cholesterol levels to 150 mg/dL. The meat and dairy recommendations for protein intake that the healthcare organizations are making will not bring the cholesterol count down to that level. It will, however, keep many people at risk for heart disease and stroke.[32]

A diet of fruits, vegetables, grains, and legumes can reduce the blood cholesterol count to 150 mg/dL and below, and do it rapidly. Additionally, this kind of diet will reduce free radicals, and add antioxidants for fighting disease. It will also easily replace the protein that needs to be restored to the body daily while eliminating harmful excess protein by-products, as we shall see in chapter 17, and it will be free of toxic pesticides and chemicals that are found in meat and fish.[33]

Fish, however, serve as one of the main sources for the omega 3 fatty acids which are considered essential. Omega 3 fatty acids have been widely promoted as an important nutrient for reducing heart disease ever since around 1980 when it was discovered that the Inuits, who consume a high-fat diet, had a low incidence of heart disease. This was attributed to their high consumption of fish which contain copious amounts of omega 3 fatty acids.

The ACS, the AMA, the Mayo Clinic, and Johns Hopkins Hospital advise eating seafood, as do the USDA and the AICR. The American Heart Association recommends eating fish at least twice a week, stressing recent research which shows that eating oily fish containing omega 3 fatty acids (for example, salmon, trout, and herring) may help "lower the risk of death" from coronary artery disease.

Eating fish, however, could conceivably "raise the risk of death" for other reasons. According to the Physicians Committee for Responsible Medicine, omega 3 fatty acids in fish are highly unstable molecules that decompose quickly and unleash free radicals in the process. Fish and shellfish also can contain toxic chemicals and high levels of methylmercury at concentrations as high as nine million times those found in the water in which they swim. Methylmercury is associated with rises in blood pressure, impaired neurological function in infants, and reduced fertility in adults.[34] Chemicals and pesticides in fish are also suspected as being possible agents in promoting non-Hodgkin's lymphoma and other cancers. Besides the dangers of mercury contamination, the ACS cautions that tuna, salmon, and larger fish may also contain dioxins and PCBs (polychlorinated biphenyls).

Dioxins are toxic chemicals associated with cancer risk, the exposure to which, according to the FDA, occurs most often through the consumption of animal fats. PCBs are probable human carcinogens that may cause liver cancer. Some studies also show that farm-raised fish have more toxins than fish caught in the wilds because they are fed other fish that have ingested contaminants like PCBs.[35,36]

For those who want to include omega 3 fatty acids in their diet but do not want to endanger their health by consuming fish, other sources are available, though they are not widely known or publicized. These include beans, nuts, soybeans, walnuts, black currant seed oil, flaxseed oil, soybean oil, pumpkin seed oil, walnut oil, Purslane (an exotic weed (a vegetable)), and seeds like flax seeds, hemp seeds, and pumpkin seeds.[37] [However, see footnote 39 for possible dangers in regard to alpha-linolenic acid (ALA), the only omega 3 fatty acid found in vegetable sources.]

In regard to oils, a word of caution should be sounded for not only animal oils but also vegetable-based oils, including monounsaturated oils such as olive oil and canola oil, which the media refers to as heart healthy oils. According to Dr. Esselstyn, however:

> ...nothing could be further from the truth. They are not heart healthy. Between 14 and 17 percent of olive oil is saturated, artery-clogging fat — every bit as aggressive in promoting heart disease as the saturated fat in roast beef. And even though a Mediterranean-style diet that allows such oils may slow the rate of progression of coronary artery disease, when compared with diets even higher in saturated fat, it does not arrest the disease and reverse its effects.[38],[39]

It should be evident that in recommending the consumption of meat and dairy foods, even when it is lean meat and low-fat dairy products, the healthcare establishment is providing the public with contradictory and confusing advice for meeting daily protein requirements. For one, as we have seen, animal products contain cholesterol and saturated fats that can increase blood cholesterol levels that in turn can create atherosclerosis that can lead to stroke, heart attacks, and coronary artery disease. Confusion also prevails because the entire mainstream medical establishment has set 200 mg/dL as the safety threshold for avoiding cardiovascular disease and heart attacks when it is not a safe level at all, as the evidence unmistakably shows.

The monumental question that arises from this nearly inconceivable practice is, why would all the healthcare organizations and the majority of doctors charged with protecting the public health want people to believe that they are heart attack safe if their total cholesterol level is between 150 and 200 mg/dL when convincing evidence shows that they are still considerably at risk — in fact, so much at risk that this cholesterol range is the same in which 35% of all heart attacks occur?

One very plausible explanation lies in that a total cholesterol level of 200 mg/dL makes room for the moderate consumption of meat and dairy products, which is the recommendation for meeting human protein needs that the healthcare organizations have unified behind. This is nothing but obeisance to the Protein Gods who have demanded this tribute from the people. Simply put, the healthcare establishment does not want to give up the consumption of animal foods. As long as our healthcare profession can pretend that 200 mg/dL is the safety level for cardiovascular disease and heart attacks, people can continue consuming animal protein if they keep their cholesterol below that level oblivious to the ceiling above their heads that may cave in at any moment — and all too frequently does.

For studies such as the one referred to in the previous chapter by Dr. Ronald Krauss, which attempts to discredit saturated fat as a causative factor in heart disease, it almost seems like their real purpose is to keep the habit of consuming animal protein alive at all costs. Those who prefer truth over fiction, however, need only to turn to the words of Dr. Castelli who said: "We've never had a heart attack in Framingham in 35 years in anyone who had a cholesterol level under 150. Three-quarters of the people who live on the face of this Earth never have a heart attack. They live in Asia, Africa, and South America, and their cholesterols are all around 150."[40] This simple fact is paramount in the debate over the pros and cons of fats and cholesterol as the cause of heart disease and is directly in line with Dr. Campbell's report on "diseases of affluence" and "diseases of poverty" where poorer countries are not subject to heart disease because they do not consume animal protein.[41]

No matter what might be brought to light pertaining to the chemical metabolism of saturated fats and LDL cholesterol, or how fascinating the comparisons of heart disease rates vs. cholesterol between indigenous populations like the Spaniards, the Swiss, and the Australian aborigines may be, the facts indicate that a total cholesterol count of 150 mg/dL is the level above which people may be at risk for cardiovascular disease. The surest way to reduce this risk is to reduce the total choles- terol count below 150 mg/dL. Dr. Bill Roberts, the editor of the prestigious medical journal Cardiology agrees as do Dr. Campbell, Dr. Castelli, Dr. Esselstyn, Dr. McDougall, and Dr. Ornish.[42] According to all these experts, the only real heart attack threshold level of safety for total cholesterol count is 150 mg/dL.

For people to protect themselves against stroke and heart attack, the science indicates that switching from an animal-based diet to a plant-based diet is one of the best steps to take. The average cholesterol level in the United States is 210. The average vegetarian has a cholesterol level of 161, and the average vegan has a cholesterol level of 133.[43]

The medical establishment may not like to admit it, and the Protein Gods may fulminate and fume, but the outlines of the road ahead for those who want to live free of statins with a heart-safe cholesterol level is clearly visible.

Chapter 10

The Treatment for Heart Disease

Are Surgery and Drugs Necessary?

Current research suggests that death from cardiovascular disease is on the decline. However, the incidence of people who get heart disease remains the same, and risk factors may be increasing.[1] (Cardiovascular disease includes stroke, high blood pressure, heart failure, and other conditions like arrhythmias, atrial fibrillation, cardiomyopathy, and peripheral arterial disease.) Discoveries that isolate the cause of heart disease and offer cures like the remarkable breakthroughs made by Dr. Caldwell B. Esselstyn, Jr. and Dr. Dean Ornish should, consequently, excite cardiologists. Yet in spite of the proved effectiveness of these new treatment options, most mainstream cardiologists and cardiovascular treatment facilities have ignored them.

Dr. Esselstyn began a twelve year cardiac disease arrest and reversal trial in 1985. Five years into the study he published his first findings and the complete report seven years later. Dr. Dean Ornish began his first clinical trial in 1986, issued his first report a year later, and then in 1990 published the results of his study in a widely acclaimed book, *Dr. Dean Ornish's Program for Reversing Heart Disease*.[2]

Both trials showed conclusively that heart disease can be prevented and reversed though a low-fat, plant-based diet.[3] Prior to these trials the field of cardiology considered coronary heart disease to be irreversible.

Dr. Ornish's plan calls for a diet of no meats and no added fats with an emphasis on whole grain foods, vegetables, fruits, and beans. It permits the consumption of egg whites and nonfat dairy products. Ornish combines his diet with exercise, stress management, and group support. With this plan he was able to reverse severe coronary artery disease without statins or other drugs.[4] Praise for Ornish's work, however, is often accompanied by negative criticisms on how difficult the plan is to follow or some other comment that casts it in a less than favorable light. The *Mayo Clinic Heart Book*, for example, offers a generally favorable review, but comments that "many people find that the program...requires substantial lifestyle changes."[5]

Dr. Esseltsyn's program, described in his book *Prevent and Reverse Heart Disease*, calls for avoiding oils, meat, fish, fowl and dairy products.[6] His trial involved 18 patients who in the eight years prior to the trial had experienced 49 coronary events such as "angina, bypass surgery, heart attacks, strokes and angioplasty." After 12 years on Dr. Esselstyn's program, these 18 patients experienced only one coronary event, and that particular patient had dropped out of the program for two years. After he came back and resumed Esselstyn's plant-based diet he had no further cardiovascular disease occurrences.

The medical establishment does not react to heart disease arrest and reversal programs like those Dr. Esselstyn and Dr. Ornish have set up with great enthusiasm. Dr. Campbell, for example, recalls the kind of responses he witnessed from his colleagues steeped in surgical and drug treatment procedures when the evidence began accumulating that nutrition could prevent cardiovascular events from occurring.

I remember when my superiors were only reluctantly accepting the evidence of nutrition being able to *prevent* heart disease, for example, but vehemently denying its ability to *reverse* such a disease when already advanced. But the evidence can no longer be ignored. Those in science or medicine who shut their minds to such an idea are being more than stubborn; they are being irresponsible.[7]

Dr. Esselstyn practiced at the Cleveland Clinic, called by some the "best medical center for cardiac care" in the country, if not the world. Patients fly there from all across the globe for advanced heart disease treatment. It was during Dr. Esselstyn's work there that he conducted the trial described above.[8]

Besides winning an Olympic gold medal in rowing and a Bronze Star for military service in Vietnam, Esselstyn was President of the Staff at the Cleveland Clinic, member of the Board of Governors, chairman of the Breast Cancer Task Force, and head of the Section of Thyroid and Parathyroid Surgery. He was also the president of the American Association of Endocrine Surgeons, author of over 100 professional scientific articles, and he was included on a list of the best doctors in America in 1994 – 1995.[9]

After he had completed his trial with the eighteen coronary patients and after his retirement in the year 2000, Esselstyn proposed to the Cleveland Clinic that he set up an arrest and reversal dietary cardiac program like the one he had done, as an option to be offered to every patient in the clinic suffering from heart disease.[10] The program cost little and presented no risk for patients. The Clinic rehired him as a consultant in 2009 to direct the Cardiovascular Disease Prevention and Reversal Program at the Cleveland Wellness Institute.

Many people at the Clinic were excited about Dr. Esselstyn's work. Staff members and trustees of the Clinic who had developed coronary disease themselves were approaching him for treatment.[11]

Esselstyn notes that work is presently being done with "stem cells to try to make new blood vessels grow."[12] He asks if it would not just be easier to prevent the disease in the first place.[13]

Campbell concurs. "We, the public, turn to doctors and hospitals in times of great need," he says. "For them to provide care that is knowingly less than optimal, that doesn't protect our health, doesn't heal our disease and costs us tens of thousands of dollars is morally inexcusable."[14]

It is worthwhile noting that in contrast to heart disease arrest and reversal programs, in 1996 a team of surgical specialists from the Cleveland Clinic flew to Brazil to investigate a new operation that an unknown surgeon, Dr. Randas Batista, had developed to treat heart failure by strengthening the heart muscle. It involved removing a wedge-shaped piece of tissue from the left ventricle, the main chamber of the heart. Batista had 400 patients under his care and claimed the operation was hugely successful.[15]

After consulting with Dr. Batista, the surgical team returned to the Cleveland Clinic and tried out this procedure for themselves on 62 patients, all of whom gave their consent. But the operation turned out to be a dismal failure. Within three years more than a third of the patients had died, and only a quarter were free of heart disease.[16]

When surgery was involved, the Cleveland Clinic flew a team of experts to Brazil which subsequently operated on 62 patients in an experimental procedure that was highly dangerous, involved intense pain, cost enormous fees, failed to provide perceived benefits for three-quarters of those operated on, and ultimately proved fatal for more than a third of the participants.

The bias favoring surgery and drugs over treatment by means of nutrition could hardly be more apparent. If the patients who were operated on unsuccessfully with the Brazilian procedure could go back and do it over again — especially those who died — can any rational person doubt that they would choose heart disease arrest and reversal treatment over the one offered by the Cleveland Clinic, the best cardiovascular clinic in the world?

Cutting open patients' chests and splicing in new blood

vessels to bypass clogged arteries costs $13 billion a year. One-half of all bypass procedures clog up again within 10 years. One-third of all angioplasty procedures clog again within four to six months. In contrast, the patients who participated in Dr. Esselstyn's program were still disease free two decades after they had finished the program, and never experienced one spasm of pain.[17]

It costs considerably less per year, obviously, to undertake a low-fat, plant-based diet as the sole treatment for cardiovascular disease. But while that is great for the bank accounts of patients, it is also a part of the problem. Medical facilities are not anxious to forego their cut of that $13 billion a year heart bypass industry which open heart surgery provides.

Cutting open someone's chest, it goes without saying, is a surgically complicated, serious, and painful procedure. As Dr. David Eddy, a professor of health policy at Duke University noted, "a coronary artery bypass may change the life expectancy of a 60 year-old man with triple vessel disease, but it will also change his joy of life for several weeks after the operation, the degree and severity of chest pain, his ability to walk and make love, his relationship with his son, the physical appearance of his chest and his pocketbook. Pain, disability, anxiety, family relations, and any number of other outcomes are all important consequences of a procedure."[18]

Patients should not have to endure this kind of suffering without at least being informed that other possibilities exist.

As for Dr. Esselstyn, his goal remains untarnished. He has glimpsed the possibilities and he forges ahead as do all pioneers when faced with mainstream status quo rejection.

I have an ambitious goal: to annihilate heart disease — to abolish it once and for all. Your arteries at the age of ninety ought to work as efficiently as they did when you were nine....We have shown that [this] number one killer in Western civilization can be abolished, through consumption of a plant-based diet. But we can do much more. If the public adopted this approach to preventing disease, if, by the millions, Americans abandoned their toxic diets and learned a truly healthy approach to eating, we could largely limit all those diseases of nutritional extravagance — strokes, hypertension, obesity, osteoporosis, and adult-onset diabetes. Meanwhile, we would see a marked reduction in cancers of the breast, prostate, colon, rectum, uterus, and ovaries. Medicine could relinquish its primary focus on pills and procedures. Prevention, not desperate intervention, would become the order of the day.[19]

Most medical facilities ignore the work of Dr. Esselstyn and Dr. Ornish in favor of more traditional approaches. At the Los Angeles Cedars-Sinai Medical Center, Dr. John Young, director of comparative medicine and chairman of Americans for Medical Progress, a pro-animal testing organization, and his staff work on research projects that include vivisecting pigs in the study of cardiovascular disease. He makes the same pitch all animal researchers make when they want public sympathy and support: the research is exciting; we're right on the verge of a cure; it's just around the corner.

In an interview on PBS early in 2009, Young showed off a magnificent, lean and muscular, black-and-cream-colored pig confined in a small holding pen and said: "The cardiovascular system of a pig is almost identical to that of a human being, okay? The coronary arteries, the heart muscle — virtually identical, so pigs are a favorite model for cardiovascular disease."[20]

It seems a terrible waste that Dr. Young and the staff of the Los Angeles Cedars-Sinai Medical Center work on experimental heart disease operations that take away the lives of beautiful pigs, like the one Dr. Young displayed, when the exemplary trials completed by Dr. Esseltsyn and Dr. Ornish have scientifically demonstrated that heart disease can be prevented, arrested, and reversed through diet. Undoubtedly, to Dr. Young and others involved in heart surgery, like those at the Cleveland Clinic who participated in the Brazil experiment, heart disease arrest and reversal treatment, no matter how successful, does not meet their standards. We should take a closer look, then, at why, from the standpoint of logic, heart disease arrest and reversal therapy is far superior to drug and surgical procedures.

For a person standing with his/her arm extended into a furnace, the best way to prevent that person's arm from being burned to a crisp is to have him/her remove it from the furnace. Healing can then begin. That is essentially what the Esselstyn/Ornish treatment does. Since animal protein is the underlying cause of heart disease (and stroke) because it puts saturated fat and cholesterol into the digestive system leading to atherosclerosis and high blood pressure, the best way to halt the progression of the disease and to begin reversing its effects is to stop the cause, which is the consumption of animal protein. It should be apparent that neither Dr. Young nor any researcher at the Cleveland Clinic is likely to surpass this simple method of saving someone from "burning their arm to a crisp." Remove their arm and the burning stops. Reduce the cholesterol count to 150 mg/dL or below and the heart disease stops. Then start the healing, which includes complete rest from the original cause.

Apparently, though, this is not a satisfactory method for Dr. Young and mainstream medical practitioners more attracted to complexity. In general they seem intent on finding some way in which a person can remain with his/her arm in the oven without burning it, or, in the case of heart disease, can continue consuming animal protein with the accompanying high cholesterol it produces. To many people, that is a farfetched dream that after decades of failure no longer deserves public tax funding, nor should innocent animals be forced to sacrifice their lives to try to achieve a goal that is essentially unethical. It is unethical because 1) it is just plain egotistical arrogance to insist that human beings should be able to put poisons (animal protein) into their bodies and get away with it just because they have a craving for the poisons, and 2) a treatment has now been developed by Dr. Esselstyn and Dr. Ornish to treat heart disease so that research to find other treatments that scientists like Dr. Young continue to work on are not necessary, especially when they involve operating on and killing innocent animals.

In comparing his method of cardiovascular treatment to conventional medicine, Dr. Esselstyn described it this way. "All the interventional procedures carry considerable risk of morbidity, including new heart attacks, strokes, infections, and for some, an inevitable loss of cognition... And the benefits of intervention erode with the passage of time; eventually, you have to have another angioplasty, another bypass procedure, another stent... Mine carries none."[21]

Heart disease has been the number one killer in America for 100 years. Every day nearly 3,000 Americans will have heart attacks and 2400 will die of heart disease.[22,23] It costs 30 billion dollars a year for heart disease for drugs to control cholesterol, blood pressure and other risk factors. Patients pay $46,000 for bypass operations in which one out of every 50 patients will die of complications. Angioplasty is a simpler procedure but also expensive, and one in about every sixteen angioplasty patients will experience "abrupt vessel closure" which can lead to death, heart attack, or an emergency bypass.[24] Angioplasty patients cannot feel very secure walking around knowing that at any second they may become one of those 1 in 16 who experience "abrupt vessel closure." Similarly, it cannot be very reassuring for bypass patients lying on the operating table just before going under knowing that they could be among those 1 in 50 who will die of complications from the operation.

All of this can be prevented. But champions of animal research and surgery and drugs would rather continue in the direction of painful open heart surgery in needless bypass operations causing patients unwarranted suffering. According to long-term studies, bypass patients do not even have fewer heart attacks than those who do not have surgery.[25]

The clinical trials conducted by Dr. Esselstyn and Dr. Ornish have proved incontrovertibly that cardiovascular disease can be arrested and reversed through nutrition. Ornish has even widened his research to include prostate cancer and has shown that prostate tumors can also be arrested and reduced through a nutrition program.[26] But even though the success of Dr. Esselstyn and Dr. Ornish has by now been widely reported, few hospitals and medical centers have made an effort to include nutrition arrest and reversal treatments in their cardiac programs. The Ornish program has, fortunately, been picked up by a few hospitals and with great enthusiasm in West Virginia, Pennsylvania, and Connecticut, including Stamford Hospital in Connecticut, which is affiliated with the New York Presbyterian Health System, a teaching affiliate of no less than the Columbia University College of Physicians and Surgeons, one of the top medical schools in the country.

If more hospitals were to start using cardiovascular arrest and reversal programs it would be possible to begin reducing expensive surgical, radiological, and chemotherapeutic treatments for cardiovascular disease. However, this is just not a priority for heart surgeons and animal researchers who are content with the high salaries and peer prestige they receive for their work. They also get enormous grants in public funding plus quid pro quo employment security for bringing in huge sums of money for the facilities that employ them through patient fees and federally funded tax grants, of which their employers get from 50% to 75%. A further obstacle to the success of arrest and reversal therapy for heart disease are the drug and medical corporations responsible for producing the expensive drugs and equipment for surgical procedures and pre- and postoperative care. Continuing the status quo can only benefit these companies.

Simply put, the healthcare establishment does not want to seriously consider the preponderance of evidence that shows beyond all sustainable doubt that heart disease can be arrested and reversed through nutritional procedures.

Today we are privileged to live in a world of technological advance. Modern science is a marvel to behold. Scientists have developed complex prosthetic body substitutes that respond to electrical activity in the muscles through computer sensors.[27] They are working on ways in which our own bodies might regenerate blood vessels. Research is being conducted for avoiding the risk of defects in childbirth. Exploration has begun on how to clone cells to create organs and even body parts.

In the field of cancer research, scientists are now trying to develop drugs to choke off the blood supply to tumors, thereby killing them. They are investigating many compounds including green tea and thalidomide, the drug responsible for the horrendous birth defects in the late 1950s and early 1960s. They also see promise in a drug derived from the bark of the African bush willow tree that Zulu witch doctors have used for centuries as a medicine and to apply as a poison to the tips of their arrows.[28] Yet when it comes to recognizing that heart disease could be almost totally eliminated through nutrition so that it is nearly nonexistent as a threat to human life, scientists and surgeons married to surgery and drugs plug their ears and do not want to hear one word.

Why Our Healthcare Organizations Are Not Revealing the Facts About Nutrition

Chapter 11

The Cattle Baron's Ball

Indifference to Disease

One reason why the healthcare establishment ignores the discovery that animal protein is the cause of many of our chronic diseases lies very much on the surface. It is the simple fact that the Western world loves its meat and dairy products. As a consequence, the powers that govern the healthcare establishment in Western countries do not take the dangers of consuming animal protein seriously.

Almost everyone growing up in the Western world is conditioned from early childhood on to believe that meat and dairy products are necessary for survival. Scientists, physicians, and business executives who come together to form the healthcare organizations that make up the healthcare establishment are no different. Individually, they are not anxious to change their beliefs. And for those in the establishment trained in medicine, their lack of training in nutrition has not given them a foundation from which to get overly excited about new concepts and ideas arising from nutritional studies — especially if they threaten their personal affection for meat and dairy foods.

Physicians, scientists, and business executives are as attached to their bacon and eggs breakfast as is the average person in the Western world, and they do not look forward to anything that challenges their daily consumption of animal products. They seize eagerly on reports that contradict the evidence even when those reports are based on faulty methodologies like the Nurses' Health Study and the Women's Health Initiative—anything to avoid giving up their love for meat and dairy products.

Consumers of animal protein who do become informed about the dangers of eating meat and dairy products and take them seriously are sometimes faced with a dilemma. To avoid the danger they have to give up the cause which they may not be anxious to do. This group is analogous to smokers addicted to three packs of cigarettes a day who, upon learning that smoking causes lung cancer, contemplate cutting down to one pack because they can't quite face completely giving up their addiction.

This is what has happened with the healthcare organizations. They may go so far as to publicly recommend that people cut down on meat and dairy foods, but they are reluctant to go the full distance and recommend that people give up animal protein entirely.[1] In fact, when it comes to actual practice, the most powerful of the healthcare organizations, the American Cancer Society, shows no real commitment even to its own stated guidelines of limiting the consumption of red meat and consuming only low-fat dairy products.[2] This becomes apparent upon investigating one of the ACS's most lucrative fundraising activities, the Cattle Baron's Ball, that the society sponsors around the country.

The Cattle Baron's Ball was first inaugurated by the ACS in Texas in 1970, an appropriate place if ever there was one, considering the huge cattle ranches that spread across the Texas plains and where beef advertising is everywhere. In the ensuing years the popularity of the Cattle Baron's Ball has grown, and the ACS now hosts these events in cities and towns in other states like California, Colorado, Florida, Georgia, Michigan, Missouri, and Ohio.

It is no small wonder that they are popular fundraisers. The September 2008 Cattle Baron's Ball in Dearborn, Michigan grossed $650,000. The Cattle Baron's Golf Round-up at the Michigan State Fairgrounds in August of 2008 yielded $130,000.[3] Participating cities are eager to promote the balls. They are good public relations events in which local businesses, city administrators, and town leaders get a chance to present themselves in a favorable light while having a grand time working together for a common good, raising money to fight cancer.

But the title "Cattle Baron's Ball" accompanied by subsidiary events like "Chuck Wagon" competitions in which entrée and dessert awards are presented for "Best Savory" and "Best Sweet" gives cause for reflection. Just how serious can an organization be about the role meat and dairy products play in cancer formation when it has no hesitation in soliciting funds under the banner "Cattle Baron's Ball?" It is the perfect symbol of the power of meat where American rancher barons rule majestically over their cowboy empires. And, as would be expected on royal occasions, guests at a Cattle Baron's Ball can come prepared for a feast that befits the festive supplicants of a Cattle Baron.

Attendees at the Dearborn, Michigan Cattle Baron's Ball were served with Lobster Corn Dogs, Smoked Beef Brisket Sandwiches, and Jalapeno Corn Cakes [made with eggs and buttermilk].[4] One of the main sponsors of the Cattle Baron's Ball in Youngstown, Ohio in October of 2007 was the Outback Steakhouse.[5]

Local restaurants in concert with sponsors go to considerable lengths to prepare a sumptuous feast for high profile guests and local cognoscenti attending the balls. Included on the menu of the Cattle Baron's Ball in Lubbock, Texas in 2006 was this choice of mouth-watering, high cholesterol, artery-clogging fare.

Cattle Baron's Ball
Lubbock, Texas
August 16, 2008

Main Ball

Flaming Steak Diane
Beef tenderloin sautéed in red wine and butter, served with a homemade roll and jalapeño béarnaise sauce.

Grilled White Wings
Small pieces of chicken breast with a slice of jalapeño and Monterey jack cheese, wrapped in a ribbon of Apple Smoked Bacon, marinated in white wine and spices, grilled over mesquite coals.

Hill Country Sausage Market
Smoked Hill Country Beef, Pork, Venison, Chicken, and Vegetable Sausage served with Colorful Bell Peppers on a Wooden Skewer accompanied with Grain Mustard and Don's Famous Barbecue Sauce.

Carne Guisada
A Traditional Mexican Favorite created with chopped beef cooked in a rich gravy with Mexican spices served in a hot flour tortilla.

Tacos Al Pastor
Slices of beef and pork slow roasted over open coals and served with savory sauces and toppings to include jerk sauce, ancho diablo sauce, shredded cabbage, cilantro, lime wedges and presented on a flour and corn tortilla.

South Texas Harvest Tray
Peppercorn encrusted roast beef, grilled chicken breast, venison salami, wild boar sausage served with a large variety of bread and condiments: grain mustards, jalapeño béarnaise sauce, jalapeño cranberry chutney.

Shrimp Corn Cakes
Cooked shrimp, jalapeño chiles and corn kernels, lightly fried, accompanied with a garlic lime mayonnaise.

Avocado Halves
A Don Strange tradition of half of a ripened avocado filled with fresh Gulf shrimp ceviche.

Several other dishes for gourmets were also available. About those shrimp corn cakes—. With the exception of chicken liver, beef liver, and pork liver, shrimp contains more cholesterol per serving than beef, pork, lamb, veal, chicken, and all other fish and shellfish except raw squid.[6]

But no one counts the calories or the cholesterol at a lavish Cattle Baron's Ball.

The ACS does not seem overly concerned for the welfare of their guests which include the most affluent members of society and officers of businesses capable of contributing large sums of money to the organization. When they attend a Cattle Baron's Ball they are served some of the most unhealthy cuisine it is possible to prepare.

The food judge for the 23 restaurants and caterers which donated more than $100,000 in food and beverages for the Michigan State Cattle Baron's Ball was Mike Skupin, the Vice President of Business Development at Premier Business Products. Skupin is perhaps best known for his role as a contestant on "Survivor, The Australian Outback," where he survived by feeding on cow's stomach, fish eyes and guts, wild boar, and stray bugs.[7] He came well qualified to judge the high-fat animal protein goodies served at the Michigan State Coliseum.

Besides the fun and games, costumes, music by the award-winning country band Lonestar, dancing, mechanical bull rides, slot-car racing, rodeo events from the Rodeo Ropers from Las Vegas, virtual golf, caricatures and fun photos offered for entertainment at the Michigan State Cattle Baron's Ball, there was also a serous side to the event. Many people in attendance had been touched in one way or another by cancer, and, presumably, one of the purposes of the balls is to honor cancer survivors and remember loved ones who died from the disease.

Honorary chair Ray Young, the executive vice president and CFO of General Motors Corporation at the time, said that it was a personal cause for him "to help out the American Cancer Society and do everything possible to beat cancer."[8] For fifteen years his wife, Debra, battled with cancer and had succumbed to the disease just the year before while the two were living in Brazil. She was only 42 at the time of her untimely and unfortunate death.

Gary Cowger, group vice president for General Motors and founder of the Michigan event, had felt cancer's sting six years earlier when he chaired a Cattle Baron's Ball in Austin, Texas.[9]

"I had just lost my mom to cancer," he said. "So I said yes when the American Cancer Society asked [my wife and me] to chair the event."

There is something profoundly sad yet grotesque about these extravagant fun-and-game ACS fundraisers for the well-to-do. Many who attend are survivors of cancer or people who have been victimized by the disease in one way or another, often through the loss of someone close to them. The ACS creates a feast for these dedicated and committed people and serves them animal protein and dairy foods, the very products that may have contributed to and even caused their own cancer experience or the death of their loved ones. While it is startling that this never occurs to anyone, this just demonstrates the kind of insensibility that thrives within the healthcare system.

The healthcare organizations do not grasp that they are not doing their job in communicating a strong enough message about animal protein to the public, and they are in denial about the dangers this product poses to people's health and well-being. A typical Cattle Baron's Ball serves some of the most appetizing and extravagant kinds of animal protein dishes imaginable. This food is offered thoughtlessly without concern about the message conveyed to the public, that meat and dairy products are really only rather innocuous substances that should not cause people undue alarm. The message sent is equally clear that the American Cancer Society just does not get it.

The guests of the ACS Cattle Baron's Balls attend in good faith. The balls are grand occasions for lifting the spirits of the attendees from their silent mourning as they raise their glasses to toast their hopes for a future in which cancer can no longer come knocking at their doors. They are sincere. They are earnest. And they are relying on the wisdom of the American Cancer Society to protect them from cancer. But how seriously has the agency met their hopes? Does the American Cancer Society really think they are doing a service to their donors by surrounding them with animal protein, a food about which even the agency is now beginning to acknowledge poses a serious cancer threat? Is it cynicism, ignorance, or fear that makes the ACS think that people will not contribute money unless they are fed a meal of flaming beef, pork, venison, chicken, and vegetable sausage wrapped in ribbons of apple smoked bacon sautéed with a savory butter sauce and served with smoked hickory cheese and a side dish of lightly fried shrimp accompanied with a homemade roll and a lime mayonnaise jalapeño béarnaise sauce?

With a little creativity, balls just as attractive could be fashioned with just as much fun and games, but not dependent on all the high calorie, high-fat, high-cholesterol animal protein foods. The imagination easily stirs up titles for such events like Cinderella's Shoe, or Tom Sawyer's Retreat, or Harvest Hay Ride. The menu and recipes for these occasions could be replaced with entrées and deserts just as challenging as any animal protein-based dishes. For example, how about the following fare.

Gourmet Menu
Meatless and Dairyless

Soups

Tortilla tofu with [non-dairy] sour cream, cilantro.
Cream of Celeriac & Potato grilled bread.

Appetizers

Gnocchi zucchini, shallots, cauliflower, mushrooms, tomato cashew cream sauce.

Grilled Artichoke & Wild Mushrooms trumpet royal, oyster & hen of the woods mushrooms, horseradish cream.

Hummus, quinoa tabouli, lemon-date chutney,
marinated olives, parata bread and zataar.

Salads

Chopped Salad mixed greens, cucumbers, blood orange, tofu feta, hearts of palm, onion, tomato, pineapple-mint dressing.

Tomato-Beet Tartar
avocado, chives, mache, raspberry dressing, almond cheese crostini.

Soba Noodle Salad
Soba noodles, ginger grilled tofu, shiitake mushrooms, edamame, julienne carrots, radish and sesame seeds.

Entrées

Ancho-Chocolate Seitan Tamales julienne vegetables, mole sauce, grilled asparagus, mango-jicama salsa.

Porcini Crusted Tofu
herbed garlic-potato mash, grilled oyster mushrooms, sautéed haricots verts, mushroom gravy.

Chili-Lime Grilled Seitan
spanish rice pilaf, sautéed greens, avocado salad, black bean sauce.

Pan Seared Cabernet Tempeh sautéed
swiss chard, radicchio, shaved fennel, mushrooms, celeriac purée, balsamic reduction.

Tuscan Lasagna
Grilled zucchini, peppers and onions, tofu basil ricotta, soy cheese and seitan ragout topped with tomato sauce. Served with sautéed greens.

Desserts
Chocolate Peanut Butter Pie w/chocolate sauce

Mexican Chocolate Cake w/chocolate sauce

cinnamon ice cream (non dairy)

Coconut Cheesecake (non dairy) w/strawberry topping.[10]

From the story above, it should be apparent that forces exist within the ACS that do not fully comprehend the dangers of consuming animal protein just like they did not grasp the danger when tobacco began to be know as a cancer risk. If they

did, they would make and follow the same kind of recommendation the organization now makes in regard to tobacco and
lung cancer.

...the best advice to reduce the risk of lung cancer is to
avoid tobacco use and environmental tobacco smoke...[11]

The same kind of statement needs to be made in regard to meat
and dairy products.

...the best advice for significantly reducing the risk of
many forms of cancer is to avoid eating animal flesh and
dairy products.

The American Cancer Society hosts spectacles like Cattle Baron's
Balls when a proper warning about the foods they celebrate
might have caused a change in diet that could have prevented
some guests from ever getting cancer and might have saved the
lives of some of those mourned.

It is time for the American Cancer Society to reengineer their
Cattle Baron's Balls so that instead of feeding their guests with
cancer-causing products, they feed them with foods that significantly reduce the danger of getting these deadly diseases. That
would send a message that gets the entire world-wide healthcare
establishment to sit up and take notice. And so would the guests
who attend these balls.

Chapter 12

The Cult of Self-Interest

Resistance to Change

In the early 1990s the office of the national president of the American Cancer Society sent out a memo to local ACS offices around the country alleging that the scientific chair of the American Institute for Cancer Research (AICR) was "heading up a group of 'eight or nine' discredited physicians, several of whom had spent time in prison."[1] The National Dairy Council picked up on the memo and distributed its own version to its district offices nationwide.

Fortunately, this story was a lie. The "scientific chair" of the AICR was T. Colin Campbell, and the purpose of the ACS memo was to try to discredit him and the AICR which together were investigating the link between animal-based diets and cancer risk. The AICR also posed a threat to the ACS as a competitor for funding.[2]

The memo came to light purely by chance. Campbell was lecturing in upstate New York to a local chapter of the American Heart Association. During the question and answer period the host for the lecture, who did not know that Campbell was the chair of the American Institute for Cancer Research, innocently referred to the institute as an organization of quacks. When Campbell inquired how she knew that, the host replied that she had received the memo described above. After the lecture Campbell asked the host if she would send him a copy. She did.

One might not be surprised to learn that a corporate power had done its best to discredit someone it regarded as an enemy who was working against its better interests. However, it is unexpected that a nonprofit health organization, like the ACS, would engage in actions that were so underhanded they could, in effect, impede progress in preventing disease. It is worthwhile to try to determine if this deliberate lie was part of a consistent pattern of deception or if it was just a deviation from the norm. We need to know if some of our healthcare organizations are misleading the public and ignoring facts related to healthcare just because they don't serve the interests of the organizations or of persons occupying positions of power within the organizations. This could be part of the reason why the information concerning the connection between animal protein to cancer, heart disease, stroke, and diabetes is not reaching the public.

In 1982 after the National Academy of Sciences (NAS) issued its report on *Diet, Nutrition, and Cancer* that suggested a possible link between high protein intake and increased cancer risk, the chairman of the Food and Nutrition Board (FNB), who was also a professor of nutrition and biochemistry at the University of Wisconsin, took exception. During an interview he referred to the NAS report and said, "we don't know enough about diet and cancer to make recommendations that will either create hopes that are unlikely to be fulfilled or apprehension because of the inability to achieve the recommendations."[3] But the chairman's motives in belittling the report were questionable. He derived 10% of his income from food company consulting, mostly from Pillsbury, a major producer of bakery goods, and Kraft, a major producer of processed cheese foods.[4]

The words of the FNB chairman could be substituted for the attitude that prevails in the major healthcare organizations today concerning reports about the dangers of consuming animal products. "We don't know enough so it would be irresponsible to do anything except to ignore it." Meanwhile, people go on consuming meat and dairy products and they are dying as a result.

T. Colin Campbell was a co-author of the NAS report to

which the chairman objected, and the chairman wrote Campbell a stern letter in which he declared that Campbell had "fallen on [his] own petard," (a kind of medieval incendiary device that could be used to break down walls).[5] Clearly, the chairman was distressed by findings that ran contrary to his own ideals. Unyielding ideals, however, should have no place in an arena where the right and wrong facts can spell the difference between getting disease and eliminating disease, and between life and death. That the chairman's ideals were likely supported by the food companies that employed him, creating the appearance of a vested interest, cannot be overlooked. The opportunity for a conflict of interest was undeniably present.

On the other hand, the ACS memo described above and the events with the FNB chairman happened long ago. Perhaps these are just unpleasant incidents that might better be forgotten. Many businesses and organizations have skeletons in their closets someplace. Nobody is perfect, and the mistakes of one individual or a few should not tarnish the image of a company, an agency, or an entire industry. So why raise ghosts from the past?

That is a point well stated — unless a pattern of this kind gets carried over into the present where it happens consistently so that it becomes engrained in the fabric of the organization. And if it happens in many organizations within an industry, then it becomes an industry-wide characteristic. It is worthwhile, then, to spend some time examining a little of the history of some of our major healthcare organizations in contrast to their present day activities. A comparison of the past with the present should offer some insight into how these organizations operate and how serious their commitment is to keeping the public fully informed with the most current and beneficial healthcare information available.

Prior to the McGovern Senate Select Committee on Nutrition and Human Needs that was organized in 1969, the National

Cancer Institute devoted none of its budget to nutrition. That did not sit well with the parents of children with cancer who pressured Congress to force the NCI to set aside some of its budget for nutrition research. That happened in 1974. The figure agreed upon, though, was a minimal 1% of the NCI's total budget, and the agency sometimes did not even use up the total amount.[6]

This was a period in which most Americans happily embraced the American diet and that included pork chops and T-bone steaks. What could possibly be better in a world in which many of the nations on the planet were half starving than a malted and a hamburger with pickles and ketchup and a few potato chips sprinkled on the side? This was nutrition at its *a la Americain* best, and it produced a nation of people filled with vigor and health, or at least messages like these were favored by the food industry.

But there is always room for improvement and many in the medical field did not share such a rosy assessment of American health. Their concerns contributed to ushering in the McGovern commission. When the McGovern report came out linking cancer with nutrition in 1977, in spite of the uproar (see chapter 16), healthcare organizations that depended on Congress for funding had no choice but to climb on board. Experts who had denounced the link between cancer and nutrition quietly crept away to some corner either to eat their words or to mumble imprecations against the upstarts who dared challenge their cherished beliefs.

By 1979 the USDA was on board and the National Cancer Institute issued new *Dietary Guidelines* in the same year followed by the National Academy of Science's report, *Diet, Nutrition, and Cancer*, in 1982. The writing was on the wall and could be dismissed by no one in the healthcare establishment. The ACS reluctantly clambered aboard too and in February of 1984 for the first time in its history issued diet recommendations specifying that enough inferential information existed about nutrition to make recommendations that would "likely produce some measure of reducing cancer risk."[7]

But what was life like back in the dark ages before nutrition and disease were linked? Going back a little further in time we see that prior to the McGovern commission the medical establishment was unified in declaring that the nutrition/cancer connection was nothing but pure quackery. "There is no diet that prevents cancer in man," wrote Dr. Morris Shimkin in a 1973 National Cancer Institute primer. "Treatment of cancer by diet alone is in the realm of quackery."[8] The AMA stated: "There is no scientific evidence whatsoever to indicate that modification in the dietary intake of food or other nutritional essentials are of any specific value in the control of cancer."[9]

Historian Nat Morris in describing those times wrote "to stress the nutritional approach to cancer eventually became the surest way to become branded a quack."[10] The same could be said for any unconventional approach to healthcare which automatically got labeled as quackery. The AMA, for example, covertly tried to discredit alternative medical practices it regarded as competition for patient care on more than one occasion on the grounds that the competitors were quacks.

The AMA was founded in 1847 by Nathan Smith Davis who was elected president of the organization during the Civil War.[11] It is the largest association of physicians and medical students in America and publishes the prestigious Journal of the American Medical Association (JAMA). The organization also lobbies to advance the interests of physicians and patients and to acquire funding for medical education. It advertises that its mission is "to promote the art and science of medicine and the betterment of public health."

That was not its mission in the 1960s, however, when the AMA began a campaign to destroy chiropractic under the banner of its Committee on Quackery.[12] As pointed out by John

Robbins in his revealing book *Reclaiming our Health*, documents exposing the scheme surfaced which resulted in four chiropractors suing the AMA. After years of litigation they won their case in 1987 when "U.S. District Court Judge Susan Getzendanner ruled that the AMA and its officials were guilty of attempting to eliminate the chiropractic profession."[13] She ordered the AMA to admit the "lawlessness of its conduct," to mend its ways, and to publish her order in JAMA. The 1990 Appellate Court upheld the ruling and the Supreme Court let the ruling stand. [See also footnote 21.]

Back in the 1940s, a long time supporter of smoking during tobacco's heyday, Dr. Morris Fishbein, editor of JAMA for 25 years, zeroed in on Max Gerson, a name that may sound familiar. Fishbein was one of the most famous doctors in America and the conservative responsible for coining the term "socialized medicine" as a weapon for discrediting the political movement toward creating a universal healthcare system. The term was so potent in its dimensions that it has been used ever since to defeat healthcare reform whenever the issue is raised and was employed even as late as 2009 to try to defeat President Barack Obama's healthcare initiative.

Gerson was a Jewish German physician famous for treating tuberculosis in Austrian, French, and German sanatoriums. His dietary treatment for the disease was widely known in Europe.

Tuberculosis, like cancer today, was the great disease to be feared in Europe and the United States in the 19th century and also the early 20th century. It was a subject on everyone's mind as exemplified in Thomas Mann's symbolic masterpiece *The Magic Mountain* (1924) which takes place in a tuberculosis sanatorium in pre-World War I Switzerland.

When Hitler came to power Gerson fled Munich for Vienna and then fled to Paris finally settling in New York City where he began treating cancer patients through nutrition. He had already been trying this treatment with some success in Germany.

According to historians, Gerson was a modest man who said "that he did not yet have enough evidence to say whether diet could...alter the course of an established tumor. He claimed only that the diet...could favorably affect the patient's general condition, staving off the consequences of malignancy."[14] To Fishbein, however, Gerson was a quack nutritionist physician whose treatment included a nutrition regimen and coffee enemas and who also spoke out against the hazards of tobacco. At this time Philip Morris cigarettes was the "AMA Journal's chief source of advertising, and one of Fishbein's main sources of income."[15] Gerson had testified before a United States Senate committee investigating cancer. He was gaining in prestige and receiving considerable publicity in newspapers and on the radio. The Gotham Hospital, with which he was affiliated, praised his work. Author John Gunther credited Gerson's treatment for a temporary remission of his son's brain tumor and wrote a best-selling memoir about it called *Death Be not Proud*.[16]

Fishbein decided he had had enough and went on the offensive. After the Senate Committee hearing he attacked Gerson in the AMA Journal for "treating cancer patients with diet and warning against cigarettes."[17] Soon Gerson found his affiliation with the Gotham Hospital revoked. In 1953 he lost his malpractice insurance forcing him to open his own sanatorium in order to keep on practicing. Then on March 4, 1958, a panel of physicians of the New York County Medical Society met behind closed doors and suspended Gerson "from the rights and privileges of membership, as a result of personal publicity" for a period of two years.[18],[19]

Contrasting starkly to the treatment Gerson received in the United States, the University of Vienna had offered him the position of Chair in its Department of Nutritional Medicine the previous year. Vienna had a different view of Max Gerson than the healthcare establishment in the United States.

Max Gerson died discredited on March 8, 1959 at the age of 78 in New York City, one year after he was suspended by the New York County Medical Society.

Albert Schweitzer, Nobel Prize winner, missionary, author of *Reverence for Life*, and acclaimed organist, issued the following statement upon learning of Gerson's death.

> I see in him one of the most eminent medical geniuses in the history of medicine...he has achieved more than seemed possible under adverse conditions. He leaves a legacy which commands attention and which will assure him his due place. Those whom he cured will now attest to the truth of his ideas.[20]

Gerson's daughter, Charlotte, opened the Gerson Institute in Mexico where she could continue her father's treatment without being harassed by the American medical establishment. The clinic still operates in Tijuana today in an advisory capacity to interested patients.

Whether or not the Gerson treatment is a legitimate cancer treatment has never been scientifically tested, and Gerson's detractors never conducted any trials to determine the efficacy of his work when he was alive. Most people agree that charlatans and frauds deserve to be dealt with in a manner that prevents them from harming the public. But the biased manner in which Max Gerson was treated with none of his accusers ever testing his method may have denied people a cancer treatment that should have been their right to choose or reject. While Gerson's methods were always controversial, his work brought him acclaim and fame in Europe for his treatment of tuberculosis where he published dozens of papers in prominent European medical journals. In the United States he could not get one paper published.

Gerson spoke up in favor of nutrition, which the AMA

opposed, and he spoke out against tobacco, which the AMA favored. The AMA is remembered even today for having backed the tobacco industry when it was under siege by an avalanche of medical documentation showing that tobacco use caused lung cancer.[21] By refusing to condemn tobacco when it was in a position of authority that influenced the health decisions people made, the AMA was surely responsible for people getting diseases related to tobacco use including lung cancer and heart disease. It is difficult to call the AMA stand on tobacco back in those days anything other than a betrayal of the American people.

No doubt today the AMA wishes the ghosts representing the stand it took on tobacco and the manner in which it treated Max Gerson would fade away. The American Cancer Society would also probably prefer not to be reminded of the letter that was dispensed by the president's office of the organization trying to discredit Dr. Campbell and the AICR. And agencies like the NCI, which were quick to brand the link between nutrition and disease as quackery, have quietly closed their doors on their former views about nutrition. But for many people the earlier history of organizations like these continues to tarnish their reputation even decades later. Are these people just being unforgiving, or do they have legitimate reasons which run far deeper? That is a subject to be pursued in the next chapter.

Chapter 13

Living with Ghosts

Kenny Ausubel's father was diagnosed with cancer at the age of 56 and succumbed to the disease six months later. After his father's death Kenny learned by chance about an alternative cancer therapy. This started him on a trail in which a "subterranean netherworld of purported cures [for cancer] using a variety of therapies — from nutrition and mental imaging to herbs and immunology" began to emerge.[1] One of these was the so-called Hoxsey treatment which caused Ausubel to begin asking the question of whether "'unorthodox' treatments [were] being politically railroaded instead of scientifically tested."

John Hoxsey the elder was a Southern Illinois Quaker farmer who in 1840 discovered that a malignant tumor on the right hock of his prize stallion had dried up and dropped off after the stallion had eaten a certain kind of weeds and plants growing in a corner of his pasture. From this discovery he developed a cancer cure with which he treated horses that had developed the disease. His grandson took the treatment a step further and began applying it to people. In 1925, the great grandson, Harry Hoxsey, went even further and founded the Hoxsey Cancer Clinic in Dallas for employing his Grandfather's treatment for which "orthodox medicine branded [him] the worst cancer quack of the century." However, two federal courts upheld the therapeutic value of the treatment and even the American Medical Association (AMA) and the Food and Drugs Administration (FDA) admitted it cured certain forms of cancer.[2]

By the 1950s, however, the National Cancer Institute (NCI), the AMA, and the FDA were all trying to "restrict" Hoxsey's clinic. Morris Fishbein [Max Gerson's nemesis referred to in chapter 12] said Hoxsey was a ghoul who "fed on the bodies of the dead and the dying."[3] John Heller, the Director of the NCI, in referring to the anti-Hoxsey campaign, wrote:

Our efforts in cancer control are directed toward reduction of the intervals between onset and diagnosis of cancer, and between diagnosis and the application of effective treatment. People who fall victims to quacks are diverted from this narrow course for the best clinical management of cancer.

The ire of the FDA was fully aroused, and though it had always refused Hoxsey's request for a scientific test, in 1960 it succeeded in having the Hoxsey treatment banned from the United States. That occurred after an undercover inspector from the FDA visited the Hoxsey clinic where he was told he had cancer that would take a long time to cure. The problem for Harry Hoxsey was that the inspector did not have cancer at all.

In 1963, Hoxsey's chief nurse, Mildred Nelson, moved the operation to Tijuana, Mexico with Hoxsey's blessings. He even chose the location. But Harry Hoxsey was out of the cancer business. He remained behind in Texas to work in the oil field. In 1967 he developed prostate cancer which his own treatment was unable to cure, forcing him to opt for conventional treatment, including surgery. One might surmise that it was a difficult and humiliating choice to make. He died seven years later in 1974 at the age of 73.

The Hoxsey clinic remains open in Tijuana to this day.

Claims have been made on both sides as to the Hoxsey treatment's effectiveness. A controlled study with mice showed that the Hoxsey tonic did not reduce tumor growth. On the other hand, a United States Department of Agriculture botanist, James A. Duke, in his own tests, concluded that the "Hoxsey tonic ingredients showed very significant chemical and biological anticancer activity."[4]

The battle over whether or not Harry Hoxsey was operating as a charlatan for financial gain is one matter, although it should be noted that Hoxsey won a lawsuit against Morris Fishbein and the Hearst newspapers in 1949 for libel and slander.[5] Whether the Hoxsey treatment has a legitimate function as an anti-cancer agent is another matter. It has never really been tested with any seriousness, and though it failed to cure Harry Hoxsey's prostate cancer, its value as a cancer treatment remains undetermined.

The Hoxsey story represents another ghost lingering about telling tales about questionable conduct from our healthcare organizations and challenging the healthcare establishment's claim that it has the right to condemn targeted cancer treatments as being inappropriate, especially considering that the failure rate for conventional cancer treatment is so extraordinarily high. Scientists are happy to go to Africa to investigate an African bush willow tree that Zulu witch doctors have used for centuries as a medicine in the hopes of finding a cure for cancer, as we saw in chapter 10. At the same time they consider horse grass discovered by a Southern Illinois farmer in the 19th century to be unsuitable for scientific testing.[6]

If someone has been told he or she has incurable cancer and they have six months to live, surely they should have the right to a treatment concocted from horse grass if that is their choice, especially if the science establishment is permitted to go out testing Zulu witch medicine. The manner in which science ranks priorities when it comes to cancer treatment is not only questionable, it further reveals the science establishment's proclivity for doing almost anything to avoid investigating alternatives to disease prevention that differ from its own institutional ideologies, including the role animal protein plays as a cause of disease.

Before he began his investigation of the Hoxsey treatment, Kenny Ausubel described his own encounter with conventional cancer healthcare as follows:

> My own direct experience with cancer had been the horror of my father's death. Visiting him in Memorial Sloan Cancer Center in New York, the flagship of conventional cancer treatment, branded my psyche with the indelible imprint of a medical concentration camp. Hopeless patients in blue smocks hovered like phantoms, their emaciated bodies ravaged by radiation and chemotherapy. A skeletal cluster of bald-headed children looking strangely like old men and women formed a macabre audience around a color TV spewing out violent cartoons and commercials for sugar-coated cereal. The place smelled of death and despair. The doctors, aloof and cold, seemed to have hardened themselves against the incredible pain of their own hopelessness.

Should people, if faced with cancer in their families, be left with no other choice than the nightmare described above or should they be allowed to choose a nutritional regimen like Max Gerson prescribed that included coffee enemas?[7] A growing number of Americans believe that they should not be forced to live with the kind of paternal protectionism the healthcare system has forced on them. They think people should be allowed to choose for themselves what cancer treatment they want and that to be prohibited from making that choice helps to create a close-minded approach to cancer research.

Dr. Lawrence Burton was another victim of institutional bias. On July 17, 1985 his cancer clinic in the Bahamas was shut down for supposed HIV blood contamination. The report turned out to be false, and another ghost materialized.

Burton had developed a blood serum drawn from healthy people and people with cancer while working as a senior investigator in the Hodgkin's Disease Research Laboratory at St.

Vincent's Hospital in New York City. He contended that his serum shrank tumors by restoring the body's immune system. Burton set up public demonstrations for his serum that amazed the press, though medical experts claimed (without proof) that he had to be deceiving people. His work was attacked by the AMA, the American Society for Clinical Oncology (ASCO), and the NCI.

(The NCI had once offered to do clinical trials on Burton's serum, but he refused because half of the patients would have been required to take a placebo which could have led to their deaths.)

Burton's enemies, especially in the National Cancer Institute, were responsible for shutting the Bahamian clinic down. Congressman Guy Molinari of Staten Island, New York, who had heard favorable reports about the Burton treatment, visited the clinic in the Bahamas and conducted an investigation. At a public hearing on January 15, 1986 he said:

> In my investigation I have found inconsistencies, and in some cases actual untruths, on the part of the various agencies which I contacted, especially on the part of Dr. Gregory Curt of the NCI.[8]

It took seven and one-half months of testimonials, lobbying, and picketing by Burton's own patients and supporters to get his clinic reopened. In the interim he had to sneak into his laboratory in the middle of the night to get supplies for treating his patients who had been shut out. If he had been caught the Bahaman police would have thrown him in jail. During the time in which the clinic was closed, 60 of Burton's patients died. Whether or not any of them would have lived, or how many, had the clinic remained open, can never be known.

Dr. Lawrence Burton died on March 8, 1993 at the age of 66. His clinic remains open in Freeport in the Bahamas today. The cancer serum which he claimed shrank cancer tumors has never been tested by the mainstream medical establishment to determine its effectiveness, and very sick people continue to travel to Freeport in a desperate last bid to find a cure for their cancers.

Ralph Moss points out in his book *The Cancer Industry*, that Benjamin Rush, M.D., one of the signers of the Declaration of Independence, described the same conditions in his time that Americans face today, where they are controlled by a powerful bureaucracy which is backed by courts that together deprive the people of their freedom to choose their own medical treatment. Rush wrote the following:

> The Constitution of this Republic should make special provisions for medical freedom as well as religious freedom. To restrict the art of healing to one class of men and deny equal privileges to others will constitute the Bastille of medical science. All such laws are un-American and despotic.[17]

A health crisis exists in our times that requires an adequate response by our healthcare organizations. Are they providing the most beneficial healthcare information to the public or are they busy pursuing their own institutional agendas like they have done with Max Gerson, Harry Hoxsey, and Lawrence Burton.

The healthcare organizations are responsible for reporting the true facts about discoveries in disease prevention. As we have seen, however, a cult of self-interest seems to have governed some healthcare organizations. It has even prevented cancer treatments from being tested that showed signs of promise.

Stories like those examined in chapters 12 and 13 raise compelling questions concerning the extent to which some of our major healthcare organizations have put their interests above the needs of the people sometimes losing their objectivity in the process. It is difficult not to wonder if they are playing the same game today. Are they just looking out for themselves without the necessary concern required to really stand up for the people? How far off course might they go? Claims have been made that they are playing ball with the financial beneficiaries of the healthcare crisis to the detriment of the public. In the next chapter, we will pursue this line of inquiry as we try to determine whether the ghosts of the past can be put to rest or if they need to continue to haunt the hallways of the American healthcare system rattling their chains in the attic at night clamoring for change.

Chapter 14

The Complicity of the Major Healthcare Organizations with the Drug Industry

Even though some healthcare organizations have damaged their reputations by the manner in which they have tried to destroy their competitors, time heals old wounds. The public assumes these agencies will benefit from their mistakes and soon forgets. Life moves forward, new faces fill old positions, and as long as no one seems to be getting hurt most people see little point in clinging to the past. On the other hand, some critics insist that while it may not be obvious on the surface, our healthcare organizations are still engaged in the same old tactics of putting their own interests above the legitimate needs of the people. They claim this is the reason why these agencies are not reporting important information to the public such as the role of nutrition in the prevention of disease.

One way to find out the truth of these kinds of allegations is to ask what kind of judgments the healthcare organizations are making in today's world. How, for example, are they handling one of the biggest problems that confronts the country, the use of prescription and over-the-counter drugs by an ever-increasing percentage of the population.

Accusations have been made from many corners that the drug companies are manufacturing a drug culture by creating counterfeit diseases that require their drugs. Should this be true, then we need to know if our healthcare organizations are doing anything about it. Have they been out investigating and trying to expose the danger, if it is indeed there, or, have they been doing what the AMA did with tobacco, cooperating with the industry and looking out for their own welfare ahead of the public good.

The kind of relationships our nonprofit healthcare organizations and government healthcare agencies build with the drug companies can have far-reaching consequences. For this reason it can only benefit us to try to determine just how much influence the drug industry has on the healthcare system. Specifically, we need to investigate whether a quid pro quo might exist between the healthcare organizations and the drug industry that could influence the communication of facts like that the consumption of animal protein is a major risk factor for getting one of the killer diseases.

The problem of prescription and over-the-counter drugs is a serious one. Statistics indicate that eighty-one percent of Americans take at least one medication during any given week and fifty percent of Americans take at least one prescription drug during any given week.[1] A study done by the National Center on Addiction and Substance Abuse at New York City's Columbia University in 2005 found that an estimated 15.1 million abusers of prescription drugs exceeded the combined number of people abusing illegal drugs like cocaine, ecstasy, marijuana, amphetamines, crack, and heroin (the possession of which can result in prison sentences). Of these abusers, 2.3 million were teenagers.[2]

Is this excessive use of drugs by the non-criminal public an indication that the drug industry is creating diseases in order to be able to sell drugs? People who think so point out that our TV commercials are filled with drug advertising and that the drug industry seizes on every human trait that deviates from the norm and tries to turn it into something for which they can develop a drug treatment. We are going to examine this claim and whether or not some of our most respected healthcare organizations have resisted or are going along with drug companies which might be engaging in these kinds of practices.

One critic of the drug industry, the late medical journalist

Lynn Payer, a graduate of the Columbia University School of Journalism, wrote in her book *Disease-Mongers: How Doctors, Drug Companies, and Insurers Are Making You Feel Sick*, that disease mongering consisted of "trying to convince essentially well people that they are sick, or slightly sick people that they are very ill." She called it "big business," and said that "disease mongering is the most insidious of the various forms that medical advertising, so-called medical education, and information and medical diagnosis can take."[3]

University of British Columbia researcher Barbara Mintzes put it this way: "Not content with providing a pill for every ill, the drug companies now push an ill for every pill."[4]

A Professor of Bioethics at the University of Pennsylvania at Philadelphia, Arthur Caplan, remarked on the CBS show *60 Minutes* that "if you want to stir up worry in the public, and you've got the advertising dollars to do it, you can turn almost anything into a disease."[5] Howard Wolinsky, a freelance scientific and medical writer from the journalism faculty of Northwestern University, reports that "critics such as Payer and Caplan maintain that the routine human condition...is increasingly being re-defined as disease."[6]

Payer's objections arose out of her concerns that the drug companies were wasting resources on the healthy that could be used for those who were genuinely sick. She noted that drug companies exaggerated mild problems like premenstrual syndrome and used unrepresentative examples to describe conditions like thinning bones [osteoporosis].[7]

Disease mongering may well play a role in the treatment of osteoporosis. Most people will lose some mineral density in their bones as they age. But how much of the treatment prescribed by the medical community is necessary? The value of expensive bone density tests for osteoporosis is controversial and the drugs used to treat osteoporosis provide only very modest increases in bone density which critics contend are disproportionately magnified compared to what they actually accomplish. A group of researchers and doctors at the University of British Columbia stated that pushing bone density testing as extensively as it has been done was a case of the "marketing of fear" to women.[8] The drugs used to treat osteoporosis can also have serious side effects.

One of the most transparent examples of drug company "exaggeration" concerns the condition of shyness, a state of mind with which everyone is familiar. It is now dubbed a 'social phobia' or a "social anxiety disorder" and is connected to symptoms like fear of public speaking, eating in front of others, or using public bathrooms. GlaxoSmithKline, a United Kingdom drug company, got approval by the FDA to extend its antidepressant drug Paxil to include the treatment of "social anxiety disorder." Sidney Wolfe, executive director of the Washington based Public Citizen's Health Research Group said:

> Shyness is a new disease invented by Glaxo. In a pathological way I'm sure that people are so shy it can be a disease. It can be a real downside for people. A lot of these people are depressed. A number of these people are shy because they have been physically or sexually abused when they were younger. Shyness is generally a symptom of something else and to gloss over finding the cause and to just throw a drug at someone is doing a disservice.[9]

In its campaign to market Paxil, GlaxoSmithKline distributed pamphlets suggesting that one in eight Americans had a social anxiety disorder. Australian journalist Ray Moynihan, a visiting editor at the *British Medical Journal* and co-author of the book *Selling Sickness: How the World's Biggest Pharmaceutical Companies are Turning Us All into Patients*, called that an "absurd fiction." He said "the point of that is to try and make ordinary people feel sick."[10]

Metabolic syndrome, aka syndrome X, a so-called precursor condition for heart disease and Type 2 diabetes, supposedly results from having multiple medical disorders like high blood pressure, obesity, high cholesterol, and insulin resistance. This is another "disease" critics accuse the drug companies of manufacturing.[11]

If a drug company wants to create a disease in 30 days without really trying, the process is straightforward enough. Find a condition and develop a drug to treat it, or, better yet, take an old drug like Benzedrine, and give it a new name. Next find a citizen's group that believes it has the disease, and then make a deal with the group. (CHADD, for example, a citizen's group for Children and Adults with Attention Deficit Disorder, gets paid $700,000 annually from drug companies which is a little over one/fourth of its annual income of $3 million.)[12] Then start a journal named after the condition. After that get government funding from the NIH to research the condition. Finally, launch an education program about the disease with the help of a major healthcare organization. You have now created a new disease.[13]

The *60 Minutes* report cited above focused on the emergence of a market for a new kind of attention deficit disorder. This was Adult Attention Deficit Disorder (Adult ADD). The story of Adult ADD is fascinating to follow.

Ritalin, which is composed of methylphenidate, a chemical relative of amphetamine, a stimulant found in some nasal inhalers and a dangerous drug pedaled by drug dealers, has been used to treat children with the disease called Attention Deficit Disorder (ADD) since the 1960s. Many people believe that the drug companies have got away with murder in marketing Ritalin. They question the legitimacy of ADD as a disease, at least to the extent to which it has been diagnosed, and view Ritalin as little more than "kiddie cocaine." Some doctors who believe that ADD truly is a disease, however, are confident that the brains of children with ADD are smaller. They believe this is the true cause of ADD. Opponents remain suspicious.[14] They say that if that turns out to be the case, every child who is prescribed Ritalin for ADD should have a brain scan to confirm the diagnosis. That is because, according to them, Attention Deficit Disorder is often misdiagnosed and frequently is nothing but the result of hard-sell advertising. They claim that schools and teachers rely far too much on drugs like Ritalin as a tool for dealing with disciplinary problems and for bending students to conform to academic and social standards that have nothing to do with disease.

From 1990 to 2000 the manufacture of Ritalin increased by 800 percent.[15] This accompanied information that Americans, with 5% of the world's population, were consuming 80% of the stimulants manufactured worldwide. America was obviously a fertile place for selling stimulant drugs. Did statistics like these provide an incentive for the drug industry to create a new disease, Adult ADD, to be treated with stimulants on the order of Ritalin? Up to this time, it had been widely accepted that all children afflicted with ADD would grow out of the condition once they left adolescence and entered adulthood. In order to create Adult ADD, however, the concept that children outgrew ADD would have to be revised. Otherwise, it could not be maintained that adults could get ADD. With the right kind of revision, though, and publicity, companies that wanted to market ADD drugs to adults could stress that ADD was a lifelong disorder. ADD would no longer be just a childhood condition treated with Ritalin and other stimulant drugs that children grew out of once they left adolescence and became young adults. The new disease could extend into adulthood as a lifelong disease. This would open a fabulous new market for drugs to treat adults with ADD.

Lilly was the first company to market a drug for Adult ADD, called Strattera, that unlike Ritalin and Adderall (to be discussed momentarily), was not an amphetamine. Lilly sold more than a million prescriptions of Strattera in its first six months in 2003 and achieved sales of $370 million in its first year.[16] This was one of Lilly's advertisements for Adult ADD:

Distracted? Disorganized? Frustrated?
Modern Life or Adult ADD?

Many adults have been living with Adult attention deficit disorder (Adult ADD) and don't recognize it. Why? Because its symptoms are often mistaken for stressful life.[17]

Suddenly the usual stresses which the majority of people encountered in their day to day interactions with the world were no longer "usual." They were symptoms of a disease called Adult ADD. Voila! A new disease had been born.

Unfortunately, whether Adult Add was legitimate or whether it was nothing but fakery and hype went uncontested by the healthcare establishment.

Shire, one of the world's leading biopharmaceutical companies, was next in line. Its drug for treating Adult ADD was called Adderall. It has proved to be a huge best seller and constitutes "more than 40% of Shire's total revenues."[18] Adderall was a mixture of four amphetamine salts that had been on the market since 1996.

Amphetamine was first synthesized in Germany in 1887.[19] It was sold as the over-the-counter nasal inhalant Benzedrine to treat asthma, hay fever, and colds in the 1930s. At the same time it made its way into the drug culture as a "high." During World War II, American troops used amphetamines to keep going with little sleep and for its drug effects. Amphetamines can activate a state of euphoria and a sense of empowerment. They can also induce paranoia. During the 1950s and 1960s, Benzedrine and amphetamine derivatives like Dexedrine and Methedrine (the trade name for methamphetamine) were popular as substance abuse drugs in the counter culture and acquired a variety of drug culture names like "speed," "bennies," "dexies," "meth," and "crystal." "Speed freaks," as illicit amphetamine users were sometimes called from the 1960s onward, were known for staying awake for days and nights after taking amphetamines. Some amphetamine users had a tendency toward violence, aggressiveness, and criminal behavior. Speed users often got the drug through a friend or an acquaintance who would obtain it from a drug dealer. The use of amphetamines continues to be a serious drug problem today.

Like Ritalin, Shire's Adderall was used to treat ADD for children before Adult ADD became an official disease. Even prior to being marketed for Adult ADD, Adderall sales surged from $10,000 in 1996 to $520,000,000 in 2003. In the same period Shire sold more than 37 million prescriptions of Adderall worldwide.

During this time 12 American boys, aged 7 to 16, who were taking either Adderall or a more potent variant, Adderall XR, died. Concerned, the Canadian government banned the drug. The FDA, however, took the position that "just because a child died while on Adderall doesn't mean the drug was the cause. It could have been 50 different causes."[20] Consequently, sales of the drug continued and eventually the Canadians were convinced to lift their ban on the drug.

Because of the extensive problems that accompany drugs, the public has the right to expect, or at least hope, that their major healthcare organizations will be out in front promoting their best interests. But the reaction of the healthcare organizations to the drug crisis and to the perception that drug companies are creating diseases in order to sell their products has been muted and questionable. For example, it took little time for Shire biopharmaceuticals to establish a profitable relationship with the American Medical Association in its marketing of Adderall for adults. That occurred as follows.

Two weeks after Adderall was approved by the FDA to treat

Adult ADD, the American Medical Association began "bombarding" medical journalists with e-mail alerts advising them about two important AMA media briefings. The first of these briefings was about Adult ADD and medications. The sponsor of this event was Shire, the manufacturer of the drug, which "supplied the AMA with an 'unrestricted educational grant for the event.'"[21] The second event was the AMA's science writer's conference, billed as bringing journalists news about "the most urgent medical issues" of the day. At the top of the list in the AMA e-mail alert was the topic "ADD." The keynote speaker was a paid consultant for Shire whose vested interest could scarcely have been more apparent.

No matter whether people believe Adult ADD is a legitimate condition or a fantasy creation invented by the drug companies to make money, it seems clear that healthcare organizations should not be promoting drugs or drug companies, especially when the drug companies pay them to do so, as Shire did with the AMA. Adderall contains dangerous, addicting amphetamines. They can be especially bad for the heart with devastating health consequences. It would seem that this is the kind of drug the AMA should have been helping people get off of, not urging them to get "on."

And what about some of the other healthcare organizations we have been discussing? Where was their demand for some oversight for this lethal mixture of amphetamines that was being pushed out into the marketplace? They were nowhere to be seen.

From the above description, the idea that the AMA may have changed its tune from the days when JAMA's editor Morris Fishbein was heralding the benefits of smoking while its biggest advertising client was Phillip Morris cigarettes, comes into question. Not long before Shire introduced Adderall into the marketplace, the AMA was busy being cozy with another industry whose products are dangerous to the public health, the beef industry. That occurred as follows.

In 1991 the USDA was in the process of revising its Four Food guidelines, as it does every five years.[22] The Physicians Committee for Responsible Medicine (PCRM) asked the USDA to consider a new Four Food guidelines consisting of Grains, Fruits, Vegetables, and Legumes to replace the old Four Food guidelines of milk; meat; fruits and vegetables; and bread and cereals. This was a proposal the meat, dairy, and egg industries wanted no part of and quickly criticized the plan for containing no animal products. The BIC (Beef Industry Council) Meat Board, however, was strangely silent on the matter and presented no opposition to the PCRM plan.[23]

But another critic was not so quiet. This was the AMA which issued a press release that found the recommendations of the PCRM to be "irresponsible and potentially dangerous to the health and welfare of Americans."[24]

To the AMA, grains, fruits, vegetables, and legumes were "irresponsible and potentially dangerous to the health and welfare of Americans." Meat and dairy products were not.

It seems clear enough that the AMA memo was speaking on behalf of the BIC Meat Board. When asked why BIC held back from protesting the PCRM's attempt to replace the USDA Four Food guidelines with a new set of guidelines minus meat, BIC Public Relations Chairman Ivan Kanak responded as follows:

The meat board prepared no formal release nor issued any statement to the press, but instead chose to do a lot of work behind the scenes. By working closely with other organizations such as the American Medical Association (AMA) and the American Dietetic Association, we were able to get a responsible, credible message to consumers.

[Donna] Schmidt, the BIC meat board's director of public relations added:

That's the kind of response the meat industry could not

deliver to consumers with the same impact and believability.

It might be argued that in 1991, when this scene transpired, the
existing evidence on the dangers of eating meat was not as well
known as it is today. Even if that argument were to be accepted,
it can hardly be overlooked that in the days in which the
evidence of the dangers of smoking were not quite known, the
AMA took the side of tobacco. Here it was once again taking the
side of another industry against the better interests of the public
health, this time aligning itself with the meat industry. And it
did so behind the scenes where no one could see what was going
on, the same tactic it employed in sponsoring Shire's Adderall.

Deceptive practices continue to be a problem for the AMA.
According to a story that appeared in the May 22, 2007 edition
of the Washington Post, the AMA earns millions of dollars each
year by licensing data-mining companies to access the AMA
masterfile database containing names, birth dates, addresses,
educational background, prescribing data, and specialties for
more than 800,000 doctors. Data-mining is the process of
extracting hidden patterns from data that can be used in various
marketing strategies. Drug companies, for example, contract
with data-mining companies to learn what medicines physicians
prescribe and in what quantities. Armed with this information
they can then target specific physicians or institutions that
employ them with a customized sales pitch.

In response to complaints about the practice, the AMA instituted a doctor opt-out in which doctors could shield their
individual prescribing data in the masterfile, but critics contend
the opt-out is not publicized and is not nearly tough enough.[25]
Some people see the AMA practice of licensing data-mining
companies to access information to be sold to drug companies as
a form of collusion with the drug companies.

The Journal of the American Medical Association (JAMA)

was also "caught red-handed" for failing to disclose the financial relationships between its drug study authors and companies that might benefit from such studies, according to a 2004 report issued by the Center for Science in the Public Interest. The CSPI noted that one author published a study on kidney disease but did not disclose that he was a consultant paid by Merck, Bristol-Myers Squibb, GlaxoSmithKline, and Pfizer. These companies all sold "products that could be marketed to the public based on the information presented in the study." The report also noted that a review of JAMA articles revealed that 11.3% of the authors writing the articles had not disclosed a conflict of interest.[26]

Two years later, in 2006, Catherine DeAngelis, editor-in-chief of JAMA, rejected calls for JAMA to ban authors who did not reveal their financial links to drug makers. DeAngelis said that such action "would only encourage that author to send his or her articles to another journal; it cleans our house by messing others."[27]

The admission that these authors' conflicts of interests would "mess" whatever journal they published in (including JAMA), seems to have escaped Ms. DeAngelis.

Mike Adams, an editor at Natural News.com and a frequent critic of pharmaceutical industry practices, responded as follows:

This is classic behavior characteristic of the incestuous relationship between medical journals and drug companies. With this announcement, the American Medical Association is openly declaring its unwillingness to meet even the most basic standards of journalistic integrity...It is difficult to find a clearer example of the collusion between Big Pharma and JAMA than this astonishing announcement which says, essentially, 'We refuse to operate with scientific integrity.' Today, JAMA has designated itself the official propaganda mouthpiece of

Big Pharma, something that independent observers have known for years.[28]

It would appear that the AMA does not see anything wrong in permitting authors with financial ties to drug companies to publish articles favorable to those drug companies in JAMA, nor does it recognize the perception that the AMA is on the side of the drug companies that must in one way or another be compensating the AMA for its loyalties.[29]

Judging from the above examples, serious questions remain as to whether the AMA has learned from its mistakes of the past in the halcyon days of Morris Fishbein v. Max Gerson.

If health organizations like the AMA are not on the side of the public whenever the opportunity for some conflicting agency gain is at hand, how can they be counted on to deliver the most current information about disease prevention unless they get some kind of financial or corporate benefit in return? Just how deep does this thirst for profit undeterred by the needs of the public go? On whose side do these organizations stand? These are the questions that need to be answered.

Like the AMA, the ACS also stands accused of ignoring the tobacco/cancer link earlier in its existence. How has this organization been doing when it comes to looking out for the best interests of the people?

Dr. Samuel Epstein, who claims that he "had the distinction of being number one on the [1983 White House Enemy's] list with an appellation next to [his] name: 'perfectly horrible,'" said in the year 2000 that the American Cancer Society had a close "interlocking relationship" with the drug industry, examples of which were then ACS trustees David R. Bethune and Gordon Binder. Bethune was also the President of Lederle Labs, a division of American Cyanamid, which makes chemical fertilizers and herbicides, as well as the anti-cancer drug Novatrone. Binder was the CEO of Amgen, the world's foremost biotechnology company, whose product Neupogen was enjoying enormous success from the increase in cancer incidence.[30]

Ties like these pose conflicts of interest. Bethune, for example, though not presently a trustee of the ACS, has always been and still is connected to pharmaceutical companies as a top officer who promotes and markets drugs as a part of his responsibilities. He is presently the interim CEO and Chairman of the Board of Zila Pharmaceuticals.[31],[32],[33]

It is difficult for people to have confidence that their healthcare organizations are advocating on their behalf and not the drug companies when their top officers and trustees are intimately connected with drug companies as high-ranking, high-salaried executives. Karen Katen, who was the president of Pfizer Global Pharmaceuticals and executive vice president of Pfizer Inc., was also an Advisory Trustee on the ACS Foundation Board of Trustees. Robert A. Ingram was a chairman of the ACS Trustees who served as Vice Chairman of Pharmaceuticals for GlaxoSmithKline, the manufacturers of Paxil, the "shyness" drug. No matter how innocent relationships like these are represented to be, a bond between the two sides can hardly fail to get established. But a bond of any kind between a drug company and a healthcare organization by its very nature undermines the independence healthcare organizations require in order to report the truth to the public, such as that some drug companies are manufacturing nonexistent diseases. To insist otherwise just defies common sense.

All too frequently conflicts of interest surface raising suspicions. In March 2006, for example, the press reported that John Seffrin, CEO of the American Cancer Society, had endorsed Andrew von Eschenbach to lead the Food and Drug Administration. Referring to Eschenbach, Seffrin said, "You have [in him] a mixture of talent, experience and sensitivity that make [him] uniquely qualified to be a regulator at an agency as important as the Food and Drug Administration."[34]

A problem of perception was immediately raised, however, because the ACS had fundraising ties to the companies Eschenbach would regulate that included Amgen, Novartis, Quest Diagnostics, and Pfizer and from which the ACS receives over $100,000 a year in contributions. According to the Center for Science in the Public Interest, in 2005 the ACS had also helped launch a major cancer prevention and treatment initiative called the "CEO Cancer Gold Standard" that was put together by the ACS and officials from major drug companies.

These actions could hardly avoid raising eyebrows. Why was the ACS surrounding itself with drug companies from which it raised considerable sums of money some of which were busy planning treatment and intervention programs for cancer that might benefit from future support from the ACS?

Meanwhile, Eschenbach endorsed the CEO Cancer Gold Standard initiative while he was the head of the National Cancer Institute as well as interim head of the FDA. This also raised eyebrows. Why, as the interim head of the FDA, the top regulatory agency for drugs in the nation, would Eschenbach be involved in endorsing a drug industry initiative that also involved the ACS, a nonprofit organization, which was taking the lead in the implementation of the program? The subsequent endorsement Seffrin made for Eschenbach hardly escapes the suspicion that this was just another instance of a "good old boy" type payback and networking of the "keep it all in the family" variety.

The ACS endorsement of Von Eschenbach by its CEO Michael Seffrin and other conflicts of interest between ACS executives and the drug industry do not look good, but are appearances that important? Healthcare organizations do not appear to think so, considering that they take no steps to change direction. Dr. Michael Thun, chief of epidemiology and surveillance research of the ACS, did not deny the ACS ties with business interests when asked about them, but said candidly,

"The American Cancer Society views relationships with corporations as a source of revenue for cancer prevention."[35]

Thun's view that it was not necessary to condemn red meat even though eating red or processed meat over a long period of time could raise colorectal cancer risk, was discussed in chapter 4.

In defending possible conflicts of interest, Thun's comment represents a certain industry point of view. What is wrong with healthcare organizations collecting a little corporate help, even if some possible conflicts of interest exist just below the surface? Surely, that is sometimes unavoidable.

Unfortunately, besides creating the appearance of wrong-doing, conflicts of interest all too often lead directly to considerable harm to the public. The ACS coziness with the drug industry and its fundraising ties to drug companies, such as those noted above, may be a part of the reason why the ACS is so ambivalent about condemning meat and dairy products. After all, a decline in the consumption of animal protein could lead to a reduction in the incidence of the killer diseases and also a reduction in the demand for the drugs needed to treat the killer diseases. A result like that could only mean less profit for the drug companies which might impact negatively on financial relationships with the American Cancer Society. Would, for example, drug companies which donate money to the ACS be so generous with their contributions if the ACS had built a reputation for taking a tough stand against animal products in order to reduce the incidence of cancer nationwide, a consequence of which could only be a reduced need for drugs to treat cancer?

In 2009, the Corporate Social Responsibility Wire reported that Pfizer pharmaceuticals had supported the ACS with $1.7 million in grant funding. [36] It should be apparent that with donations like this neither the ACS nor any other organization is likely to seriously investigate a drug like Pfizer's Lipitor to determine whether or not it should be shelved because of its negative side effects and its failure to provide advertised benefits. These kinds of financial arrangements seriously subvert the honesty required to serve the public needs. Laws and regulations that cannot be manipulated that have real teeth need to be enacted to control this kind of corporate giving.

Another pharmaceutical company contributing more than $1 million to the ACS was AstraZeneca Pharmaceuticals LP. It does not seem likely that the ACS will be issuing any reports to the public about the negative aftereffects of AstraZeneca's Crestor (a statin) either, though, as we shall see, tough warnings against the use of statins are more than warranted by all the healthcare organizations.

Healthcare organizations that go along with drugs manufactured by companies with which they have ties just to get along in an unspoken quid pro quo relationship can also cause considerable damage to the public when those drugs have dangerous side effects. The injury gets compounded even further if other treatments without side effects, such as the cardiac disease arrest and reversal treatments developed by Dr. Esselstyn and Dr. Ornish, are ignored just because they do not financially benefit the healthcare industry or various drug companies with whom the healthcare organizations are joined in an unspoken pledge of loyalty. When this happens, the public does not get adequately informed that alternative, inexpensive, safe treatments in disease prevention are not only available but advisable. Eliminating animal protein as a means for reducing the risk of the killer diseases must certainly be counted among such treatments. But that kind of plan requires no drugs, reduces the need for conventional medical treatment, and can only lead to a reduction in the overall use of drugs and visits to healthcare professionals by the public. This means less profit for the drug companies, healthcare insiders who profit from drug company relationships, healthcare professionals, and healthcare organizations involved in advising the public about catastrophic diseases.

Exploring the extent to which conflicts of interest pose a threat to the public health will be an adventure for the next chapter. There we will take an even closer look at the inter-locking chain of "good old boy" type relationships where one hand is always busy washing the other. It will lead us to a fuller understanding of why some of our healthcare organizations are ignoring the facts about proper nutrition, most notably that the elimination of meat and dairy products from the diet can vastly reduce the risk of getting cancer, heart disease, stroke, diabetes, and other chronic diseases.

Chapter 15

The Good Old Boy Network Hard at Work

Wherever one turns there seems to be some suspicion of complicity between the country's healthcare organizations with the drug industry. It is through connections with the government that the drug industry was able to turn statins, the treatment for high cholesterol, into a best seller. That happened in 2004 when statins got a big boost from the National Institutes of Health which issued a report saying that a good eight million more people could benefit from taking the drug.

This was good business for Pfizer's Lipitor and Merck's Zocor, both statins, two drugs that, according to IMS Health, a global healthcare information company, ended up being the top sellers for the year. Lipitor sales were at $10.6 billion, up 13.9% over 2003.[1] The NIH report also could not have hurt the other popular brand-name statins: AstraZeneca's Crestor, Bristol-Myers Squibb's Pravachol, Merck's Mevacor, and Reliant Pharmaceuticals' Lescol.

But the story does not end there. As reported by CBS News correspondent Sharyl Attkisson, the NIH advice raised serious concerns. It turned out that almost all of the NIH experts recommending statins "had financial ties to statin drug companies."[2]

Attkisson was not the only one to notice. The *New York Times* reported that "consumer groups, including the Center for Science in the Public Interest in Washington, asserted that many of the experts on the panel that drew up the guidelines had received consulting fees, money for research, or other money from companies making statins." The Times further reported that the NIH "has acknowledged that eight of the nine experts on the panel that issued the recommendations had received financing from one or more of the companies that make statins."[3]

Not only did the NIH have a serious conflict of interest to explain, but any justification for the recommendation based on the science also had to be questioned. John Abramson, a clinical instructor at Harvard University, whose objections to statins was noted in chapter 9, said of the NIH advice, that it "flies in the face of science."[4] Abramson and 30 other doctors and scientists requested that the NIH make an independent review of the cholesterol guidelines promoting statins and cited one study showing that women using statins got slightly more heart disease, not less. And, as reported in chapter 9, no studies have been done to show any benefits for statins use for people over 65 or people under 65 who did not have diabetes or had not already had a heart attack. Moreover, eight percent of people whose cholesterol was reduced with statins developed coronary problems like a heart attack or angina.

It appears that the NIH panel threw all caution to the winds when issuing the report. Frequent complaints by the public about the use of statins indicate that the drug can pose substantial health risks to the user and that some side effects are permanent. Travis Raiborn took Merck's Zocor on the recommendation of his doctor just to avoid the risk of a heart attack, even though his cholesterol was not high. As a consequence he suffered severe loss of muscle function and nearly died. "My muscles were not muscles, they were just tissue you slapped back and forth," Raiborn said of the side effects. "There's no way I can get myself up." Today he cannot function normally and he battles constant pain.[5]

Duane Graveline, a former astronaut, said that of the two times he was put on Lipitor he "descended into the black pit of amnesia." He wrote a book and created a website on the adverse side effects of statins.[6]

Problems for seniors who take statins can also be an issue.

While taking Lipitor, Jane Brunzie, at age 66, had "senior moments" so severe that her daughter refused to let her babysit for her granddaughter, and the family began looking into finding a home for her convinced she was suffering with dementia.[7] The senior moments stopped when she stopped taking Lipitor.

Some doctors believe that symptoms of muscle aches and cognitive problems affect up to 15 percent of people taking the drug. As to be expected, however, Merck and other statin makers insist serious side effects are extremely rare. Dr. Scott Grundy, the lead author of national guidelines for statins use who has received honoraria from Pfizer, said: "You need to look at the big picture rather than worrying yourself to death over individual trials."[8]

High powered statin promotions by the drug companies backed by government agencies have put the message of the danger of uncontrolled high cholesterol front and center in the public's consciousness. In an article that appeared in the January 17, 2008 issue of Business Week, "according to the official government guidelines from the National Cholesterol Education Program (NCEP), 40 million Americans should be taking [statins]."[9]

This is an astonishing figure considering the increased scrutiny on statins because of their adverse side effects and because of the legitimate concerns that have been voiced about their failure to provide any real benefits for a large number of people. The point of the criticism made here is not to resolve the conflict about the use of statins. The facts do that. But the question that needs to be asked is why the NIH felt it was necessary to state that 8 million more people could benefit from taking statins and why the NCEP would put out guidelines saying that 40 million people should be taking the drug considering that it is so controversial. For that matter, the word *corruption* is difficult to evade for the members of the NIH panel endorsing statins who had financial ties to the manufacturers of the drug. What is the liability of the panel if members of the public suffer severe side effects from taking statins based upon their recommendation? It seems clear that they should not be permitted to do and say whatever they please without penalty just because they sit on a panel of the NIH.

If the NIH and the NCEP really want to make recommendations that will help from anywhere between 8 to 40 million people, they should advise that everyone try to reduce their total cholesterol level to 150 mg/dL. As we have seen, that advice, if followed, would not only practically assure protection from heart attack and cardiovascular disease, it would present no danger of aftereffects like the debilitating muscle condition that created so many health problems for Mr. Raiborn, the senior moments that almost put Jane Brunzie into a nursing home, the amnesia that caused Astronaut Graveline to literally lose his mind, or any of the other documented cases of harm arising from the use of statins.

In the interests of the public health, perhaps a nationally televised public debate could be arranged with the NIH panel of experts seated at the debate table who had financial ties to the statin drug companies and who recommended statins to 8 million people. Maybe the NCEP could also join in and tell the American people how it decided that 40 million people should be taking statins.

Sometimes conflicts of interest are so extreme they almost defy the imagination, as shown in the following example. At an American Heart Association seminar, Dr. Bryan Brewer, a senior official at the NIH, described AstraZeneca's Crestor as safe and effective. His talk was published in a special supplement by the American Journal of Cardiology, which is read by prescribing physicians. This coincided with the launch of Crestor into the American market. At that time, however, Brewer was a paid advisor for Crestor. According to later congressional hearings, he earned $200,000 from outside public interests while holding down the position of branch chief at the NIH. On top of his ties to AstraZeneca, Brewer was "financially tied to eight other drug companies."[10]

The NIH is not the only healthcare agency that has entertained questionable relationships with the private sector. One of the frequent criticisms made against the FDA is that the agency is a puppet of the drug industry. It does not seem to mind. For example, on September 15, 2008 the Center for Science in the Public Interest reported that the FDA was setting up a website to help customers separate fact from fiction about drug ads. A problem of perception existed, however, in that the FDA hired Shaw Science Partners to develop the website, a public relations firm specializing in launching drugs like Viagra, Celebrex, Zoloft, Cymbalta and the now-withdrawn Rezulin.[11] Suspicions were immediately raised. The FDA is so powerful, apparently, that it does whatever it pleases without concern about appearances.

Like the NIH, the American Heart Association (AHA) is not averse to recommending drugs made by companies with which it has financial dealings either. In the year 2000 the AHA guidelines panel gave Altephase, a clot buster drug for stroke manufactured by Genentech, its Class I recommendation without publishing a dissenting report on the panel by a prominent critic, Dr. Jerome Hoffman, a clinical epidemiologist at UCLA. He dissented because "the Class I recommendation for the use of Altephase was based on only a single clinical trial."

Hoffman argued that "the risk of bleeding outweighs any benefits of Altephase if the drug [had to be used in a setting where it could not be] used as precisely as it was in the highly organized and rigidly controlled structure of the [one single] clinical trial.[12]

His interpretation "was shared by many physicians and more

than one emergency medicine professional organization." The AHA, however, did not regard Hoffman's dissent as being important enough to include in their promotional guidelines for Altephase.

Jeanne Lenzer, a freelance medical investigative journalist, saw it differently. She published a piece in the British Medical Journal pointing out that the AHA had received $11 million from Genentech (the maker of Altephase) in the previous ten years and that six of the eight Altephase guideline panelists had ties to Genentech or its partner Boehringer Ingelheim.[13] The President of the AHA vigorously denied a conflict of interest.

The American Heart Association has also found a lucrative market in endorsing drug companies, though it would prefer not to call them endorsements. Bristol-Myers Squibb paid $600,000 to the AHA for the right to display the AHA name and logo in ads for its cholesterol-lowering drug Pravachol. Although nonprofits like the AHA deny an endorsement is involved in arrangements like this, O'Dwyer's PR Services Report says that "[public relations'] pros view those third-party endorsements as invaluable ways to build goodwill among consumers for a client's product line." O'Dywer advises, however, not to "use the word 'endorse' when speaking to executives from non-profits about their relationships with the private sector. The preferred non-profit vernacular is: recommended, sponsorship, approved, or partnership."[14] As was the case for the ACS in regard to the $1.7 million donation it received from Pfizer, does anyone think that the AHA would ever utter even one word of criticism of Bristol-Myers Squibb's Pravachol (a statin) after receiving $600,000 for an AHA endorsement?

Our healthcare organizations often seem overly eager to profit without adequate concern for the loss of independence that goes into the bargain as well as the potential harm to the public good the loss of independence can bring. In the year 2002 the American College of Cardiology (ACC), a non-profit organization that advocates for better cardiovascular care and disease prevention for the public, conferred on Pfizer pharmaceuticals their Diamond Heart Award for a donation of $750,000. They presented Avenis, Bristol-Myers Squibb, GlaxoSmithKlein, and Procter and Gamble Pharmaceuticals the Gold Heart Award for their more than $250,000 each in donations. Six more drug and device companies received the Silver Heart Award for donations greater than $100,000 each.[15]

It is difficult to believe that after this kind of patronage the ACC or any other organization would do other than promote the interests of these drug companies should the need arise. And even if no corruption were involved, the potential for corruption could hardly be more conspicuous. Almost everyone agrees that nonprofit health organizations should not be receiving money from drug companies that can profit in some way from these kinds of relationships. The payback need not even be visible. A quid pro quo understanding not to criticize or obstruct in any way the path the drug company intends to pursue can be just as profitable.

It is not just the drug companies with which healthcare organizations partner for money. For instance, besides drugs, the AHA also endorses food companies, provided they are able to pay. In 2001 Steve Millay, a biostatician, lawyer, and adjunct scholar at the conservative Cato Institute, said that food manufacturers pay $7,500 for each product approved by the AHA, and $4,500 for renewals. He noted that:

> There's gold in the AHA's credibility. Several hundred products now carry the heart-check logo [the logo of the AHA]. You do the math. Adding insult to injury, consumers pay up for the more expensive brands that can afford to dance with the AHA. Pricey Tropicana grapefruit juice is 'heart healthy' but supermarket bargain brand grapefruit juice isn't?[16]

Government agencies have also been caught in conflicts of interest with the food industry. In December of 1999 the Physicians Committee for Responsible Medicine sued the USDA and the Department of Health and Human Services (DHHS) in order to ensure, among other matters, that in the future they "choose members for all dietary guidelines advisory committees who do not have inappropriate relationships to any food industries; and to ensure...that they operate dietary guidelines advisory committees in accordance with the public disclosure requirements of the FACA [Federal Advisory Committee Act]."[17]

The suit was necessary because of the eleven members who had been chosen to serve on a USDA Advisory Committee, six had had (or had recently held) financial ties to the meat, dairy, or egg industries. In addition, the Deputy Undersecretary of Agriculture, who was participating in the advisory committee meetings, had had a business relationship with the Dannon Institute, manufacturers of yogurt and other dairy products.

The USDA guidelines that were being developed by this advisory committee were for the purpose of establishing "the basis for all federal food assistance and nutrition programs, including the National School Lunch Program, the National School Breakfast Program, the Food Stamp Program, and the Special Supplemental Nutrition Program for Women, Infants, and Children." Yet in spite of the obvious need for appointing an impartial committee to make these important nutrition recommendations that would affect the health of millions of Americans, especially children, the USDA and the DHHS had set up a committee of which more than half of its members had ties to the meat and dairy industries.

As a result of the suit, the USDA Dietary Guidelines Advisory Committee for the first time ever advised that "soy-based beverages (soy milk) are on a par with cow's milk as a source of calcium" and that "the foundation of a healthy diet is plant food."

Cornered, as they were, and embarrassed by the law suit that was looking over their shoulders, the committee members with the conflicts of interest had little choice but to do the right thing.

We have now examined several examples of the way some of the more prominent government and nonprofit healthcare organizations have conducted business from the distant past to present times. In this investigation we have tried to determine if they are functioning in ways that best serve the well-being of the public. Some important concerns have emerged, notably the conflicts of interest that seem to play an integral part in the operating procedures of several healthcare organizations.

In the past certain of these organizations tried to smear the opposition as they did with Dr. Gerson, Harry Hoxsey, and Dr. Burton in order to try to silence them. But there are different ways of trying to silence opposing views such as ignoring them as if they did not exist, the hope being that ignored long enough they become irrelevant. This seems to be one of the primary strategies the healthcare organizations are using in regard to the evidence that animal protein is the major cause of the killer diseases. Why they would do this, as we have seen, can often be linked to profit relationships such as with the drug industry or other financial interests. At the same time, organizations become concerned about protecting their own turf. Other motives also enter the picture including resistance to change, jealousies, pride, institutional prejudice, personal biases, and individual appetites and inclinations toward consuming animal protein.

The ghosts of the past stand guard over the public good because the healthcare industry frequently does not. It is time for the healthcare organizations to begin doing their job by telling the American people the facts:

1) Overwhelming evidence shows that animal protein is a cause of many forms of cancer, heart disease, stroke, and

diabetes.

2) Thirty-five percent of people with a cholesterol level between 150 and 200 mg/dL are at risk of having a heart attack. People can practically eliminate the risk of heart disease, heart attack, and stroke by keeping their total cholesterol levels at 150 mg/dL or lower. The way to do that is to stop consuming animal products.

3) Heart disease, some cancers, and diabetes Type 2 can be reversed through nutrition.

4) Dairy products are a direct link to prostate and other cancers as well as Type 1 diabetes.

5) Breast cancer risk can be greatly reduced by avoiding animal protein and eating a plant-based diet that keeps estrogen levels under control.

6) Dairy products raise the risk of osteoporosis by increasing metabolic acid which draws calcium from the bones which is excreted in the urine.

7) It is also possible that the elimination of animal products from the diet can significantly reduce the risk of Alzheimer's Disease, multiple sclerosis, and other chronic diseases and conditions including kidney stones.

8) A nutrition regimen that excludes animal products can be effective in the treatment of arthritis.

The nation eliminated tuberculosis as the number one killer and heart disease took its place. Now cancer is on the verge of overtaking heart disease as the number one killer according to a 2008 report by the International Agency for Research on Cancer. Douglas Blayney, the president of the American Society of Clinical Oncology, reports that "on the world scene cancer is one of the greatest untold health crises of the developing world."[18] And he is right. In the next few years the cancer rate is expected to double worldwide with new cancer cases increasing from 12 million to 27 million by the year 2030.[19] By then it is anticipated that 75 million people will be living with this dreaded disease. Among the most important factors motivating the increase in cancer incidence is the adoption of Western habits by the developing countries. [This is discussed more thoroughly in chapter 24.]

If there is any good news in this bleak forecast it is the possibility, at least in the United States, of eliminating both cancer and heart disease as the top killers they are today just as happened with tuberculosis. The means to do it are here, right now. Communicating the truth about the dangers of consuming animal protein can contribute dramatically to that goal. But the country needs the American Cancer Society, the American Heart Association, the American Medical Association, the Food and Drug Administration, the National Institutes of Health, the National Cancer Institute, the United States Department of Agriculture, and all the other healthcare organizations to step up to the plate and do their part too.

How We Got to Where We Are

Chapter 16

A Century of Government Research in Nutrition

The Long Trail Toward Health

Wilbur Olin Atwater (1844 - 1907) earned his Ph.D at the Sheffield Scientific School at Yale University in 1869 with a dissertation on feed corn, the first modern analysis of food in the United States.[1] After graduation he traveled to Germany where he studied physiological chemistry for a year in Leipzig followed by a further year in Berlin.

When Atwater returned to the United States he taught for two years at East Tennessee University and then for a few months at Maine State College before he was appointed as the first Professor of Chemistry at Wesleyan College in Middletown, Connecticut, a position he would hold for the remainder of his life.

At Wesleyan, Atwater, worked with his former teacher, Samuel W. Johnson (1830 - 1909), to help establish the first agricultural experimental station in the United States for the purpose of studying and solving problems associated with food and agriculture. Johnson, who had studied in Munich with the famous chemist Justus von Liebig (1803 - 1873), was the primary force in founding the Sheffield Scientific School at Yale.[2]

In 1882 Atwater took a year's leave to travel back to Germany to study the metabolism of mammals in the class of Karl Voit (1831 - 1908), with whom he had become acquainted during his first trip. Voit had been credited with setting the first daily standards for protein consumption at 118 grams.[3] Years later Voit's influence would be reflected in Atwater's own recommendation that the daily consumption of protein should be set at 125 grams. This decision would have major ramifications for nutrition in the United States.

After completing Voit's class, Atwater returned home where he continued to teach at Wesleyan and also directed program development at new agricultural experiment stations across the nation.

Not too much was known about nutrition in the late 19th century other than that carbohydrates and fat provided energy to maintain body temperature and do muscular work, and that protein built and repaired tissue.[4] Specific vitamins were unknown, and only a few major minerals like calcium and phosphorus had been isolated, though their purpose was not clear. Atwater was a passionate and tireless investigator in the pursuit of knowledge about nutrition and approached his work eagerly. The training he had acquired in Germany for measuring respiration and metabolism provided the ideal background for hundreds of food studies he would undertake along with studies involving dietary evaluations, energy requirements for work, the digestibility of foods, and the economics of food production.[5]

Atwater was aided in his efforts by his own invention, the respiration calorimeter, one of the more advanced scientific instruments of the 19th century. He used it to quantify the dynamics of energy metabolism, measure the balance between food intake and energy output, and evaluate the effects of diet and muscular activity on metabolism.[6]

A friend of Atwater, Edward Atkinson, who had corresponded with Atwater for years about their common interest in persuading the poor to adopt a more nutritious diet, happened also to be a personal friend of the U.S. Secretary of Agriculture, J. Sterling Morton. He spoke to Morton about Atwater and his ideas with the result that Morton issued a $10,000 grant to Atwater to establish a laboratory for food investigations at the

Department of Agriculture. It would be called the Office of Experiment Stations, and it was the first government office for nutrition in the United States.[7]

The office opened in 1894. In the same year Atwater issued the very first dietary recommendations by a government agency which he called the Farmer's Bulletin.[8] Four years later he published chemical analyses of 2600 American foodstuffs he had been working on his entire career.[9] But he never forgot his concern for the poor:

> The individual man is coming to realize that he is his brother's keeper, and that his brother is not only of his household but may live on the other side of the world. With all these thoughtful people the conviction is growing that there is one fundamental condition of the intellectual and moral elevation of the poor, the ignorant, the weak, the destitute, namely the improvement of their physical condition.[10]

Atwater worked in four areas: 1) the types and amounts of foods consumed by different population groups, 2) the chemical composition of foods, 3) the effects of cooking and food processing on nutritional quality, and 4) the amounts and types of nutrients people needed to function at their best; this entailed studies of human metabolism and respiration. The diet he recommended was based on the content of protein, carbohydrates, fats, and mineral matter.[11] Atwater defined food as consisting of:

> … material which, when taken into the body, serves to either form tissue or yield energy, or both. This definition includes all the ordinary food materials, since they both build tissue and yield energy. It includes sugar and starch, because they yield energy and form fatty tissue. It

includes alcohol, because the latter is burned to yield energy, though it does not build tissue. It excludes creatin, creatininin, [sic] and other so-called nitrogeneous extractives of meat, and likewise thein [sic] or caffein of tea and coffee, because they neither build tissue nor yield energy, although they may, at times, be useful aids to nutrition.[12]

By 1902 Atwater had become aware of a causal connection between diet and disease:

Unless care is exercised in selecting food, a diet may result which is one-sided or badly balanced — that is, one in which either protein or fuel ingredients (carbohydrate and fat) are provided in excess....The evils of overeating may not be felt at once, but sooner or later they are sure to appear — perhaps in an excessive amount of fatty tissue, perhaps in general debility, perhaps in actual disease.[13]

It was at this time that Atwater set the recommendation for the daily consumption of protein at 125 grams.[14]

By 1904 some of the views to which Atwater subscribed were being challenged. He thought, for example, that fruits and vegetables were luxury foods, not foods with special nutrient qualities. His view that all digestible proteins were of equal nutrient value was also losing favor, and Russell Henry Chittenden (1856 - 1943), a mid-career biochemist who, like Atwater, had attended the Sheffield Scientific School at Yale, was trying to challenge Atwater's daily recommendations for protein intake. (The importance of Chittenden's work will be reviewed in chapter 17.)

Unfortunately, not enough was known about nutrition at the time that might have helped Atwater lower the high blood pressure that would cost him his life. In November of 1904 at the age of 60 he suddenly suffered a severe stroke. He was confined at home for the remainder of his life, cared for by his wife and daughter, where he died three years later in 1907.

Wilbur Olin Atwater was one of the first major pioneers in nutrition in the United States. He succeeded in putting the "subject of human food and nutrition on a quantitative basis in the U.S."[15] Some call him the father of nutrition in the United States.

In 1917 Caroline Hunt, a nutritionist at the USDA, in concurrence with Atwater's work, put out diet guidelines based on five food groups: 1) cereals, 2) milk and meat, 3) vegetables and fruits, 4) fats and fatty foods, and 5) sugars and sugary foods. Hunt had issued similar USDA guidelines for children the previous year. In 1921 the same guidelines were published with an addition that recommended how much food a family of five should purchase. Two years later different sized families were added to the guidelines. These kinds of guidelines were popular with the public in the 1920s. Then in 1933, in response to hardships caused by the depression, Hazel Stiebeling, a USDA food economist, identified four cost levels interlaced with 12 different food groups to help people shop for food.[16]

World War II prompted President Franklin D. Roosevelt to convene the National Nutrition Conference for Defense in 1941. Drawing on the expertise of nutritionists from the Food and Nutrition Board of the National Academy of Sciences, the conference produced the first set of RDAs (Recommended Daily Allowances) and offered recommendations for calorie intake plus nine essential nutrients: protein, iron, calcium, vitamin A, Vitamin D, thiamin, riboflavin, niacin, and ascorbic acid (vitamin C).[17]

Two years later the USDA published a Basic Seven foods guide called the National Wartime Nutrition Guide that took into account food limitations caused by the war.[18] The guide was revised in 1946 after the war as the National Food Guide and was used for the next decade.

Then in 1956 the USDA issued a new guide based on four food groups. 1) milk, 2) meat, 3) grain products, and 4) fruits and vegetables. Known as the "Basic Four," this served as a nutrition guide for the next two decades.

In the meantime, a 1964 panel of experts at the World Health Organization (WHO) linked diet and metabolism to chronic disease and reported that:

The potential scope of cancer prevention is limited by the proportion of human cancers in which extrinsic factors are responsible. These include all environmental carcinogens (whether already identified or not) as well as modifying factors that favour [sic] neoplasia of apparently intrinsic origin (e.g. hormonal imbalances, dietary deficiencies, and metabolic defects).[19]

The search for dietary and metabolic connections to cancer had begun.

In 1968 Senator George McGovern of North Dakota was appointed to chair a Senate Select Committee on Nutrition and Human Needs with a mandate to eradicate malnutrition in the United States.[20] Before it was finished the committee would create laws to assist the poor, including the creation of the Food Stamp program. In 1969 the committee organized a White House Conference on Food, Nutrition, and Health which discussed matters such as how many calories people should consume and how much fat, cholesterol, salt, sugar, and alcohol in the American diet should be considered excessive.[21] By 1970 the committee's work was drawing to a close, but some members wanted to extend the committee's work to include overnutrition and excesses in diet. McGovern, who with his wife had gone through Nathan Pritikin's low-fat diet and exercise program, was in sympathy and agreed.

Cardiologists were already doing research on nutrition. They were impressed by the absence of heart disease in societies in foreign lands that lived on plant-based diets. The McGovern committee was aware of their studies and urged the NIH to support nutrition-based research that might assist in the prevention of disease. In 1973 the McGovern committee held hearings on nutrition and in 1974 issued a report on diet and chronic diseases. New hearings were held in 1976 titled "Diet Related to Killer diseases" at which witnesses testified that the "wrong kinds of foods would increase the risks for cancer, cardiovascular disease, and obesity."[22]

Then in January of 1977 the committee released a bombshell report titled *Dietary Goals for the United States* that recommended Americans consume more fruit, vegetables, whole grains, poultry and fish and reduce consumption of meat, eggs, foods high in fat, butterfat, sugar, and salt, and substitute nonfat milk for whole milk.[23] A storm of protest followed from cattle ranchers, egg producers, sugar producers, and the dairy industry which foresaw declining profits if people started following the advice offered in the report.

"All hell broke loose," recalled Mark Hegsted. "Practically nobody was in favor of the McGovern recommendations." (See chapter 5 for Professor Hegsted's views on dairy products in relation to osteoporosis.) The meat and egg producers demanded new hearings and the American Medical Association got in on the act arguing that physicians giving out advice to individuals was far better than Congress giving out advice to everyone.[24]

Under the barrage of criticism, the McGovern committee revised its report and made changes in the wording that suggested cholesterol guidelines could be relaxed so that pre-menopausal women, young children, and the elderly could get the "nutritional benefits of eggs in the diet." The advice the committee wanted to include in the report that read "reduce consumption of meat" was changed to read "choose meat, poultry, and fish which will reduce saturated fat."[25],[26] Pressure from the food industry had succeeded in changing congressional diet guidelines to the detriment of the American people. But even though the report did not go as far as the committee would have liked, it still represented a major turn in protocols from concentrating on obtaining the right amount of nutrients, to avoiding excessive consumption of the wrong foods (saturated fats and too much salt). It introduced new ideas into the discussion about diet and health and shifted the focus of the healthcare organizations that controlled and disseminated diet guidelines to the public.

Organizations move according to evolving ideologies and ideas were beginning to change. The National Cancer Institute published new dietary guidelines in 1979, and though the USDA had been slow to sense the new focus on nutrition, it too climbed on board in the same year with a publication titled *Food* in which it addressed the role of fats, sugars, and sodium in relation to chronic diseases.[27] In 1980 the USDA issued another report, this time in conjunction with the Department of Health and Human Services, titled "Nutrition and Your Health: Dietary Guidelines for Americans." Momentum was not to be stopped. In 1982 a panel of experts from the National Academy of Sciences appointed by Congress issued the first report that deliberated on the association of dietary fat with cancer and recommended a "maximum fat intake of 30% of calories for prevention of cancer."[28] The report attributed as much as 90% of cancer to environmental factors and diet.[29] It was co-authored by T. Colin Campbell who 23 years later would publish *The China Study*. With this report the national debate about the connection between diet and disease was in full swing and has continued ever since with the government sponsoring significant research projects every few years.

By 1984 the American Cancer Society had joined the procession as scientists increasingly targeted the role dietary fat intake plays in cancer and heart disease formation. In 1988 the United States Surgeon General called on leading authorities in the field of nutrition and health to prepare a textbook on how nutrition could prevent different diseases, including cancer. Some scientists said that diet was the cause of cancer in men in 30% to 40% of cases and for women, 60% of the time. Two epidemiologists suggested that "diet could significantly prevent cancer."[30]

Two years later the Congress of the United States put out its own textbook titled "Unconventional Cancer Treatments" through the Office of Technology Assessment. It stated emphatically that:

It is our collective professional judgment that nutritional interventions are going to 'follow' psychosocial interventions up the ladder into clinical respectability as adjunctive and complementary approaches to the treatment of cancer.[31]

The Cancer Treatment Research Foundation invited experts from around the world to participate in a an international symposium concerning the role of nutrition in comprehensive cancer treatment in 1993. Along with American institutions like the National Institutes of Health, Harvard University, the University of Pennsylvania and other prestigious universities, these authorities agreed that diet and supplements "could play a major role in improving the quality and quantity of life for medically treated cancer patients."[32]

A new organization (1982) that quickly established credentials among the elite healthcare organizations was the American Institute for Cancer Research. It issued its First Expert Report on *Food, Nutrition and the Prevention of Cancer: A Global Perspective* in 1997. Focusing on the causes of cancer, among the recommendations the panel of 16 experts made, was to consume "predominantly plant-based diets rich in a variety of vegetables, fruits, pulses (legumes) and minimally processed starchy staple foods," and to limit red meat "if eaten at all" to less than 3 ounces a day.[33] T. Colin Campbell was the co-chair of this panel.

Dr. Campbell and his son Thomas published *The China Study* in January of 2005 which presented undeniable evidence in the national press pointing to a causal link between eating animal protein and diseases like cancer, heart disease, stroke, diabetes, and many other chronic diseases. It further showed that "advanced heart disease, relatively advanced cancers of certain types, diabetes and a few other degenerative diseases could be reversed by diet."[34]

Then in 2007 the AICR together with the World Cancer Research Fund issued a Second Expert Report on *Food, Nutrition and the Prevention of Cancer: A Global Perspective*. In this study it directly linked body fat to six cancers, including colorectal and post-menopausal breast cancer.

It has taken a century of scientific research and discovery to establish a new order of healthcare organizations intent on discovering the links between diet and disease from the time W.O. Atwater took the reins of the first government office on nutrition at the USDA with a budget of $10,000. One hundred years later, the Federal government provides funding of more than $400 million dollars annually for nutrition and food research.[35]

Nutritional research began with an investigation of the amounts and types of nutrients people needed which resulted in the recognition that too much food is a risk factor for disease. This evolved into recommended dietary allowances including calorie and nutrient intake. As this became a standard part of the nutritional lexicon, research brought mounting evidence of the connections between dietary intake and disease to light. The role dietary fat played in the promotion of disease next emerged as a key player while complex carbohydrates and fiber continued to gain acceptance as the guardians of good health and warriors against chronic disease. Evidence continued to mount that it was not just dietary fat scientists needed to be investigating in the etiology of nutritionally-related disease, but, specifically, saturated fats, trans fats, and cholesterol so that by the dawn of the 21st century, the finger of accusation pointed directly at red meats, processed meats, and dairy products as the undeniable agents responsible for specific cancers, heart disease, stroke, diabetes, and other chronic conditions.

The scientific nutritional research of the 20th century led to one inescapable conclusion resulting from arguably the most significant discovery ever made about the origins of chronic disease: the consumption of animal protein including dairy products is the cause of the major killer diseases.

Not everyone is thrilled when new evidence like this arrives for a variety of reasons, as we have seen. Some scientists by disposition are change resistant, some are biased, others are envious, and still others don't believe the new evidence that the world is round when they know with absolute certainty that it is flat.

Institutions as well as individual scientists also have vested interests that keep them from accepting the new. In 1982, for example, it was growing ever more apparent that new research in nutrition linked dietary fat with cancer. Yet even while the National Academy of Sciences was preparing the congressionally funded report titled *Diet, Nutrition, and Cancer*, one of the leaders of the Food and Nutrition Board (FNB) at the National Academy of Sciences appeared on a TV news program with Tom Brokaw to discuss a different report he and some friends at the FNB had prepared titled "Toward Healthful Diets."[36]

In the ensuing discussion, the FNB officer, who had strong connections to the meat, dairy, and egg industries, praised "the health value of McDonald's hamburgers."[37]

Back in 1982 not many people knew as much about fast food burgers as is today common knowledge, thanks to reports like Eric Schlosser's monumental study, *Fast Food Nation*, which reveals that hamburgers are an amalgamation of unhealthy products including bacteria-laden manure as well as chunks of dirt and intestinal spillage, and that one hamburger will be likely composed of the parts of hundreds of different slaughtered cows.[38] But even then an FNB officer should have known enough about the high-fat content in fast food burgers to be cautious in recommending them to several million viewers.

The FNB officer was, of course, expressing the consensus view about nutrition still held by an old guard of scientists during that period. Those were times in which the USDA nutrition guide of 1979 recommended two servings of milk or cheese and two servings (2 to 3 ounces per serving) of meat, poultry, fish, or beans a day. By 1984 this amount had even increased from two servings to two to three servings.[39] New research findings about dietary fat were not yet strong enough to coalesce into the firm recommendations the healthcare organizations follow today, which is to limit dairy intake to low-fat dairy products and to restrict red meat consumption to low-fat and lean meats while limiting or avoiding processed meats.

Back in the early 1980s, those bold enough to suggest that red meat was unhealthy would certainly not have been added to the guest list of many of the officers of the Food and Nutrition Board. In fact, to get around their entrenched views, the president of the National Academy of Sciences (NAS), the parent agency of the FNB, had to appoint an independent panel of experts to write the landmark 1982 report on *Diet, Nutrition, and Cancer*.[40] James S. Turner, the chairman of the Consumer Liaison Panel of the NAS at the time, wrote that "we can only conclude that the [FNB] Board is dominated by a group of change-resistant scientists who share a rather isolated view about diet and disease."[41]

Reflecting on just how far off the FNB officer was in espousing support for an unhealthy product like McDonald's burgers to millions of viewers on Tom Brokaw's program, one can hardly avoid comparing just how up-to-date today's healthcare experts are in making their recommendations for what they consider to be the most current and healthy dietary guidelines available. Why, for example, does the entire healthcare establishment continue to advocate the consumption of meat and dairy products when ample evidence now indicates that they are cancer-causing, heart attack-promoting, diabetes-advancing substances?

It is easy with hindsight to look backwards and find fault with those whose entrenched views resisted the progressive discoveries of approaching times. But today the same indifference to new research findings exists within the entire healthcare establishment as that held by the FNB officer who appeared on Tom Brokaw's show and recommended McDonald Burgers.

This is the way of progress. It is a kind of game. The new wages a battle with the old and once it is victorious, it settles in and becomes comfortable and complacent, basking in the new ideals its job is to govern. As the new ideals spread they gain increasing power, and a kind of "group think" takes over and reigns supreme, gradually becoming the old. Meanwhile, another round of newer ideas and ideals is brewing in the ever fertile and expansive human mind. Soon the stage is set for the next fight. And that is what is happening today in the battle over the rights and wrongs of meat and dairy food consumption.

In the future historians will look back on this battle just as today we look back on the battle against tobacco. Those involved, whether they have grasped it or not, are in the middle of a fight and have no choice but to choose on which side they stand. Are they for the consumption of animal protein and dairy products which detractors insist lie at the root of the major killer diseases, or are they against the side of the meat and dairy industries which deny the threat. These are the people whose turn it is today to stand up and be counted. And history will judge which side is right and which side is wrong.

Chapter 17

Creating the Myth

The History of Protein

Most people have heard many times in their lives that animal food is the best source of protein. It can come in the form of meat, poultry, fowl, or seafood and includes animals like cows, pigs, sheep, rabbits, chickens, turkeys, ducks, geese, quail, pheasants, frogs, salmon, tuna, trout, carp, herring, sardines, lobsters, mussels, clams, oysters, scallops, squid, and octopus.

In some countries the fare includes cats, dogs, horses, goats, camels, llamas, mice, rats, snakes, snails, squirrels, pigeons, and bats, though in the Western world people are not eager to hear those stories. In America the public in general tolerates deer, elk, and moose on the menu, but grows queasy at the thought of consuming catfish, eel, or opossum.

We learn from early childhood on that protein is synonymous with animals and dairy products. We want a breakfast of bacon and eggs, a chicken, fish, or cold-cuts sandwich for lunch with maybe a milk shake or ice cream added on, while a cup of yogurt or possibly some cheese crackers will do nicely for a mid-afternoon snack. For the evening meal, steak and potatoes with beef gravy or pork chops serve nicely with some pie or cake for desert, made with eggs and cream, of course, and a tall glass of milk before bed. Into this mix we might throw a few miscellaneous fruits or vegetables here and there. This is the typical kind of protein paradise with which we grow up. It is filled with an abundant supply of milk and dairy products and meat and animals of every kind.

But paradise has begun to lose some of its charm in recent

years as animal protein has increasingly become the prime suspect for stealing our health and the health of those we love. Even so, the protein message continues to get passed along in our homes, in our schools, in our universities in our communities, in our churches, at work, and from on high from our most respected healthcare organizations. The odds are heavily stacked in favor of continuing the banquet which effectively keeps the suspicions about the dangers of consuming animal protein in check.

Surprisingly, milk and eggs are said to "represent the best amino acid matches for our proteins" and stand at the apex of the protein hierarchy, even above meat.[1] That point notwithstanding, it is the kind of protein "as in beef" that we turn to when we think of strong bodies, robust health, and athleticism. There is nothing like steak and hamburger to build big, strong-boned, sleek-muscled children who grow up to be vibrant, physically empowered adults, or so goes the dream.

Plant protein? That is another matter. We hear tales that small amounts of protein are embedded in vegetables, and that if they are combined in great enough numbers they can even furnish enough low-quality protein to ensure survival — barely.

There is a very good reason why these kinds of stories seem credible. It is because protein consists of about 20 amino acids of which eight cannot be manufactured by the body, and animal protein contains all eight of these amino acids leading to their informal classification as "complete" proteins. Because the eight amino acids are not all contained in individual plants, plant proteins are called "incomplete" proteins. Amino acids are vital to life because they are metabolized in the liver into forms that are used to build protein in the body tissues. But if one or more of these eight amino acids are missing in great enough quantity, the protein building system will not function properly and will grind to a halt.[2]

People who do not eat animal protein can get these essential eight amino acids from plants, but since plants singly do not contain all eight amino acids, different kinds of foods, like beans and rice, need to be combined to produce these eight essential amino acids which the body will convert to protein for its own use. At least this is what we are told. How should we know differently? Not being nutritionists, and if we are like most people, being somewhat nutritionally ambivalent, we are not likely to know just what plants contain or which ones to combine to get those eight essential amino acids, that is if food combining is really necessary. And so the premise that animal protein is superior and plant protein is inferior continues to be widely circulated and accepted.

Fortunately, this explanation does not tell the true story. In fact, it turns out that the body can get all the essential amino acids that it needs from common plant protein through its own "enormously complex metabolic" system without undue worry about combining different foods. Even better, plant protein "allows for [a] slow steady synthesis of new proteins [and] is the healthiest type of protein."[3] And, as we shall see momentarily, the right kinds of common plants produce all the essential and nonessential amino acids we need.

The body can also consume enough plant protein to grow just as big and muscular as if it had consumed animal protein as reported by Dr. Campbell in his studies on rural China. There, the protein consumed was mostly plant protein, not animal protein.[4]

For those who want more proof that plant protein can produce strong muscular bodies, try vegans like Carl Lewis, the track and field star, Ricky Williams, the professional football player, Salim Stoudamire, the professional basketball player, Martina Navratilova, perhaps the greatest woman tennis player of all times, or Brendan Brazier, professional Ironman triathlete and two-time Canadian 50km Ultra Marathon Champion. Many other athletes are also vegans.

When it comes to losing weight and dealing with the obesity epidemic, a low-fat, plant-based, low-protein diet wins hands down over a high-fat, animal-based diet. That is because diets high in animal protein convert calories into fat that finds a home in our waists, arms, and buttocks. A low-fat, low-protein diet, on the other hand, causes calories to be lost as body heat so that fat takes leave of our waists, arms and buttocks.[5] Protein that comes from animals is high in fat. Plant protein is low in fat.

We live at a point along a continuum in time where we strive for greater understanding. It is there that we get our basic knowledge about medicine according to the conventions of the day. Back in the mid-19th century our forefathers were living along that continuum in 19th century terms. They came to a fork in the road where one direction pointed toward an animal-based, high-protein diet under the heading: "The maximum quality of good health!" The other direction pointed toward a plant-based protein diet under the banner: "Don't be fooled. This is the true path!"

Proponents of the path toward greater animal protein consumption posted well-muscled men at the crossroads looking strong and virulent to flex their biceps, puff up their chests and urge people forward along the path toward eating more animal protein. But many misrepresentations were posted on the direction sign the public read as it took the turn and followed the well-muscled men of strength and virulence.

For example, the public did not know that protein needs had been hugely exaggerated by researchers whose research methods were superficial and unscientific. These researchers were the ones posting the well-muscled men at the crossroads.

Back then, no one took into account that after humans stopped growing and entered adulthood their protein needs were minimal so that there was no need to rush into diets that were high in protein, which meant animal-based foods. Perhaps it was just that no one thought of it at the time. Researchers have since determined that humans lose only about one-third of an ounce (10 grams) of protein a day.[6] We really only need a small amount of protein daily to replace the protein that has been lost. Humans have no need for excessive amounts of protein that the body cannot use. Facts like these are not widely publicized and are not widely known.

We also do not hear that animal protein intake between 10% to 20% (as a percentage of calories) is firmly associated with many health problems.[7] (The average protein intake in the United States is from 15% to 16%.)[7] Excessive protein consumption is harmful to our health, and since most people get too much protein, the health of many people is compromised as a result. One reason is that unlike fat, the body does not store protein, and over-consumption can cause an "accumulation of toxic protein by-products."[8]

Details like these are mostly ignored, and we are urged to eat huge portions of animal protein. Compared to the Chinese in rural China, for instance, Americans consume between 70 and 100 grams of protein a day, most of which is animal protein, while the Chinese average only 7.1 grams of animal protein a day.[9] (Seven grams of animal protein is equal to about three chicken McNuggets. Seventy grams of animal protein is equal to about an eight ounce porterhouse steak.) The high consumption of animal protein has lead the nation down the path to the national health disaster with which it now lives.

How the country arrived at the animal vs. plant protein juncture is worthwhile examining.

Looking to the past we see our ancestors struggling to achieve some sense of comprehension about what food was about in relation to human health. In China, at the beginning of the Han dynasty (202 BCE to 220 CE), Taoism and Confucianism were the dominant belief systems. Confucius (551 BCE - 479 BCE) had handed down basic dietary guidelines such as that food should be clean and not overcooked and he had warned against overeating. The Taoists followed the teachings of the legendary Lao Tse (author of the Tao-Te Ching (The Way)) who is thought to have lived sometime during the 6th and 4th centuries BCE. The Taoists wanted to return to simple egalitarian communities of ancient times where the people "lived in common with birds and beasts, and formed one family with all creatures."[10] They governed themselves according to the universal forces of Yin and Yang (polar opposites as in black and white or high and low) where Yin was the female principle, passive and dark, and Yang was the male principle, active and light. Yin and Yang served as manifestations of Qi (pronounced chee), which the Taoists believed was the cosmic life force in all things. They sought to isolate Yin and Yang principles chemically and in the process developed alchemy and pharmaceutics. In the field of nutrition they developed dietetics.[11] For the Taoists, some foods were Yin, steamed foods, for example, and others were Yang, like grilled foods. Taoists believed that a balance had to be maintained between Yin and Yang foods which would help keep the life force (Qi) in the body in a healthy state and lead to longer life.

Medicine has been concerned with the metabolic processes of food for centuries. Not too long before the Han dynasty was drawing to a close, Galen, who grew up in the ancient Greek city of Pergamum but practiced medicine in Rome, was making his own nutritional observations. He wrote that "our bodies are dissipated by the transpiration that takes place through the pores in our skin that are invisible to us; therefore we need food in a quantity proportionate to the quantity transpired."[12] Galen's doctrines on anatomy and physiology were followed for centuries until Ibn al-Nafis (1210 - 1288), an Arab physician, arrived on the scene. Working in Cairo he made his contributions to anatomy and physiology and discovered pulmonary circulation, though for many years the discovery was credited to William Harvey (1578 - 1657).

Ibn Al-Nafis was a prolific writer who wrote on a wide range of medical subjects as well as religion and made commentaries on the work of Galen, Hippocrates, and other early physicians. He also wrote an extensive medical encyclopedia and a book on nutrition and health in which he placed greater emphasis on the importance of nutrition compared to the use of drugs. Additionally, he wrote about metabolism noting that "both the body and its parts are in a continuous state of dissolution and nourishment so they are inevitably undergoing permanent change."[13],[14],[15]

In 1659 Walter Charleton, who as a young man had been one of the physicians of King Charles I of England, made his contributions to the still fledgling field of nutrition and ultimately to our own ideas about protein by writing a book titled *The Natural History of Nutrition, Life and Voluntary Motion*. To him the first function of nutrition was the "continuous assimilation of equivalent particles from our food" and the second was "to provide fuel (or oil) from the vital flame burning within us, which can be extinguished either by suffocation or want of sustenance."[16]

The man who has been called "the father of Nutrition Science," Antoine Lavoisier (1743 - 1794), was falsely accused of trying to defraud the public by adding water to tobacco products and of committing other crimes. He was guillotined in Paris in the last year of the French Revolution. Lavoisier was also honing in on the processes of metabolism and how the body used energy. He worked on trying to show that the amount of heat to the quantity of carbon dioxide produced by animals was equal to the ratio of heat to carbon dioxide produced by candle flame and reasoned that the heat of living creatures came from the chemical energy of the combustion of their food.[17]

Finally, in 1838 a Dutch physician, Gerrit Mulder (1802 - 1880), wrote to Jakob Berzelius (1779 - 1848), a Swedish chemist [today considered one of the "fathers" of chemistry], that he had analyzed egg albumin, serum albumin, fibrin, and wheat gluten and that they contained a common radical [an atomic grouping].[18] Berzelius replied enthusiastically and suggested the name "protein" be given to the "organic oxide of fibrin and albumin." It was a name derived from the ancient Greek God Proteus who had the power to change into different shapes.[19]

Thus the name "protein" as a designation for the structural material in plant and animal tissue was born. Within a century "protein," particularly animal protein, would acquire nearly Godly status as the most important dietary component necessary for maintaining a healthy body.

Following in Berzelius' footsteps, Justus von Liebig (1803 - 1873), one of the leading chemists of his day [the teacher of Samuel Johnson], embraced the new concept and declared that protein was the only true nutrient capable of forming or replacing tissue and provided the only energy source for muscle contraction. It was therefore "essential for both body building and physical activity."[20] He developed "a method of determining the amount of protein in plant and animal tissue."[21]

Soon, however, Liebig found fault with Mulder's research and turned against it. Mulder staunchly defended his work. The debate about protein was underway. It has continued throughout the 19th and 20th centuries and is still going on today.

Another debate involving protein was also underway. This concerned the ethical question about consuming animal protein. By the start of the 19th century a vegetarian (vegan) movement had begun in Europe and the United States. Like many Greek and Roman philosophers and poets such as Pythagoras (?580 - 500 BCE), Plato (427 - 347 BCE), Ovid (43 BCE - 17 or 18 CE) and later thinkers, artists, and poets like Leonardo da Vinci (1452 - 1519), Margaret Cavendish (1623 - 1673), William Wordsworth (1770 - 1850), and Percy Bysshe Shelley (1792 - 1822), the vegans declared it was morally wrong to kill animals. Jean-Jacques Rousseau (1712 - 1778), who had argued that kindness was more important than knowledge, was an inspiration for the movement.

John Newton (1725-1807), composer of the hymn *Amazing Grace*, was an early vegan who wrote: "man of all races is diseased" because he had "quit the nutriment on which alone Nature had destined him to enjoy a state of perfect health...man was commanded to eat, not fish or meat, but the Fruits of the earth of every sort."[22]

This was a minority viewpoint. Writers and researchers on nutrition judged protein needs in terms of their digestibility and their ability to replace tissue. Morality was not a feature of their inquiry.[23]

By this time the move toward greater animal consumption was gradually growing, and protein was increasingly becoming equated with consuming animal flesh. In England, during the Napoleonic wars, the sentiment was that the higher meat diet of Britain made "one Englishman equivalent to at least two Frenchman."[24]

One of the first persons to begin setting daily standards for protein intake was Dr. Karl Voit, considered by many to be the father of modern dietetics. We first met Voit in chapter 16. He was one of Atwater's teachers. Before becoming a professor of physiology at the University of Munich, Voit had worked in Liebig's laboratory as one of his assistants.

When Voit began his work on protein no means had yet been devised for quantifying the amount of protein the body needed. Voit did not find one either. But he had an imagination and he had thoughts. One was that people with enough money to buy any kind of food they might choose would instinctively select the food that gave them the right amount of protein.[25] Voit observed that laborers consumed about 3100 calories a day and since these were big, hefty fellows, he deduced that people needed 118 grams of protein daily if they were to become big and strong. This was the only research Voit did and it was his method of quantification.

Voit's laborers were the well-muscled men positioned at the crossroads leading to greater protein consumption.

The recommendation for protein intake based on laborers become known as the "Voit standard." It caught on and set the standards for high protein intake that the public followed for decades.[26] Other scientists followed Voit's methodology, but also added soldiers to their calculations. Their recommendations for daily protein intake ranged from 110 grams in France to 146 grams in Italy to 180 grams in Sweden.[27] Thus a sociological rationale provided the foundation for the myth that humans need a huge amount of protein for optimum health.

Besides faulty methodology (the absence of a factual basis for assuming that laborers would instinctively consume the right amount of protein), another problem existed with Voit's standard. In reality, he believed that humans needed only to consume 48.5 grams of protein per day. In keeping with the "cultural biases" of the times, however, in which protein meant meat and more and more people wanted meat, he upped his recommendation to 118 grams.[28]

This is not the first instance where faulty methodologies in research have paved a way that generations of scientists would accept and follow without testing the original hypothesis for themselves. One of the most notorious examples occurred in the 17th century with the work of the French scientist René Descartes (1596 - 1650). It was he who declared "Cogito, ergo sum!" (I think, therefore I am.) Based on a vision he said he had received from the Mother of God, Descartes proclaimed that the entire universe was mechanical.[29] Only humans possessed a soul.

Descartes' vision for how humans should relate to the earth and the universe was an extreme departure from the animistic views of earlier cultures that had held for centuries. Aristotle (384 - 322 BCE), for example, believed that life could be divided into three categories. The first was vegetable which grew by virtue of a vegetable soul, the second was animal which moved by virtue of a sensitive soul, and the third was human which possessed intelligence by virtue of a rational soul.[30] These kinds of views of the relationship of living entities with the world and the universe lasted until Descartes and his generation ushered in his new mechanistic worldview which, until present-day revolts, has generally been followed by science ever since.[31]

In a Descartian world, animals, unlike humans, are not informed by a soul. Therefore, being a part of a mechanical universe, they have no emotions and are just things which scientists are free to use in their research as they desire.

Descartes' followers declared a dog could be kicked and would feel no more pain than a church organ did when a key was depressed. They reasoned that since an organ was a mechanical object which, a priori, could feel no pain, an animal, which was equally a mechanical object, also could feel no pain.[32] Unfortunately, they neglected to test the latter part of their thesis — that an animal could feel no pain. After Descartes, vivisection increased considerably.

Sitting in on Voit's classes was Wilbur Olin Atwater, who, as referred to previously, would become the first head of a government nutrition laboratory in the United States, the USDA Office of Experiment Stations. Atwater took Voit's protein standards back with him to the United States and in 1902 raised Voit's protein recommendation for daily consumption from 118 grams to 125.[33] This became the standard for almost 40 years until Franklin D. Roosevelt's National Research Council cut the Recommended Daily Allowance (RDA) for protein down to 70 grams for men and 60 grams for women.[34] Today it has been set at 56 grams for men and 44 grams for women by the National Academy of Sciences.

As discussed above, the average amount of protein consumed daily by Americans is somewhere between 70 and 100 grams.

This is way over any possible human requirements since, as we have seen, the body only needs a small amount of protein every day for maintenance. In rural China the people consume 7.1 grams of animal protein daily and have no health problems associated with protein intake. Since 1974 the World Health Organization has recommended a diet with 5% of protein from calories which calculates to 37.5 grams of protein for a man burning 3000 calories [3000 x .05 = 150/4 (1 gram of protein = 4 calories) = 37.5]. It comes to 29 grams for a woman burning 2300 calories.[35] And, as should be apparent, official dietary recommendations like these need to be set higher than necessary in order to accommodate people who naturally fall outside the average range. This means that the 37.5 and 29 grams standard for men and women set by the WHO might be higher than necessary.

Another American pupil who had studied German physiology was Samuel Johnson. As noted earlier, he had studied in Liebig's laboratory in Munich and was instrumental in founding the Sheffield Scientific School at Yale University where Atwater studied[36] Yale was also the place where Russell Henry Chittenden went to study. The world was not ready for the discoveries this scientist would make or it might have turned back from the road toward greater protein consumption down which it had rushed with such reckless abandon.

Chittenden did put Voit's hypothesis to a test to see if it was correct. He explained his reasons.

We are all creatures of habit, and our palates are pleasantly excited by the rich animal foods with their high content of proteid [sic], and we may well question whether our dietetic habits are not based more upon the dictates of our palates than upon scientific reasoning or true physiological needs.[37]

According to Chittenden, too much protein could only have a negative physiological effect.

> With proteid (protein) foods...when oxidized, (they) yield a row of crystalline nitrogenous products which ultimately pass out of the body through the kidneys. (These nitrogen-based protein by-products) — frequently spoken of as toxins — float about through the body and may exercise more or less of a deleterious influence upon the system, or, being temporarily deposited, may exert some specific or local influence that calls for their speedy removal.[38]

For nine months Chittenden lived on a diet consuming 40 grams of protein a day, one-third of Voit's recommendation.[39] At the end of that period he described his health as being with "greater freedom from fatigue and muscular soreness than in previous years of a fuller dietary." The arthritis in the knee as well as headaches and abdominal pains with which he had suffered all his life disappeared.

Chittenden next conducted three trials lasting six months on three different groups to confirm the results of his experiment upon himself. This included a sedentary group from Yale University, eight Yale Athletes, and volunteers from the U.S. Army Hospital Corps. All groups remained healthy during the trial and the athletic group improved its performance by 35%.[40] The evidence showed Chittenden that Voit's and Atwater's protein recommendations could not be correct.

In 1904, two years after W.O. Atwater upped Voit's protein recommendations from 118 to 125 grams daily, Chittenden revealed the final results of his studies. They showed that only 30 to 50 grams of protein daily were necessary for adults to maintain good health.

Today Chittenden is often called the "father of American

biochemistry." His home in New Haven, Connecticut is a National Historic Landmark. But the world to date has paid little attention to his trial studies on protein. Ironically, the highest range for protein intake in his well-planned scientific experiments (50 grams) was close to Voit's original hypothesis. (Remember, Voit really believed that people needed only 48.5 grams of protein daily.) Voit's subjective raising of his protein standards from 48.5 grams to 118 grams carried on by Atwater at 125 grams has had the unfortunate consequence of leading the Western World down a merry trail that has been very good for the meat and dairy industries, but not very good for the health of people living in Western societies.

The promotion of a high protein content diet coincided with a steady increasing rise of meat eating in the 20th century. Prior to this time nations around the world were still not consuming that much meat. Several factors came together to motivate the meat increase in America besides the high protein standards set by scientists like Voit, Atwater and a few European scientists following Voit's lead. For one, increased prosperity brought on by the industrial revolution and improving transportation and refrigeration techniques made it easier to mass transport livestock products and helped create a market for meat. As Dean Ornish reports:

> Until this century [20th], the typical American diet was low in animal products, fat, cholesterol, salt, and sugar, and high in carbohydrates, vegetables, and fiber.... Early in this century [20th], with the advent of refrigerators, freezers, good transportation, mechanized agriculture, and a prosperous economy, the American diet and lifestyle began to change radically.[41]

Nutritional factors were also responsible. In 1914 Lafayette Mendel and Thomas Osborne, two biochemists, conducted studies on the protein and amino acid requirements of rats which showed that rats grew better on animal protein than on vegetable protein. This led to the suspicion that vegetable foods could not meet normal growth requirements because they contained insufficient amounts of amino acids.[42] This and other animal-based experiments brought a classification system into existence in which meat, eggs, and dairy foods were classified as superior "Class A" proteins, and vegetables were classified as inferior "Class B" proteins.[43]

In 1940, Dr. William Rose of the University of Illinois showed that the removal of any one of the essential amino acids from the food of growing rats led to a rapid decline in weight, loss of appetite, and death. But when the rats were fed with meat, poultry, milk, and eggs they were healthy and energetic. That experiment led to broad assumptions that a diet low in animal protein intake was unhealthy. As a result of these kinds of studies, the amino acid pattern in animal products was "declared to be the gold standard."[44] This kind of information made its way out into the world and created a general fear with the public about not getting enough animal protein in the diet.

The research that followed, however, showed that it was a mistake to compare rats to human beings because infant rats mature much faster than humans and therefore need much more protein than human babies which mature more slowly. For this reason rat breast milk contains ten times more protein that human breast milk.[45] Armed with this information, Dr. Rose reevaluated his work and conducted further experiments on humans which determined that they needed only eight of the amino acids required by rats. He further discovered that the highest requirements for human protein needs were easily met with any starchy vegetable. Rose published the results of this research in sixteen papers in the Journal of Biological Chemistry in the spring of 1952.[46] His work reveals that the "incomplete protein" classification automatically assigned to non-animal protein is a myth.

Dr. John McDougall sets the record straight about this myth as follows:

> Fortunately, scientific studies have debunked this compli-
> cated nonsense. Nature designed and synthesized our
> foods complete with all the essential nutrients for human
> life long before they reach the dinner table. All the
> essential and nonessential amino acids are represented in
> *single unrefined starches* such as rice, corn, wheat, and
> potatoes in amounts in excess of every individual's needs,
> even if they are endurance athletes or weight lifters.
> Common sense tells you this would have to be true for the
> human race to have survived on this planet. Throughout
> history the food-providers went out in search of enough
> rice or potatoes to feed their families. Matching beans
> with rice was not their concern. We have only the hunger
> to relate to food; there is no drive to tell us to mix and
> match protein sources to make a more ideal amino acid
> pattern. There is no need for such a drive because there is
> no more ideal protein and amino acid composition than
> that found in natural starches. [emphasis in original][47]

This says it all. It is not necessary to combine plant-based proteins in order to try to match the amino acid compounds of animal-based food.[48] The myth keeps getting reinforced, unfortunately, by accounts such as a 2001 American Heart Association report on the Atkins, Zone, and Sugar Busters diets. This report contained the statement that: "although plant proteins form a large part of the human diet, most are deficient in 1 or more essential amino acids and are therefore regarded as incomplete proteins."[49]

Stories like this can hardly be viewed as other than an attempt to disparage plant-based protein products and promote animal-based protein foods. The AHA could scarcely have failed to recognize that this kind of information misleads the public as indicated by the following account.

Dr. John McDougall strongly objected to the AHA report and voiced his objections in correspondence to the AHA in which he referred to the Rose studies cited above and pointed out that:

A careful look at the founding scientific research and some simple math prove it is impossible to design an amino acid-deficient diet based on the amounts of unprocessed starches and vegetables sufficient to meet the calorie needs of humans…A vegetarian diet based on any single one or combination of these unprocessed starches (eg. rice, corn, potatoes, beans), with the addition of vegetables and fruits, supplies all the protein, amino acids, essential fats, minerals, and vitamins (with the exception of vitamin B12) necessary for excellent health. To wrongly suggest that people need to eat animal protein for nutrients will encourage them to add foods that are known to contribute to heart disease, diabetes, obesity, and many forms of cancer, to name just a few common problems.[50] [Note: Vitamin B12 is not found in plant-based foods and needs to be obtained through supplements or other non-animal sources.]

The AHA was forced to back down. In a reply to Dr. McDougall, Barbara V. Howard, Ph.D, of the MedStar Research Institute wrote that "we do not suggest that people need to eat animal protein exclusively for nutrients." While trying to make a case that "it is difficult [for a non-animal-based diet] to maintain essential amino acids at optimum quantity and distribution," without providing any examples why, Dr. Howard acknowledged that:

"We certainly agree with Dr McDougall that a vegetarian diet based on the AHA guidelines of 5 to 6 servings of whole grains and 5 or more servings of vegetables and fruit would, in fact, supply all of the amino acids necessary for health."[51]

With this face-saving statement ["a vegetarian diet based on the AHA guidelines..."], Howard admitted that Dr. McDougall was right. The idea that animal protein is required for optimal health is a myth and simply untrue.

Once started, a myth is hard to live down, and sometimes it even gets repeated unintentionally by those holding the alternative point of view. For example, Francis Moore Lappé's *Diet for a Small Planet*, which she published in 1971, was a phenomenal success that benefited millions of people but at the same time perpetuated the myth that plants needed to be combined to provide all the essential amino acids the body requires.[52] Ms. Lappé, realizing her mistake, did her best to correct the record in the 1982 10th Anniversary Edition of the book in which she wrote:

In 1971 I stressed protein complementarity because I assumed that the only way to get enough protein...was to create a protein as usable by the body as animal protein. In combating the myth that meat is the only way to get high-quality protein, I reinforced another myth. I gave the impression that in order to get enough protein without meat, considerable care was needed in choosing foods. Actually, it is much easier than I thought. With three important exceptions, there is little danger of protein deficiency in a plant food diet. The exceptions are diets very heavily dependent on fruit or on some tubers, such as sweet potatoes or cassava, or on junk food (refined flours, sugars, and fat). Fortunately, relatively few people in the world try to survive on diets in which these foods are virtually the sole source of calories. *In all other diets, if people are getting enough calories, they are virtually certain of getting enough* protein. [Emphasis in original][53]

In light of their agreement about what they perceive today's nutrition needs to be, our government healthcare agencies and nonprofit healthcare organizations continue to cling to animal protein as a staple of their diet recommendations. Over the years, fortunately, as differing facts about the dangers of animal protein consumption have emerged, these organizations have all downgraded their guidelines from recommending a high animal-based protein diet to suggestions to limit the consumption of red meat and processed meats, as we have observed. In regard to dairy foods, they now recommend switching from regular dairy products to low-fat or nonfat dairy products. These recommendations are a vast improvement, but our healthcare organizations are still unwilling to completely give up their addiction to animal protein.

The tales about the supposed dangers of not consuming enough animal protein are difficult to shake. That is unfortunate because the opposite is true. "Increasing scientific evidence links diets high in animal fat not only with obesity but also with coronary heart disease, stroke, breast cancer in women, prostate cancer in men, colon cancer, osteoporosis, diabetes, hypertension, [and] gallbladder disease."[54] It has also been reported that eating too much protein can damage the liver and kidneys by causing them to work too hard to convert the protein into urea and then filter it from the blood.[55] Dairy foods, as we have seen, are also suspects as a cause of excessive urinary excretion of calcium leading to osteoporosis.

In its general dietary guidelines for cancer prevention the American Cancer Society refers to meat as "high-quality protein."[56] Many other healthcare organizations and medical professionals do the same. But T. Colin Campbell says that the "concept of quality" in regard to protein really refers to the "efficiency with which food proteins are used to promote growth."[57] This efficiency, of course, is severely jeopardized if the product to which it refers, animal protein, promotes cancer, heart disease, and other debilitating conditions. That is not "efficiency." It is "inefficiency." If all apples were rotten they would no longer be thought of as promoting the kind of good health that "keeps the doctor away." It is only logical, then, that meat, which has been shown conclusively to be a source of disease, should not be referred to as a source of "high-quality protein." Let us call it what it is, "a source of disease." To continue to refer to meat as high quality protein is to just mindlessly repeat a convention that has become fixed in the public's mind.

Long ago the country made a choice for a high protein animal-based diet. The information justifying the diet was supplied by some well-intentioned but mistaken scientists who were just novices themselves in the budding field of nutrition. It has turned out to be a long, hard journey. Will we continue to live with a myth that has controlled the dietary habits of Americans for generations bringing with it significant disease, illness, and death? Or will we turn back to that fork in the road at which we arrived more than a century ago and now take the path not yet trodden? This is the trail calling for a plant-based diet which proponents insist leads to greater health and longer life. And they have the evidence to back up their claim.

Part II

The Revenge of Nature

The Consequences of a Meat and Dairy-Based Diet

Chapter 18

How Humans Fashioned Societies Founded on the Exploitation of Animals

In the long march from the stone age to civilization humans moved from a life style of hunting and gathering to one of domesticating plants and animals for their personal use. This meant herding animals together. But for the animals this was not a cooperative venture in which they willingly complied. In order to bend animals to their will, humans had to use cunning and deception while resorting to some of their most brutal capabilities. To avoid overpopulation of their herds, for example, the herders would have needed to sterilize some of the male animals. As Charles Patterson describes in his illuminating book *Eternal Treblinka: Our Treatment of Animals and the Holocaust*, the herders would likely have accomplished this in the same way some herders in various parts of the world are still doing it today, by holding the animals down and either cutting out or crushing their testicles.[1] Other means by which herders have controlled captive animals are whips, chains, collars, and branding to show individual ownership.

The domestication of animals and plants changed the relationship to the world to which people had become accustomed over the centuries. Taking a clue from the worldview of the ancient Greeks, it is possible to conceive how early humans may have grown up regarding everything that lived, including the rocks, the trees, the grass, the rivers, the lakes, the hills, and the mountains, as being participants in a living cosmos in which plants, animals, and all living creatures possessed intelligence and interacted as soul possessing entities.[2] After domestication, the partnership with animals and nature would have gradually faded into memories of a long gone era that would have become increasingly difficult to recover. Herding brought a change in the status of animals from one of respect and equality to one in which they were ruthlessly subjected to the selfish interests of the herders.

As noted by Mr. Patterson, Sigmund Freud wrote that:

> ...in the course of his development toward culture man acquired a dominating position over his fellow-creatures in the animal kingdom. Not content with his supremacy, however, he began to place a gulf between his nature and theirs. He denied the possession of reason to them, and to himself he attributed an immortal soul, and made claims to a divine descent which permitted him to annihilate the bond of community between him and the animal kingdom.[3]

During the hunting and gathering era, before herding became a fixture of life, warfare was rare. Societies had little interest in controlling land spaces, did not own much property, and were not strongly organized by means of a centralized leadership.[4] Because they had little stored food they could not wage wars at any great distance. The wars that did occur were usually family feuds or revenge raids for some alleged witchcraft plot. It was not until societies began to live in fixed geographical locations that they began to develop more skilled military methods. Then tribal battles for stealing a neighboring tribe's wealth in combination with population growth evolved into ever larger and more complex wars. The techniques early humans were acquiring in domesticating animals were also employed in waging these wars: shackles, chains, castration of males, separation of females from males, whipping, branding, confinement, and killing.

Before tribes settled down to a more sedentary life, slavery seldom occurred, but when it did, it usually was an offshoot of tribal warfare.[7] The organized enslavement of animals, also known as herding, connected directly to the enslavement of human beings. The follow-up, war, was a logical consequence, for it is not likely that one group of human beings is going to sit idly by while another group subjugates and enslaves it. Unlike animals, humans have the capacity to organize wars of retaliation and the desire to seek revenge.

Just as Freud described, enslaving animals destroyed the sense of kinship early humans felt toward their four-legged, fellow earth travelers, opening the door to redefining the status of other species in the new world over which humans were gradually taking ownership. Once these species were fully consigned to an inferior rank as mere beasts suitable only for the purpose of meeting human needs, it takes little imagination to envision our ancestors corralling and clubbing an animal to death whenever they needed it in some way for their personal use, such as for clothing and food. This process could also be applied to neighboring tribes in waging wars.

The core ingredient in the process of one human group conquering another is that of dehumanization. This is accomplished when the group that wants to wage war transforms the image of the group it wants to conquer to the image of nonhuman animals or beasts of some kind. As Patterson describes it, the ideal is to select animals that are particularly repugnant to the tribe preparing for warfare. It then becomes easy to rationalize using the most appalling and barbaric kinds of actions in conquering the neighboring tribe.[5] This has been the pattern of conquest throughout human history and it still continues today. The conquerors mentally demonize their enemies, turning them into animals, insects, or wild beasts, describing them as monkeys, gorillas, swine, whining curs, mad dogs, and termites.[6] Once the enemies have been relegated to less than human status, they can be humiliated, raped, tortured, shot, blown up, and murdered. For example, Hutu leaders described Tutsis as cockroaches and snakes during the 1994 Rwanda massacres.

Thus the abuse and use of animals for clothing and food was one of the primary factors that started human beings down the long road to war that they have travelled the last 10,000 years and still travel today with little letup.

The Greek philosopher Socrates (470 - 399 BCE) also saw the consumption of animals as being one of the central factors leading to war when he said, "if we pursue our habit of eating animals and if our neighbor follows a similar path, will we not have need to go to war against our neighbor to secure greater pasturage, because ours will not be enough to sustain us, and our neighbor will have a similar need to wage war on us for the same reason?"[8] Was Socrates being clairvoyant or stating an axiom? More than 2500 years later the consumption of animals and the increasing need for enough land space to cultivate grain to feed the animals that are needed for a growing population of meat eaters has become a major cause of global concern, as will be discussed in chapter 24, and could lead to strife between nations and even to war in the coming decades.

The mechanistic universe proclaimed by Descartes in the 17th century, after which animals were increasingly regarded as mere things with which humans could do anything they pleased, hastened the process of the human attempt to exert dominion over all species on the earth and led inexorably to university research laboratories, factory farms, fur farms, circus cruelty, zoos, and other abuses of animals.

These manifestations of human cruelty are symptoms of the attempt by human beings to set themselves apart from the rest of life and proclaim their ownership of the earth. But it is marked by a failure to recognize the interconnectedness of all forms of life, the cooperation with which is required to maintain the balance on the planet necessary for it to thrive successfully.

The human journey has brought us to a place where we now stand surrounded by the cruelty upon which we have learned to depend as a means for survival. This has created a problem that is so tremendous in its proportions that it threatens the future existence of society as we know it. There is a way out. First it is necessary to recognize that the problem does exist. Then the forces of compassion that reside within every person need to be unleashed. This is the only force that can subjugate the cruelty upon which human beings have become so dependent as a way of life.

Today, though we seldom stop to think about it, rendering plants process 40 billion pounds of dead animals a year which humans use in some way for their personal benefit.[9] The dead animals are collected from places like animal research laboratories, animal shelters, factory farms, and animal control agencies, or are scraped from roads (roadkill). They are then converted into by-products that manufacturers use in just about everything, including handcreams, hairsprays, lotions, lipsticks, nail polish, ointments, shampoos, shaving creams, soaps, deodorants, mouthwashes, and toothpastes. People are literally washing their clothing, cleaning their homes, bathing themselves, and brushing their teeth in dead animals unless they take care to buy soap brands and cleaning and hygienic products made without animal by-products. Animal by-products are also used in the manufacture of plastics and automobile tires that transport people from place to place, and in pet foods and cattle feed that is fed to livestock which humans eat.[10] These by-products are even used in the manufacture of film for making moving pictures so that the pleasure of watching a movie may in part be derived from the by-products of animals that may have been experimented upon in animal research laboratories.

[Some of the code words for animal by-products printed on the labels of the commodities listed above are Bitartrate, Caprylic Acid, Choline, Glycerin, Glycerol, Lecithin, Oleic Acid,

Palmitic Acid, Stearic Acid, Tallow, and various derivatives such as Tallowate. (There are some exceptions in regard to Tallow, like Japan Tallow and Vegetable Tallow, and also in regard to some forms of Glycerin.)]

Considering the lowly status to which most societies have relegated animals, it is small wonder that the Canadian government permits furriers to club 350,000 defenseless seals and their babies to death on the ice fields of Canada's east coast every year, skinning many of them while they are still alive and leaving thousands of half-dead seals and seal corpses to rot on the ice or in the water next to the icy shores — just for their pelts.

And we ask ourselves how people could be so ghastly cruel and sadistic. Whether this is deeply ingrained in our DNA or is more of a learned trait handed down over the last ten thousand years is a worthy question to ponder.

Fortunately, the scientific evidence increasingly suggests that humans do not come into the world as amoral creatures but are born with "a rudimentary moral sense from the very start of life." [9] This should be apparent from observing that, as shown by the scientific evidence, even our closest nonhuman relatives, chimpanzees, have a well-developed sense of compassion. (They are also capable of killing stranger chimps which they perceive to be a threat.) It is not unreasonable, then, to conjecture that some kind of opposition to the brutalization of animals based on compassion was present ten thousand years ago when early humans first began capturing and herding animals into enclosures. Some of our ancestors must have been horrified to witness their friends, neighbors, and family members brutalizing animals just as people are horrified when they witness it today.

For a few concrete examples of ancestral expressions of compassion for animals we can turn to the words of ancients like Pythagoras, Plato, Empedocles, Socrates, Ovid, Plutarch, and more recent relatives like Thomas Paine, Robert Browning, Thomas Edison, Eleanor Roosevelt, Albert Einstein, and Rachel Carson. (For a list of a few other historic notables who believed that compassion should extend to all animals see chapter 20, footnote 24.)

No matter how sadistically humans have expressed themselves in the struggle to survive, a compassionate side has also stood resolutely by to challenge that cruelty. It was present in the rise of the vegetarian movement that began in Europe in the early 19th century, and it is visible today in the rapid spread of the animal rights movement demanding fundamental change in the way society treats animals.

It can hardly be denied that the number of people in the world concerned about the welfare of nonhuman species is increasing. The question that is on many people's mind is whether the forces of compassion can increase enough exponentially to compel the herders to stop their cruelty in the near future or whether it will take more time. More time, unfortunately, means more suffering. But people armed with facts, truth, and the will to demand change can make a difference. After 40 years of fighting the Canadian government, opponents of the seal hunts have recently got the European Union to ban all seal hunt products, closing seven out of ten of Canada's main export seal markets. For the first time in Canada's history, a Canadian official, Senator Harb, has proposed a bill to ban the seal hunts.

Even the United States Senate passed a resolution to put an end to Canada's seal trade. It was sponsored by Carl Levin [Democrat-Michigan] and Susan Collins [Republican-Maine] and noted that one million seals have been killed during the past five years with 95% of them being pups between the ages of 12 days and 12 weeks old.

Carl Levin said: "Canada needs to understand that the rest of the world will not stand by and allow this slaughter to continue.

Ten countries have now either banned trade in seal products or have indicated their intentions to do so and the European Union has just enacted a prohibition on seal product trade." Susan Collins expressed similar concerns. "International opinion, as well as the opinion of the vast majority of Canadian citizens, is overwhelmingly in favor of ending the Canadian seal kill. We strongly encourage the government of Canada to bring atrocities to an end."[10]

But even with pressure like this as well as from its own citizens and from around the world, the Canadian government will not close this brutal chapter in the country's history and is even talking about subsidizing the industry to make up for the lost revenue caused by opposition to the seal hunts. This is not so surprising considering that governments are composed of people, and people frequently will do almost anything to avoid admitting they are wrong.

In the meantime, America has its own problems with slaughtering innocent animals. It is long overdue for Senator Collins, Senator Levin and other congressmen and congresswomen to sponsor not only a resolution but legislation to ban America's brutal factory farms and animal research laboratories and to begin admitting that an enormous cruelty dilemma also confronts America. While food industrialists and animal researchers do their best to hide it away, the cruelty at their facilities is undeniably present in all its manifest brutality, as we shall see in the coming chapters. And it goes on around the clock every day of the year, minute by minute, hour by hour.

We are now at the dawn of a new era at the beginning of a new century, and we are turning down new corridors of time. More and more people are waking to the realization that animals deserve the same kinds of rights that humans beings have accorded to themselves, the right not to be abused, disrespected, treated cruelly, and killed against their will. These people are the abolitionists of the 21st century who trace their roots all the way back to those early ancestors who surely stood up to oppose the captive abuse of animals even then.

As people who believe in the dignity of life for all living creatures, today's emissaries of the future reject the enslavement of animals their progenitors began some ten thousand years ago that continues in these times in animal research laboratories, on factory farms, on fur farms, and in circuses and zoos. They are fully conscious of the evidence showing that nature has not stood idly by watching humankind mistreat earth's creatures so terribly. There are consequences for wrong doing, and our societies are being paid back for their exploitation of animals in the form of cancer, heart disease, heart attacks, strokes, diabetes, and many other diseases. But it doesn't stop there. The human reliance on animals has escalated so significantly that the recompense now endangers the air we breathe and the water we drink and is responsible for the increase of poverty in the developing world. It is not an exaggeration to say that it threatens the survival of the human species and the earth, a premise that will become clearer as we examine some of these problems in chapter 24.

Meanwhile, our modern day herders corral today's animals on factory farms, in animal research laboratories, on fur farms, and in circuses and zoos where they continue to exploit them for their own ends. Unfortunately, those ends are enriching the few at the expense of the many and portend a devastating conclusion unless we start making dramatic changes in the way we treat animals.

Chapter 19

Descent Into Hell

The Cruelty on Factory Farms

The correlation of tobacco to cancer was first reported by Dr. Franz Muller, a scientist living in Cologne, Germany, in a 1939 epidemiological study published in the Journal of the American Medical Association.[1] Though it offered convincing proof of the link between tobacco and cancer, it would take another 25 years before the United States healthcare community began to accept the idea that tobacco really did cause lung cancer. As previously noted, at that point the American Cancer Society, following up on a report by the Royal College of Physicians in England, stepped forward to join the fight. (See chapter 4.) The Surgeon General's Office was not too far behind and issued its own report in 1964.

The parallel between Franz Muller's epidemiological discovery linking tobacco with lung cancer with T. Colin Campbell's epidemiological study showing that the consumption of animal protein is linked to cancer, heart disease, stroke, diabetes and other chronic diseases is unmistakable. The question that remains to be answered is how many years it will take for the American Cancer Society, the Surgeon General's office, and other organizations within the healthcare system such as the National Cancer Institute and the American Heart Association to step forward and announce that animal protein is the major cause of these diseases.

In the fight-back against tobacco, citizens' groups often waged anti-tobacco campaigns and were successful in forcing airlines to ban smoking on airplanes, getting the FDA to put labels on birth control pills warning women of the higher risk of cancer for smokers taking the pill, and prompting the Federal Trade Commission to put stricter warnings on cigarette packs.[2] Surely, it will take similar and even greater pressure to get the Federal Trade Commission to put labels on all meat and dairy products that read: "Warning: The consumption of this product may lead to cancer, heart disease, stroke, diabetes, and other chronic diseases!"

Once exposed, the tobacco industry battled back and has managed to survive and even increase its reach across the globe. The world can expect a similar fight from the meat and dairy industries if ever some respected body of health experts musters the courage to declare the facts about meat and dairy products.

No doubt remains today that many of the foods that cause human beings so much sickness and premature death are produced by the meat and dairy industries. The right arm of these industries is the factory farm that generates their products. These farms are places of enormous suffering and cruelty to animals. And though it is not a subject people are eager to talk about, it can hardly be denied that human beings who consume meat and dairy foods manufactured on factory farms share in the responsibility for the suffering it takes to produce their food.

Factory farms are notoriously cruel to animals as has been well documented thanks to whistleblowers and courageous undercover operators from animal rights organizations. The meat and dairy industries deny it, as would be expected, but it is hard to cover up undercover videos like the Humane Society of the United States (HSUS) filmed in January of 2008.

This footage showed farm workers in Southern California committing criminal acts against downed cows that were sick or had been injured while being transported for slaughter. These and other undercover videos showed workers ramming cows that were too weak to walk with the blades of a bulldozer, kicking and beating the cows to make them stand, jabbing the cows in the eyes, dragging the cows with chains, and shocking cows that had been lying in cow feces all day with electric prods to force them into the slaughter box. One video showed a man in a bulldozer riding over the face and leg of a downed cow causing it to bellow out in agony.

The Humane Society recorded undercover videos of "downed cow" abuse in the year 2008 in Maryland, New Mexico, Pennsylvania, and Texas. The inference that the entire factory farm industry is involved in systemic and widespread abuse of downed cows can hardly be avoided.[3]

In 2008 another video surfaced of a pig farm in Iowa that supplies ham to A. Hormel & Co., where one worker slammed little piglets from over his head, bashing them down on the concrete floor, and then threw them on a heap of other dying, mortally wounded piglets all writhing in a bloodied mass of cruelty and pain. A supervisor on the farm shoved a cane up a sow's vagina while workers beat other pigs with metal gate rods and jabbed clothes pins into their eyes. Another supervisor kicked a pig in the genitals and face and said: "You gotta beat on the bitch. Make her cry."[4]

Hardly had that story faded from view than another story appeared in the *New York Times* that read:

An animal rights group on Tuesday released undercover videotapes taken at the nation's premier poultry-breeding operation [The Aviagen Turkeys plant in Lewisburg, West Virginia]...The scenes show stomach-turning brutality. Workers are seen smashing birds into loading cages like basketballs, stomping heads and breaking necks, apparently for fun, even pretending to rape one... After seeing the video Tuesday, company representatives said they 'condemn the abuse of any of the animals in our care and will take swift action to address these issues.' They promised an investigation that could lead to the employees being fired.[5]

Whenever incidents like these occur, company spokespersons step forward to quell the storm of protest that erupts and to assure a queasy public that the incidents are just a momentary aberration. Fines are levied, and the public vaguely assumes that someone will get punished in some way, maybe even get suspended or fired.

Once the customary slap on the wrist has been administered, the public is pacified, assured that the steady supply of burgers, steaks, chicken wings, and pork chops will continue without any further unpleasantness, with plenty of fresh milk for the kids, low-fat yogurt and cottage cheese for the diet-minded, pizzas with cheese, ham, pepperoni or sausage for quick lunches, and frozen dinners of meatloaf at dinnertime for the harried and stressed. Everyone is at peace again.

Meanwhile, the cruelty and the carnage in the slaughter-houses continues. The public relations lies put out by the meat and dairy industries to placate a dozing public that would rather not know, fools no one except those who want to be fooled. Eventually, another incident of unspeakable brutality will be exposed, and once again the unpleasantness will be forced into the public's consciousness.

The cycle goes on. But it becomes more and more difficult for the public to hide from the awareness of what is taking place. A sense of shame already hovers over many of the more sensitive consumers of animal protein who have become aware of the cruelty that puts the food on their dinner plates. This applies especially to people of faith and others who have at their core a philosophy based on compassion. Some religious people are even beginning to organize into groups and are posting discussion websites to debate the ethics of abusing and eating animals and the effects this has on human character and the claims for leading a religious life.[6] (See, for example, www.all-creatures.org.)

The meat and diary industries have laid a feast before the American public to feed upon. But the feast has as its foundation the cruelty and abuse of animals. Many farm animals are kept in crates or stalls that are barely larger than the animals themselves. The animals are unable to turn around their entire lives. Such is the fate of sows forced to live in gestation crates where they are artificially inseminated three times a year. The floors of the crates are slotted so that urine and feces can fall through to a floor below. The stench is unbearably intense and the sows live with it 24 hours a day for their entire lives. Confining pigs in this manner means that many pigs can be assembled together in a smaller area with less time spent caring for and feeding each pig. This results in greater profits for the farmers.

When the mother pigs are ready to deliver their litters they are put in farrowing crates where they also cannot turn around. The farrowing crates are accompanied by a smaller crate that separates the piglets from their mother. Piglets gain access to their mothers' teats separated by perpendicular bars spaced every few inches apart along the length of the crate which prevents the babies from snuggling against their mothers. Keeping the mothers immobile in a reduced space is more profitable and exercises more control over the baby piglets suckling their mothers. The mothers are only allowed to nurse their babies for two or three weeks before the piglets are taken away, causing the sows and the piglets immense emotional suffering. The obvious cruelty of this practice is not a factor for consideration.

The practice of using gestation and veal crates is so loathsome that Arizona, California, Colorado, Florida, Oregon, and Maine have barred them, and an initiative to get rid of them is gaining ground in New York State. It takes bitter court battles accompanied by massive public pressure, voter initiatives, and enormous financial resources to ban the crates during which the farm industry complains on behalf of the farmers that their profits will drop precipitously and they will be reduced to poverty if gestation and veal crates are outlawed. This is nonsense, of course, and results from the old but common habit of divorcing ethics from profit.

Gestation and farrowing crates represent only a portion of the suffering factory farms have in store for pigs. At Belcross Farm in North Carolina, for example, a pig was videotaped having her leg sawed off and her skin peeled away while she was still fully conscious.[7]

It is common practice throughout the industry to engineer pigs genetically to make them grow faster and bigger than normal, which means more money for the farms. But the pigs are not anatomically strong enough to support the additional weight so that they have difficulty walking and often break their legs when they try to stand. If the pigs then are too injured to survive the journey to the slaughterhouse, workers often beat and kick them out of the way, or let them just lie where they fall and die in misery. At Seaboard Farms in Guymon, Oklahoma, dying pigs were left on freezing cement slabs for days.[8]

Pigs badly injured but not hurt enough to be spared from further torment by death are crammed so tightly with other pigs into transport trucks that they can hardly move. There without relief for their suffering they are hauled to the slaughterhouse.

Pigs are sent to slaughter after living only a few months. Left to live out their lives, they could have lived to the age of 15 years or more.

In the wintertime the skin of some pigs squashed against the walls of the transport trucks freezes against the sides. When the trucks arrive at the slaughterhouses there is no time to attend to pigs individually and workers pull the pigs harshly from the trucks, sometimes ripping their skin away from their bodies. Inside the slaughterhouse several men corral each terrified, screaming pig into a corner while a worker either slaps a tong like electrical apparatus onto its head that stuns it, or shoots it in the head with a stun gun. Either way, the device emits a bolt that is supposed to render the pigs unconscious. They are then hoisted by a hind leg chained onto a conveyor belt that transports them down a line where a man waits to stick a knife into the throat of each pig that passes by in order to kill it. But many of the pigs are still conscious, screaming and struggling upside down as they see the man sticking a knife into the throat of other pigs getting ever closer. Like the stun gun, this method is also inefficient. Sometimes the man with the knife misses because his aim is off target. At other times he misses because the pigs are struggling which causes him to miss. The pigs not killed by this method are transported still struggling to tanks of scalding water into which they are dunked screaming and still alive. There, their hell finally ends.[9]

(The tanks of scalding water serve the purpose of removing the hair from the pigs' skin.)

Researchers at Purdue University found that pigs are among the most intelligent of all animal species. Other research shows that they lead complex social lives in the same manner as primates. Pigs have a sense of direction, learn from one another, dream, and the mothers sing to their babies when they nurse.

The same basic fate is in store for cows unfortunate enough to be born and raised for slaughter for meat or for milk production. Those not born on feedlots or on large dairy farms are transported to one once they are fully grown, often without sufficient food or water during the transport from which they emerge covered in feces.[10]

[A feedlot is an enormous patchwork of holding pens containing from 100 to 1,000 cows in each pen. The feedlot in Grand View, Idaho spans 750 acres and has the capacity to hold 150,000 cows.[11] (750 acres = approximately1.2 square miles.)]

The food industrialists say to themselves, why incur the cost of feeding and giving water to animals that are just going to be killed eventually anyway, especially when regulations permit cows to be transported without food or water for 52 hours.[12] It is the bottom line at work again. Profit divorced from ethics. The same applies to transport trucks that do not have cooling or heating equipment to ease summer and winter distress for the animals they transport. Why spend the money to make cows more comfortable whose destiny is just to be slaughtered?

Cows, like all animals, are innocents and cannot comprehend the suffering they are forced to endure at the hands of humans. Sudden starts and stops during transport often causes cows to fall in the trucks, injuring themselves. Many of these cows cannot then physically lift themselves up and they become "downed cows" like those described at the beginning of this chapter.

Often cows are auctioned off and transported several times during their lives. They are then subject to extremely painful branding with hot irons and "waddling," an agonizing identification procedure that entails cutting out huge hunks of the skin that hangs under a cow's neck.[13]

At the feedlots beef cattle destined for slaughter are given growth hormones and fed enormous amounts of grain to increase their body weight and fat content (marbling). The process is referred to as a confined animal feeding operation (CAFO). At the CAFOs the cows live in a filthy manure filled environment in which the air is thick with bacteria and particulate matter that can cause respiratory problems.[14,15]

Dairy cows have their own special destiny in store.[16] In the United States millions of these cows are confined in huge barns on feces-caked mud lots. They are artificially inseminated yearly and they are also pumped full of bovine growth hormone that causes a painful udder condition called mastitis. This applies to 30 to 50 percent of all dairy cows, according to the industry's own figures. Milked by milking machines that tear at their

udders, cows are forced through genetic manipulation, antibiotics, and hormones to produce 50 pounds of milk a day. (Under
natural conditions they produce 16 pounds of milk a day.)
According to Samuel Epstein, bovine growth hormone has been
implicated as a cause of breast cancer, colon cancer, and prostate
cancer.[17]

The cows' newborn calves are taken from them generally the
day after their birth, causing the mothers tremendous suffering.
They bellow and bellow in mourning for their babies often long
after they have been separated. The new born calves are raised
to repeat the fate of their mothers, if they are females, or led to
tiny veal crates where they are caged, if they are males. The
crates are dark inside and so small that the calves cannot turn
around. On farms where the calves are permitted outside their
crates, they are chained so close to the crates that they can barely
move. The calves are kept immobile so that their flesh stays
tender, while being fed a liquid, low iron, low nutrient diet to
keep their flesh white. Frightened, apprehensive, and alone
without a mother, the calves suffer from anemia, diarrhea, and
pneumonia. They are killed after a few months.

The metabolic hazards of consuming this kind of animal
flesh are yet to be thoroughly tested, but it is not difficult to
infer that they must be substantial.

After about four years dairy cows, which normally live
between 25 and 40 years, are removed from their milking
machines and sent to the slaughterhouses to be turned into
soup, low-grade hamburger, or animal food. Forty percent of
them are worn out and lame from the confinement, forced
milking, and continuous pregnancy.

According to Eric Schlosser, author of *Fast Food Nation*:

...The animals [that are] used to make about one-quarter
of the nation's ground beef — worn out dairy cattle — are
the animals most likely to be diseased and riddled with

antibiotic residues. The stresses of industrial milk production make them even more unhealthy than cattle in a large feedlot.[18]

Dairy cows and beef cows raised for meat are slaughtered in the same way. The terrorized animals are forced down a narrow chute and into a kill box where a workman sends a bolt to the head with a stun gun that is supposed to kill them instantly but often doesn't. The kill rate is 400 cows per hour, so the kill line is not about to stop just because a cow is identified as still being alive after being hit with the stun gun. The assault on the bodies of the cows begins dead or alive and often their hides are ripped from their bodies and their feet are cut off while they are still living and conscious. This is the process that turns cows into hamburgers, T-bone steaks, and Châteaubriand cuts for human consumption.

Factory farm chickens raised for broiling or egg production also have their private hell waiting to claim them. Farmers "persuade" laying hens to increase egg production through forced molting.[19] Forced molting is a cruel process in which chickens are deprived of water, food, and light to manipulate their hormones and speed up egg production. During the molt chickens starve and pluck each other's feathers off trying to get something to eat. Food is withheld for as much as two weeks, and the mortality rate rises. It has been estimated that 300,000 chickens die yearly from forced molting in California alone, where 25 million chickens are raised for egg laying purposes.

Ten egg laying chickens are forced to live in a single cage called a battery cage that measures about 2.33 by 2.33 square feet. The battery cages are stacked one on top of the other from floor to ceiling in the facilities in which they are stored. The floors of the cages are slanted so that the eggs will roll out onto a conveyor belt. Each individual chicken lives in an area that has been estimated to be about the width and length of a sheet of typewriting paper. They are packed in so tightly they cannot spread their wings. These crates are banned in Switzerland, Belgium, Austria, Sweden, and the Netherlands. In the United States, however, according to the egg industry, 98 percent of all eggs come from hens living in these cages.[20] Before they are forced into the cages, the hens' beaks are sliced off without anesthesia with a burning, hot blade so that they cannot peck one another.

Battery cages prevent chickens from living life the way they were born to live where they dust bathe, nest, perch, and forage. Instead, the wire mesh of the battery cages cuts their feet and bruises their bodies. Feces and urine cascade from the upper cages down to the lower ones creating an unbearable stench. The hens suffer from dehydration, bacterial infections, and heart attacks, and many die. Billions of chickens live like this in an arena of filth and feces with injured or dead bodies of other chickens underfoot. After about two years, after their egg production slacks off, the hens are sent to slaughter. By then they are emaciated and sick with 29% suffering from broken bones. Their flesh is so devastated it can only be used for chicken soup, animal feed, or "canned, boned and diced meat," much of which goes to the National School Lunch program for the nation's school children to eat.[21]

Male chicks on egg farms have a different fate in store. Since they are useless as egg producers, millions of them are discarded live into trash bags where they suffocate. Others are thrown live into macerators that grind them into bits.[22]

Broiler chickens destined for the dinner table, like pigs, are also genetically engineered from the time they are chicks. They never see their mothers and grow so huge in body size that their legs and organs often cannot support their weight, resulting, also like pigs, in broken legs and other debilitating injuries. If human babies grew at the same rate they would weigh 350 pounds by the time they were two years old. But genetic engineering makes a bigger, plumper chicken for the dinner table.[23] These chickens also live in filth and cramped conditions with many dying from disease, pollution, and noxious ammonia from urine fumes.

When they reach market weight at the age of about 45 days, these chickens are taken to slaughter. During transport they are frequently thrown violently into cages where they suffer from dislocated limbs and broken bones and are given no food or water.

Whether raised for the dinner table or for laying eggs, all chickens that manage to survive their ordeal are eventually slaughtered. Their journey through hell only ends when their legs are shackled upside down to a conveyor belt and their heads are lopped off by decapitation machines. But sometimes the machines are only partially successful and do not fully decapitate the birds, in which case, like pigs, they are then dunked fully alive and conscious into tanks of scalding water.

Many people shut the cruelty to the animals they eat out of their minds and refuse to think about it, but the reality does not go away. It is always there in the subconscious destroying our peace of mind. We may not have heard specifically about the Pilgrim's Pride plant in Moorefield, West Virginia that supplies chickens to Kentucky Fried Chicken where workers were video-taped stomping on chickens, kicking them, slamming them violently against floors and walls, ripping their beaks off, twisting off their heads, spitting tobacco in their eyes and mouths, spray-painting their faces, and squeezing their bodies so hard that they expelled feces — all while the chickens were conscious and alive — but we know that this kind of abuse goes on.

After seeing the video, Dan Rather said on the CBS Evening News: "[T]here's no mistaking what [it] depicts: cruelty to animals, chickens horribly mistreated before they're slaughtered for a fast-food chain."[24] The nation is not so naïve and innocent that it can claim it is not aware that the same kind of behavior is going on someplace, somewhere all across America wherever animals are assembled together and slaughtered.

Factory farms started in the 1960s when food industrialists began moving slaughterhouses from Chicago to rural states hostile to labor unions.[25] Freed from union restraints, they built vast new feedlots and slaughterhouses and paid workers two-thirds less than they earned in Chicago. By 1971 the Chicago meatpackers' union had been broken and the stockyards had largely closed their doors. An industry that once numbered 40,000 workers had been reduced to 2,000.[26]

The new work force for the slaughterhouses in the rural countryside were immigrants made up of the low-skilled, the uneducated, and the disenfranchised. They were poor, spoke little English, and came from distant places like Central America, South America, Southeast Asia, and Mexico. Malleable and easy to exploit, they lived in old trailers and motels, slept many to a room on mattresses on the floor, and sent some of their money home to help their impoverished families.[27] Immigrant workers like these are the kind of employees who are paid to do the nightmarish work of killing one animal after the other hour upon hour, day after day, week after week, month in and month out, year after year.

How many of the cows are still living and conscious when their hides are ripped from their bodies and their feet cut off, no one knows. No one knows either, how many pigs have their throats slit while they are still conscious or how many pigs and chickens are still alive when they are plunged into scalding water. The number of immigrant farm workers who are seriously injured doing this highly dangerous work is also a mystery.

It is easy to take advantage of immigrant workers. In Iowa, for example, in the fall of 2008 the state's labor board fined Agriprocessors Inc., a kosher slaughterhouse, 9.6 million dollars for illegally deducting money for uniforms from the paychecks of 2000 illegal immigrant workers employed at the plant. In addition, Agriprocessors illegally deducted pay for sales tax and employed workers as young as 13 to operate dangerous machinery prohibited for young workers to use.[28]

The machinery is also dangerous for the consumer. As machines remove the hides from cows, chunks of dirt and manure fall from the animals to contaminate the meat. It is why Schlosser tells us there is "shit" in the hamburgers people consume. The contents of the digestive system are also prone to spill out onto the meat. It is the speed employed on the production line to meet the standards demanded by the food producers that ensures this will happen.[29] The risk of contamination is great. So is the chance that a hamburger will contain cow feces.

The same kinds of processes also apply to chickens. Slaughter machines spatter bacteria-laden feces onto the chickens' bodies so that up to 90 percent of all chicken flesh sold in the United States is swarming with salmonella, campylobacter, and other dangerous bacteria. As many as 4,000,000 Americans get sick from salmonella "flu" each year; and about 500 die.

The effects of diseased food on the consumer are well known by the factory farm industry, but not well publicized. Schlosser notes that "every day in the United States, roughly 200,000 people are sickened by a food borne disease, 900 are hospitalized, and fourteen die."[30]

Tyson Fresh Meats (formerly IBP (Iowa Beef Processors)), ConAgra, Excel, and National Beef are the top meatpacking firms that together slaughter about 84% of the nation's cattle.[31,32] Other CAFOs (Confined Animal Feed Operations) include Perdue (chickens), Smithfield Farms (pigs), and Case Vander Eyk Jr. Dairy (cows).[33] ConAgra, founded by Mike Harper, is the biggest meatpacker on earth.[34] The four biggest hamburger chains in the world are McDonald's, CKE (Carl Karcher

Enterprises), Burger King, and Wendy's, of which McDonald's, founded by Ray Kroc, is the nation's biggest purchaser of beef.

The effects of factory farms on surrounding communities can be devastating. As Schlosser points out, IBP (now Tyson Fresh Meats) has controlled prices, manipulated the market, broken unions, consorted with the mob, befouled the air of communities, and created an environment where crime cannot fail to fester in towns where their plants are located.[35]

A growing number of people are troubled by the feast the meat and dairy industries have prepared for the American dinner table. They are disturbed by the dawning recognition that the meat and dairy industrialists have become enormously wealthy at the expense of animals they have abused in the most cruel ways, by employing an impoverished work force under dangerous, substandard labor conditions, and by putting the health of all segments of the American public at risk — babies, children, adolescents, young people, adults, seniors, and the elderly.

Most troubling of all is the recognition that to partake of the American feast of hamburgers, steak, veal, ham, chicken, pork, lamb, milk, milk shakes, yogurt, cheese, pizza, and all the different kinds of cute foods like Buffalo Wings, McNuggets, and Whoppers, is to be complicit in the cruelty and abuse that produced it and to be a part of the nightmare that is spreading disease to our families, our neighbors, the country, and the world.

The kind of hell on earth that we humans have managed to create for ourselves and other species is a marvel to behold. It is time we began to invent new systems for the distribution of power and the control of resources in which at least we do not have to look into the mirror and see someone staring back at us who has been unwittingly deceived into complying with the abuse of animals.

Unfortunately, even as we begin to recognize the horrors that happen on factory farms, we can hardly draw a breath before we are forced to acknowledge that another cruel industry awaits our inspection just around the corner. This industry makes its money using animals in animal research projects. That is the next topic for discussion at the round table where it becomes evident that our permissive attitude toward the consumption of animals is responsible for the existence of the university, government, and private research facilities where animal research takes place. To get to these facilities we must enter undetected through closed doors. The operators keep the doors closed because they do not want us to see what is going on inside this multi-billion dollar industry funded by our tax dollars. If we find out, they fear a storm of protest will erupt, and they will lose their treasure trove of wealth.

Chapter 20

The Fraud Called Animal Research

How the Universities Are Taking Our Tax Dollars

The image that most people have of an animal researcher is that of a well-trained, highly skilled scientist surrounded by test tubes and flasks. Wearing an immaculately clean, white coat, the scientist looks up from his or her microscope and while stroking a plump, white rat with clean pink ears and feet, converses about the latest medical discoveries being made with the help of animals. This is an image the animal research industry has carefully cultivated for decades. It is also an image that animal researchers from the military, non-profit organizations, and the world of industry (cosmetics, household products, etc.) hide behind for public acceptance.

Since many people tolerate medical research on animals, they routinely accept all other forms of animal testing never quite realizing the differences between the two. But medical research, as commonly referred to, is funded by the public in the form of tax dollars and is intended to solve medical problems. This is distinct from industry research that is privately funded and is conducted for commercial purposes. Charities are also privately funded, though their research may be for medical reasons. Military research, on the other hand, is funded by the public but is done only to achieve some kind of military objective. (See Appendix I for examples of these different kinds of research.)

While many people sanction animal testing, they still cringe when they hear tales of animal cruelty. They do not want animals to be abused and mistreated. People agree to animal research only because 1) they have been led to believe that this

229

is the only way to find cures for cancer, heart disease, stroke, diabetes, and other chronic diseases, and 2) they are not aware of the abuses of animals that go on in secret behind the closed doors of animal research facilities.

Today our consumption of disease-promoting foods, namely meat and dairy products, provides the rationale for the existence of animal research laboratories. That is because these labs exist almost solely for the purpose of trying to find a cure for the diseases from which the public is most at risk (cancer, heart disease, stroke, diabetes, etc.). We now know with scientific certainty that these are primarily caused by consuming meat and dairy products.

Akmaeon of Croton (?510 BCE -?), who may have been a pupil of Pythagoras (?570 - 495 BCE), was one of the first vivisectors. He is principally known today for severing the optic nerve of living animals in order to study vision. Since his time medical researchers have continued to vivisect animals in the pursuit of finding cures for various diseases with little to show for their efforts. As we have discussed, Egyptian healers were contemplating cancer as early as 1500 BCE, and it was Hippocrates who finally gave cancer its name. Now nearly 2500 years after Akmaeon first cut into a living animal, researchers are still vivisecting animals hoping to find cures for one disease or another. When anyone objects and suggests that 2500 years is ample time for any project to succeed or fail no matter what it is, these researchers repeat their favorite mantra that a cure is right around the corner and continue cutting. But they don't fail to stop by at the cashier's desk on Fridays to pick up their very large paychecks from the NIH.

Fortunately, we have finally learned categorically and scientifically that the major killer diseases can be prevented if we stop putting the kind of food into our bodies that causes these diseases to develop, namely, animal protein. The rationale for continuing animal research, consequently, no longer applies insofar as it relates to these killer diseases. This is important to contemplate because if we as a nation decided to put a stop to this unnecessary animal research it would free up a vast reservoir of billions of tax dollars that could be redirected toward new horizons in healthcare explorations and disease prevention as well as other positive societal agendas.

Animal research as it is studied in this book breaks down into two main categories. The first involves research that is intended to explore medical mysteries for the benefit of humanity. This research is conducted by more serious researchers, some of whom may be on track for the Nobel Prize. We shall be meeting some of these researchers in the next chapter where we will direct a number of criticisms in their direction while considering a number of alternatives to animal testing. The second category, which we will examine in this chapter, consists of projects by researchers who claim that their work is for humanitarian purposes. When their work is examined closely, however, it becomes apparent that this research is really invented for the purpose of procuring government funding in order to build lucrative careers and create institutional wealth for the universities and independent medical research facilities that sponsor this work. Here we find the world of curiosity research, nicotine and drug addition testing, and repetition research that has already been done (often many times), but that is modified in varying ways to make it appear like it is original and different. Since much of the work has already been done, this makes it easier for the animal researchers to prepare their proposals for government grants. (For a satire piece on how to fake a grant proposal to the NIH, see Appendix II.)

The bulk of the research in this second category, examples of which will be illustrated, produces few benefits, no matter how cleverly the researchers dress their projects in scientific terminology. In fact, as shown by national statistics, two-thirds of these ventures have little human application. Most of it is done just to satisfy the curiosity of the researchers.[1] In Great Britain the figure for curiosity research has been estimated at 50%. The Canadian Advocacy Coalition of Canada statistics for 1999 calculated that "curiosity driven" research accounted for 53% of the animal testing that was done in Canada."[2] By 2001 this figure had risen to 59%. And, the Humane Society of the United States (HSUS) reports that "the great majority of animal use for experimental purposes can best be described as 'curiosity-driven.'"[3]

In spite of these kinds of criticisms, the people involved in this kind of research insist that their work does have human utility. But a large number of these projects involve drug or nicotine addiction testing, the objections to which will be addressed momentarily, or are so esoteric in their dimensions that they have no relevance to human healthcare, such as attempts to measure the manner in which the brain instructs the eyes how to control the center of gaze.

While it might satisfy our curiosity to try to answer a question like this, the subject has nothing to do with finding a cure for disease. In order to conduct this particular experiment, which took place at the University of Connecticut, the researcher drilled holes into the skulls of monkeys and then attached tiny steel coils directly into the monkeys' eyes. Two monkeys died as a result just to satisfy the curiosity of the researcher.[4] In this instance, the university at least had the courage to step forward to reprimand the researcher and put a stop to his work. But that rarely happens and researchers are seldom penalized or criticized.

Because of their wealth the affluent countries of the West have been able to spend huge sums of money on medical research searching for the causes of the killer diseases that haunt their world. The heart of this multibillion dollar industry lies in animal research laboratories owned and operated by universities and various medical facilities. Researchers affiliated with these institutions compete for billions of public-funded tax dollars in grants for animal research projects which are mostly dispensed by the National Institutes of Health (NIH), as well as lesser known government funding agencies that include the Agency for Healthcare Research and Quality, the Center for Disease Control and Prevention, the Department of Justice, the Food and Drug Administration, the Health Resources and Services Administration, the Office of Assistant Secretary of Health, and the Substance Abuse and Mental Health Services.

The NIH does its best to keep the kinds of animal projects it funds secret. In 2007 the organization, which by far has the deepest pockets of all the government funding agencies, had a budget of $28.5 billion to spend.[5,6] Even though this is public money, the agency will not reveal how much of it goes for animal research. Various sources have estimated it comes to as much as 70 percent of the total budget.[7] That means nearly $20 billion is spent to fund animal research.

The facts are that the animal research industry experiments upon tens of millions of vertebrates every year, exactly how many, no one has a clue. Mice, rats, and birds are not even kept track of because they are not protected by provisions of the Animal Welfare Act, and research facilities that use these animals are not required to register with the USDA.[8]

The 1986 estimate by the Office of Technology Assistance of between 17 and 22 million animals used in research every year is still widely relied upon for statistical data by many organizations.[9] A later study done by the Animal and Plant Health Inspection Service of the USDA estimated that between 25 and 30 million animals are used to experiment upon annually.[10] However, other figures put the number as high as 200 million.[11]

After they are used in experiments, most of the animals are either subjected to repeated experimentation or they are killed.

University medical centers and other medical facilities (hospitals, for example) apply for and get public tax dollars for

233

their research, though the public has little say about what goes on inside the laboratories. The research continues year after year at these institutions, and, like taxes, the public accepts it as a fact of life.

The motor that operates this money-dispensing machine consists of two main parts. The first is a propaganda feed that tells the public a cure is just around the corner and that all cures for disease are dependent upon animal research. The second, that is never divulged to the public and seldom spoken aloud, is the assumption that, in spite of issuing periodic reports of progress being made, cures for the killer diseases will never be found. This assures that the machine will run in perpetuity so that the funding will never dry up.

While this may sound like a cynical appraisal, as we shall see, the shallowness of most animal research in terms of its capacity to even hint at any real human significance in terms of disease that is not drug related, offers a fair indication that this is indeed the case.

Applying for grants involving drug trials and surgery on animals is one of the surest ways to get NIH funding. According to T. Colin Campbell, "almost all the billions of dollars of taxpayer money expended by the NIH each year funds projects to develop drugs, supplements, and mechanical devices. In essence, the vast bulk of biomedical research funded by you and me is basic research to discover products that the pharmaceutical industry can develop and market."[12]

Those who would like to see the medical profession stop relying on surgery and drugs in favor of nutritional procedures in curing and preventing disease are confronted with the hard fact that this would require university medical centers and medical institutions to say good-bye to billions of tax dollars that they get from the NIH in grants related to unconscionable drug development. It is unconscionable because 1) it is not necessary, 2) it creates drugs for fictitious diseases (see chapter 14), and 3) it involves nicotine and substance abuse testing. (See further below concerning the ethics of substance abuse testing.) Institutions that benefit from animal research grants are not inclined toward giving up their share of this money just because heart disease can be arrested and reversed through diet and nutrition or because cancer, heart disease, stroke, and diabetes can be prevented if people stop consuming animal products.

University medical centers and other medical institutions insist that only animal research can lead to a cure for the killer diseases. This creates a general atmosphere of prejudice that hinders alternative research approaches from making progress. And while animal research enriches the institutions and researchers that engage in this activity, it represents an enormous squandering of public money and is undeniably cruel to countless millions upon millions of innocent animals.

Just how much money is at stake is hard to determine. Figures are difficult to come by because the NIH keeps the figures secret. Government funding statistics reported by Sourcewatch Encyclopedia, however, offer a clue as to the kind of money involved. Their report, which excludes the millions of animals that are not covered by the Animal Welfare Act (mice, rats, and birds), indicates that the total amount of money paid for animal research for the year 2005 came to over $8.4 billion. This is based on 28,937 funded NIH projects for the year times an average grant of $291,502 (which was the average estimate per grant paid out by the NIH for the year 2000).[13],[14]

The animal research industry has made a concerted effort to communicate the message that animal research causes no suffering to the animals involved. However, according to a USDA Animal Welfare Act Enforcement Report released in January of 2009, 77,766 animal experiments caused animals unrelieved pain and/or distress in the year 2007, an increase of five percent over 2005.[15] This suffering does not even include experiments in which researchers made some attempt to mitigate the pain the animals endured but in which the animals suffered nonetheless.

Extrapolating from the number of animals experimented upon yearly as indicated above, can anyone with a straight face say that they believe the NIH and other government funding agencies know beyond a vague guess what has happened with the millions of different research projects that have been funded over the years, or what the results were, or, for that matter, how the results have had human applicability? Does anyone have an idea of what happened with these research projects even within the last year?

As just noted, for the year 2007 about 77,766 animals were used in experiments that caused unrelieved pain and/or distress. When that figure is multiplied by five, ten, fifteen, or twenty years into the past, it means that more than a million animals have been experimented upon in which animals were subjected to unrelieved pain and/or distress in just the past few years. It should be apparent that the NIH cannot and will not say that these animals were used in experiments that had human applicability.

When this little multiplication test is used times the rest of the estimated 25 to 200 million animals experimented upon annually, just how extensive animal medical research really is begins to register. Worldwide, scientists have conducted tests for medical research upon billions of animals in just the last 20 years.

Still they have found no cure for cancer, heart disease, diabetes, arthritis, multiple sclerosis, or Alzheimer's Disease, but insist that all these countless millions of animal experiments have had human applicability. That defies all believability.

There is good reason why scientists and their universities cling to animal research. Here is a small sampling showing typical amounts they receive in research grants annually.

University of California, Los Angeles, $194,110,000. Harvard

University, $441,273,869. Johns Hopkins University, $256,886,000. Yale University, $199,066,000. Stanford University, $164,374,000. Vanderbilt University, $170,982,000. Emory University, $239,303,364. Duke University, $162,309,000. Baylor University, $173,047,000. University of Pennsylvania, $256,060,000. University of Wisconsin, Madison, $141,655,452. University of Washington, Seattle, $418,889,748. University of Michigan, $216,825,000.[16]

Sums like these are difficult to renounce. The situation is parallel to the period of apartheid in South Africa during the 1970s and 1980s in which the universities refused to divest their South African stocks and bonds until they were forced to by student demonstrations.[17] Though some Boards of Trustees were too obstinate to admit their error and never did divest, 180 universities did. By withdrawing billions of dollars of investments from companies doing business with South Africa, these universities contributed to bringing the South African Apartheid government to a close.[18] It is never too late to do what is right and good, and the role of ethics and "right and wrong" is of particular relevance in the discussion of animal research.

Consider, for example, the ongoing research done at the Oregon Health and Science University (OHSU). There a researcher with an M.D. from the Harvard Medical School and a Ph.D. from M.I.T., has been paid $7.6 million tax dollars by the NIH since 1992 (and will continue receiving funding until 2012) to literally take baby monkeys from their mothers' breasts to study nicotine effects on infant monkeys.[19] Sometimes the baby monkeys are acquired through cesarean section, while other times the mothers are allowed to keep their babies for several weeks before a human hand reaches into the cage and tears the babies away from their mothers, driving the mothers nearly insane. The other monkeys caged in the community, who have witnessed the kidnapping, start screaming and leaping wildly around their cages as they wail in protest.

If the above description sounds like an exaggeration, this is how Matt Rossell, an undercover operator for IDA (In Defense of Animals), described what he experienced at the Oregon Health and Science University.

> Among the most horrifying things I witnessed at the lab were the times when baby monkeys were stolen away from their mothers. This was a chaotic, ugly, heart-wrenching scene. A worker wearing thick leather gloves would reach into the cage where the baby clung to her mother's breast, and snatch the baby by one shoulder and arm and rip her from her mother who was screaming and desperately fighting to keep her baby safe. Once removed, the entire room of monkeys would erupt into total pande-monium — screaming, thrashing and crashing against the sides of their cages — some even reaching out through the bars in vain to get the baby back.[20]

Losing their babies causes tremendous suffering for these primates who are operated on five times during their forced pregnancies for the purpose of implanting nicotine pumps in their backs. This is cruel, but the Oregon Health and Science University behaves as if it were as normal as a casual walk on a warm summer's day and staunchly defends the research.

The researcher claims he is trying to develop treatments for lung cancer caused by smoking and to learn how to block the effects of maternal smoking on fetal lung development.[21] But primates should not have to suffer the abuse of being held captive, being artificially inseminated, having nicotine pumps implanted in their backs, and having their babies torn from them in an attempt to find cures for lung cancer caused by smoking. Yes, it is unfortunate that people get lung cancer from smoking, but animals should not be abused, tortured, and forced to forfeit their lives to try to save human beings from their own bad habits.

That this is a question of ethics could hardly be more apparent. And if human beings pride themselves on being ethical creatures, ethics cannot be omitted from the equation when animal research is debated, especially in a university setting where morality and ethics are traditionally held in the highest esteem.

The names inscribed above the columns on the façade of the Butler Library at Columbia University read: Homer, Herodotus, Sophocles, Plato, Aristotle, Demosthenes, Cicero, Vergil, Horace, Tacitus, St. Augustine, Dante, Cervantes, Shakespeare, Milton, Voltaire, Goethe. These are the kinds of cultural heroes whose contributions to civilization are trumpeted in colleges and universities all across the land.

It seems more than apparent that these illustrious servants of humanity would agree that the morality of testing on animals in university research laboratories to cure human substance abuse is a subject that requires public debate. We know that certainly the orator and statesman Cicero (106-43 BCE) would think so as indicated by his own words: "Man is destined to a better occupation than that of pursuing and cutting the throat of dumb creatures."[22]

Certainly, too, Vergil would nod his assent, as would Voltaire along with the historian Herodotus (484 - 425 BCE) who said: "Why cause suffering, to these inferior and innocent orders of being and why take the life that only the Gods could give."[23]

And while Aristotle might have disagreed with his noble colleagues, the very fact that there is disagreement is the reason for debate — not to conceal and carry on these operations in secret as our universities today are doing. Let it be proclaimed far and wide and loudly, that those universities which refuse to engage in this debate publicly are not living up to the highest intellectual standards which the public has every right to expect.

Until they do, the officers of our universities are hiding from the responsibilities that inescapably become theirs the instant they don their scholarly robes.[24]

Cruel research on animals that attempts to find ways for human mothers to continue to smoke during their pregnancies without harming their own babies, such as that in which the researcher is engaged at the Oregon Health and Science University, would certainly be considered by a significant percentage of the national population to be morally indefensible. If this researcher and his university believe the contrary, as apparently they do, then they should be willing to engage in open, public debate. The money they receive for this research, after all, is public money. It should also be noted that smoking cessation programs for pregnant women are available as are other alternative treatment options to cure smoking. However, these cannot be used to get public tax dollars.

Until protests finally forced OHSU to stop the practice, collecting semen from the male monkeys to impregnate the females in this research was quite a spectacle. A male was strapped in a standing position so that he was unable to move any of his limbs while a laboratory attendant attached wires to his penis and shocked him until he ejaculated. If the first attempt failed, the attendant kept trying, sometimes numerous times, until the monkey produced the semen. Not only was this Frankensteinian, it was grossly obscene and constituted the rape of an innocent animal. But this is the kind of bizarre research animal researchers dream up and transform into reality with public tax money. It is only brought to a stop when undercover operators expose the abuse or whistle blowers blow the whistle.

Most people regard research like this as repulsive. They also think it is equally obscene to take a baby primate by cesarean section and then subject it to nicotine testing.

What might some of history's greatest literary figures like Shakespeare, Shelley, Wordsworth, or Voltaire have to say about these kinds of procedures? Perhaps the officers of the Oregon Health and Science University would care to engage them in a debate. We can make a fairly good guess at what Voltaire would say according to his own words in relation to a dog:

> This dog, so very superior to man in affection, is seized by some barbarian virtuosos, who nail him down to a table, and dissect him while living, the better to shew you the meseraic veins. All the same organs of sensation which are in yourself you perceive in him. Now, Machinist, what say you? Answer me! Has Nature created all the springs of feeling in this animal, that it may not feel? Has it nerves to be impassible? For shame! Charge not Nature with such weakness and inconsistency.[25]

In spite of protests against the animal research taking place at the Oregon Health and Science University by the public and various animal rights group, including the highly respected In Defense of Animals, led by its founder, Dr. Elliot Katz, DVM, a graduate of Cornell University, OHSU is not likely to give up the millions of tax dollars it takes from the American people to do this ill-considered animal research in which it is a partner.

Our universities are not acting with the highest ethical standards. They are participants in the fraudulent procurement of public funds to fill their coffers at the expense of innocent animals. We see this time and time again by examining the research projects in which universities are occupied which they conceal from public view while refusing to debate their necessity.

How many people are aware, for example, that at Ohio State University an animal researcher subjects dogs to invasive surgical procedures that constricts an artery in order to kill a portion of the heart muscle. The researcher then puts a cuff around a blood vessel which he closes off while forcing the dogs to run on a treadmill. This induces a heart attack.[26] He has been doing this for 25 years and his research has produced nothing of significance for human beings. In fact, he admits that after 25 years "the mechanisms responsible for VF [ventricular fibrillation] at the cellular and subcellular level remain largely to be determined." But not to worry. This researcher tells us that "it, therefore, is very likely that this canine model for sudden death will continue to stimulate new research and produce *interesting* results for the next 25 years."[27] [Author's emphasis] That gives him 25 more years of cozying up to the NIH to take public tax dollars to induce "interesting" heart attacks on dogs. Ohio State University, like many other major universities, is not interested in knowing that heart attacks can be prevented through nutrition. Seven hundred dogs have been killed in Ohio State University's "sudden cardiac death" experiments.[28]

Perhaps the "virtuoso" researcher and the Ohio State University trustees would also like to have a debate with Voltaire?

Let us be honest. The kind of research that we have been observing is not for finding a cure for something. This is research for the purpose of extracting taxpayer money from the government for financial gain, whether it is to build institutional wealth for universities and medical facilities, or to build lucrative careers for individual researchers. In fact, the institutions that sponsor animal research get paid 50 to 75 percent of the grant money supplied for all research projects so that it is in their financial interests to support animal research no matter how cruel and bizarre it may be.

More and more people are beginning to see that this partnership between the NIH and university and other research laboratories is nothing but an insane scheme run amuck that is literally robbing the public of billions of tax dollars every year.

A 2010 media release by In Defense of Animals listed some of the findings of 10 NIH sponsored research projects published in peer-reviewed journals. They included the discoveries that baby chimpanzees need nurturing, exercise may help people lose weight, lizards forced to fight get stressed, and female rats enjoy vaginal stimulation. This absurd nonsense, which the researchers were not even too embarrassed to publish in medical journals, was obtained at a cost of millions of dollars to the taxpayers.

Many other studies involving sexual stimulation of the genitalia of animals that has nothing to do with finding the causes of disease have been conducted at institutions like Columbia University, Dartmouth College, and the University of Virginia. Here scientists injected varying amounts of testosterone into castrated hamsters in order to define the optimum concentration for maintaining ejaculation. Researchers at the National Institute of Mental Health castrated male monkeys in order to learn that castrated monkeys exhibited more subordinate and less dominate behavior than monkeys that were not castrated. This brilliant research further showed that intact gonads were important in adolescent social behavior. And the money for this useless, unnecessary research all came out of the citizens' pockets.

Because of public "unease" about the morality of animal testing, more and more animal research scientists have begun to ask if their research is worth the few results, negative publicity, and community contempt. Far too many people keep companion animals in their homes or have some other connection with animals and are, consequently, hostile to animal research. Some just believe that it is morally and spiritually indefensible to abuse an animal in vivisection procedures. Citizens were outraged, for example, when a videotape surfaced showing University of Pennsylvania researchers laughing and ridiculing baboons upon whom they were conducting head trauma experiments.[29]

By now animal rights organizations and whistleblowers have

brought cruel animal research projects to light so often that universities are forced to defend their animal policies to the public, at least on those occasions when they get caught abusing animals. In any case, universities and medical centers that conduct animal research are now required by federal law to set up Institutional Animal Care and Use Committees (IACUCs). But a 2005 USDA audit by the Office of the Inspector General found repeated failures of IACUCs to contend with serious problems in their programs. The report noted that research laboratories were failing in their "search for alternative research, veterinary care, review of painful procedures, and researchers' use of animals." The audit also revealed that "IACUCs did not ensure that unnecessary or repetitive experiments would not be performed on laboratory animals."[30] This is an admission by the USDA that universities are knowingly engaging in repetitive research.

The replication of animal research projects is one of the more ignominious aspects of animal testing. This is the senseless repetition of painful, cruel experiments that have already been conducted just to get government grants. Researchers become adept at making research proposals appear like they are something new and different when the work is really just a copy of some project that has already been done. In the process these researchers often invent bizarre, sadistic research techniques, as we shall see, while, it cannot be said often enough, collecting millions of tax dollars from the public. (See also Appendix III for examples of vivisection techniques animal researchers copy from each other and for additional examples of bizarre, sadistic animal research.)

The University of Minnesota advertises that their Institutional Animal Care and Use Committee works to assure that research and other activities involving animals are "justified by their benefits and [that they] minimize any pain or suffering." They must have forgotten about one of their researchers who for twenty-two years at a cost of nine million dollars to taxpayers has been using food deprivation to forcibly addict monkeys and rats to drugs including nicotine, cocaine, PCP, heroin, amphetamines, and alcohol.

Reportedly, the researcher's lab subjects primates to withdrawal that causes seizures, nose bleeding, respiratory problems, skin infections, self-mutilation, incessant rocking, hallucinations, screaming, and depression. The researcher's own daily primate logs from 2004 – 2005 made the following observations about one of her subjects: "...ripping hair from the armpit area and chewing on the fur, each time he would grab a tuft of hair he would vocalize...primate jumping back and forth wildly...hypersalivating, disoriented...shows evidence of self mutilation, did bite knee after observation...extremely thin, body condition is poor, severe alopecia [loss of hair], bruising on left ankle...lost part of his tongue."[31]

Just as with the Oregon Health and Sciences University, the fact that the practice of using innocent animals in an effort to attend to the addiction problems human beings have created for themselves is unethical and unjust seems not to have occurred to this highly educated, highly paid researcher and the trustees and administrative officers of the University of Minnesota. Do the American people really want their money spent to abuse animals to learn how to treat smoking and drug addiction? Should animals have to pay the penalty because human beings smoke and take drugs? From the standpoint of ethics, is this question that difficult to answer with a resounding "No?"

Moreover, when it comes to testing for drugs, most of this research is useless. The FDA reported in 2004 that 92 out of every 100 drugs that have successfully passed animal trials fail in follow-up human trials. That means that 92% of animals used in drug testing suffer for nothing.

Like the University of Minnesota, Columbia University also uses its Standards of Care website to try to reassure a suspicious public. There, Columbia asserts that it "recognizes its scientific and ethical duty to treat animals involved in research humanely and requires that all faculty, staff and students involved in animal research maintain the highest standards of care."

However, these kinds of assurances are as much public relations as anything else and do not tell stories about experiments that have taken place at Columbia like the one in which every puppy in an entire litter was killed by cardiac puncture. Undercover videos taken in Columbia's animal laboratories in 2003 revealed that mother baboons and their babies in utero were operated on repeatedly to measure the flow of nicotine through the umbilical chord; baboons had one eye removed in senseless experiments to attempt to induce strokes before being abandoned in cages without care or painkillers; and monkeys had metal pipes implanted in their craniums driving them into a frenzy in irrelevant menstrual stress studies. The suffering these animals endured ended only when they died from the effects of these experiments or when they were killed by their researchers.

Columbia researchers were still experimenting on animals for drug and nicotine addition in 2009 so it is certain that this major Ivy League university also does not understand the moral ramifications of experimenting upon innocent animals to cure human substance abuse.[32]

The University of California San Francisco is the fourth largest recipient of federal research grants, receiving over $420 million from the NIH annually. On a university webpage the text above a photograph of a cute white mouse nestled cozily in the pocket of an empty, purple surgical glove advertises that "the University has established policies on the use of animal subjects to promote their humane care."[33] The text continues below the photograph in a statement all too similar to those made by Columbia and the University of Minnesota announcing that the university oversees all "research and instruction that involves vertebrate animals, in order to ensure that the highest ethical and animal welfare standards are met."[34]

In the real world the University of California San Francisco has frequently been in violation of the federal Animal Welfare Act, according to the U.S. Department of Agriculture, which in 2004 filed formal charges against UCSF for over 60 Animal Welfare Act violations between 2001 and 2003 resulting in a fine of $92,500.[35],[36] These charges included performing surgery on an ewe and her fetus without providing local anesthesia and post-surgical pain relief (that means cutting into an animal without anesthesia and then allowing it to suffer alone and in pain); leaving monkeys and lambs unmonitored after surgery (which resulted in a lamb frothing at the mouth and gasping for breath); forcing marmoset monkeys to breed continually and give birth while still nursing infants (one marmoset mother gave birth seven times to fourteen babies in just over three years; six of the babies died and the mother lost 70 percent of her bodyweight during that period); depriving monkeys of water, resulting in severe weight loss; performing a craniotomy on a monkey without providing post-operative pain relief; and subjecting at least one monkey to multiple injections of a brain-destroying chemical through the carotid artery.

Some of the most extreme curiosity research conducted at the University of California San Francisco has been done by a researcher who in imitator tests similar to ones in which the March of Dimes has engaged (See Appendix I), reportedly sewed closed the eyes of 22 newly born kittens, forced them to stay awake by means of a motorized floor, and paralyzed them in preparation for brain recordings.[37]

The researcher does this kind of work to test brain development without visual stimulation. He also implants chemical pumps into some of the kittens' heads so that he can inject drugs through a port into their craniums. Eventually, he reopens their eyes and cuts off the tops of their skulls to measure brain activity while they sit in front of television screens. This research that has been funded since the 1970s has made the amazing discovery that "cats brains do not develop normally when their eyes are sewn shut."[38] Since 1979, this researcher has received millions of tax dollars to experiment on cats and kittens and has received one million dollars for this research during the period of 1998 to 2000.[39]

The foregoing are examples of what the University of California San Francisco calls the "highest ethical and animal welfare standards." The NIH obviously concurs.

In July of 2007 six physicians with counsel from the Physicians Committee for Responsible Medicine filed a lawsuit against UCSF for using tax dollars to pay the fine of $92,500 referred to above for mistreating animals. Pia Salk, Psy.D., the niece of Jonas Salk, who created the first vaccine for polio, was the lead plaintiff in bringing suit.[40]

Animals at research laboratories are forced to endure harsh living conditions. They are kept in cages and isolated in extreme, cramped conditions often for months and even years at a time. Jane Goodall, in writing about her visit to a large medical research laboratory funded by the NIH, described how young chimpanzees were crammed together two at a time for more than three months in cages measuring 22 inches by 22 inches and only 24 inches high so that they could hardly even turn around. At this facility, monkeys were kept in small cages stacked on top of each other in which they "circled round and round and chimpanzees sat huddled, far gone in depression and despair."[41]

Living under conditions of such "severe sensory deprivation" eventually drives the animals insane. It is difficult to comprehend why animal researchers fail to grasp that forced confinement of any animal in a tight, closed space constitutes torture. Differences in blood pressure between caged and non-caged animals has been well documented and show that caged animals suffer. Confining animals also prevents them from living their normal lives and carrying out their usual social interactions. Unfortunately, animal researchers are not interested in information like this. In fact, they intentionally subject animals to confinement experiments, for example by putting them in tubes where they cannot move a muscle. This is done in order to test for stress. These kinds of experiments are cruel. Scientists at San Diego State University, Colorado State University, the University of Arizona College of Medicine, and many other universities have all conducted this kind of research. At the California National Primate Research Center, researchers restrained rhesus monkeys in primate chairs two hours a day for seven days. Should anyone have been surprised by the results that showed the monkeys exhibited signs of acute and chronic stress? Scientists should not be allowed to use public tax money to conduct research that has so little meaning related to finding cures for disease and is so exceedingly cruel. Anyone can invent experiments like these and claim they have medical relevance.

Animals are also often neglected in other ways that can have deadly consequences. Examples include the University of Nevada at Reno where 38 pregnant sheep died when they were locked in an area without food or water for three days, the University of California at Davis where researchers left monkeys in temperatures up to 115 degrees Fahrenheit for many hours resulting in the death of seven of them, and the University of Washington where 500 mice died when they were left in rooms where temperatures reached 104 degrees Fahrenheit.[42]

The thirst by government agencies to fund unnecessary experiments on animals seems unquenchable, and our esteemed universities continue to shovel public tax dollars into their treasuries with little sign that they are embarrassed by their display of greed as they walk hand in hand with animal abusers up to the cashier's window. They are luxuriating in one grand joyride at the expense of the taxpayers.

Let us not be afraid to call a spade a spade. This so-called research that we have been examining is cruel and it is sadistic.

And it has created a collective mindset among animal researchers that is nearly impenetrable. They will not admit that what they are doing is cruel, and they will not listen to any suggestions that could lead to a better way.

For example, birth defect experiments on animals cannot be applied to humans, so why are they done? Better pre-natal care and helping women to quit smoking can reduce infant mortality by over 35%, so why does ineffective nicotine testing on animals and their living fetuses continue? Computer technology already exists capable of putting an end to animal testing for drugs, so what is the necessity of testing for drugs on millions of animals other than to take billions of tax dollars from the public? Many other methods of nonanimal medical research are available several of which are examined in the next chapter.

Many questions remain and should be directed at the NIH and the government. Why are so few controls implemented to prevent needless repetition of the same old animal tests? Why are no standards set to assure that animal testing has human applicability? Why are no limitations placed on the kinds of animal tests that researchers are allowed to perform, thus eliminating bizarre, sadistic, and cruel research projects? Why should animal tests not be required to meet ethical specifications, the kind of which would exclude the funding of projects for smoking and drug addiction which is fundamentally and patently unethical? Why are applications for research grants not monitored to prevent curiosity research from being funded? Why will the NIH and other government agencies funding animal research not open their books to the public so that the people can see for themselves how their tax money is being spent? And finally, why should the government give the NIH far more money than it requires thus forcing the agency to fund unnecessary animal research projects in order to prove the funds are needed?

The answers to questions like these are obvious in an ideal

world. But it is not an ideal world. The way the public wealth has been used up to the present to fund animal research reveals a world of corruption in which countless billions of animals have been and continue to be unnecessarily abused and killed. If we are to protect the animals and recover this wealth so that we can use it in the most productive ways, it is crucial that we open wide the doors on this corruption so that it is fully visible to everyone.

Look to the trustees and officers of our universities and medical facilities. They are the ones who invite and permit this animal research to go on at their institutions, and they are the ones who can put a stop to it overnight — just like they did with their investments in South Africa — and they will do it, if enough people protest and demand an accounting of this useless, cruel research for which their hard-earned money is being wasted.

Chapter 21

Science at Work

The Future of Healthcare Research

In spite of the cruelty and hypocrisy associated with university medical centers and other animal research facilities, it is still undeniable that some animal researchers do engage in animal research that is intended for humanitarian purposes. These are the scientists of whom some are on track for the Nobel Prize. In some cases they make a deliberate, conscious choice based on carefully considered principles that it is moral to put human health concerns above those of the rights of animals even though it means that animals are forced to submit to a wide variety of experiments that are plainly harmful to them and often results in their death. Because they are the elite of their profession, these scientists have considerable authority in determining the course and direction research on animals takes.

One of the charges made against these researchers, however, is that they are very much aware of the animal research fraud that is being carried out by the universities and research facilities, often their own, but keep silent about it in order to avoid trouble. They seldom criticize even the most transparent cases of spurious research by their colleagues and won't publicly or privately acknowledge it exists just to protect their own funding and to avoid fights among the researchers. This attitude contributes substantially to building a "wall of silence" that helps cover up the hoax and assists in perpetuating the deceptive research that is costing tax payers billions of dollars.

Another criticism leveled at these researchers is that they ignore the suffering of the animals upon whom they are conducting experiments as though the suffering of these animals is inconsequential. Yet it would be difficult, no matter what their personal philosophies are, for even the most caring animal researcher to deny that experiments sometimes cause suffering and pain to the animals involved. Dr. Robert Kass, Department Chair, Department of Pharmacology at the Columbia University Columbia Medical Center, wrote that "we test as humanely and effectively as possible," indicating that there are times when it is not possible to test humanely and effectively.[1]

Scientists searching for humanitarian cures for disease do sometimes make discoveries that are applicable to humankind such as reported by Dr. Eric A. Rose, Associate Dean for Translational Research and Chair of the Department of Surgery at Columbia University who wrote: "The concept of cardiac catheterization was born here — animal research allowed the idea to become an applicable technique."[2]

Dr. Rose's defense of cardiac catheterization indicates he is concerned enough about the ethics of animal testing to defend it. But from the standpoint of right and wrong, critics have their side to point to when they note that the technique of cardiac catheterization might never have been necessary without the meat-based diets responsible for the arterial problems requiring catheterization. Is it ethical to slaughter animals in cruel ways on factory farms and eat them, acquire a disease in the process of digesting and metabolizing them, and then experiment upon more animals to develop techniques like cardiac catheterization in an effort to try to find a cure for the disease caused by eating them?

The continuation of cardiovascular experiments upon animals to develop more sophisticated surgical techniques also stands as a barrier to communicating the information to the public that the public needs to hear. Heart disease can be cured and prevented through nutrition regimens such as those championed by Dr. Esselstyn and Dr. Ornish. The need for cardiac catheterization and heart surgery does not exist for those who really want to avoid it.

Nevertheless, the sincerity of this elite group of medical scientists upon whom we are focusing is difficult to deny. In attempting to solve public health enigmas they use animals in their research out of a sense of compassion toward human beings. Donald M. Silver, author of over 40 books on science for children and teachers, did cancer studies on mice at Sloan-Kettering Hospital in the 1970s. He said that when doubts about his work arose, he only had to think about the terminally ill patients in the children's ward.[3] Doctor John Young, introduced in chapter 10, the director of comparative medicine at Los Angeles Cedars-Sinai Medical Center, made the same argument when he said:

> People will ask me, how can you possibly do what you do? I can answer that question very easily. I walk them over to the pediatric cancer ward and show them children with bald heads with glioblastoma, brave children who will tell you, "I am terminal." We are curing rats with the same disease at a 70 percent cure rate. I am excited about that. It would be immoral, in my opinion, not to have done what we've done in the rats.[4]

Scientists like Dr. Silver and Dr. Young invariably point to terminally ill children in justifying animal research as a moral imperative. Those who agree with this position like to pose questions to opponents like, "What if it was your own child suffering from cancer?" But few people would deny terminally ill children the best possible chance for survival with the best possible care, or, for that matter, any suffering person, even if it had been derived by experimenting upon animals. That is the direction the world has taken up to the present. However, this does not justify continuing on the same course while refusing to consider even the possibility that alternative directions exist. And that includes thorough investigations of non-biological causes of disease including environmental and nutritional factors. A categorical insistence that animal testing is the only legitimate method for medical research also does not grasp the fundamental concept that animals have the same right for life that human beings have. Only human arrogance denies the reality of that right. Sigmund Freud saw this very clearly. (See chapter 18.) The failure to recognize and understand this fundamental idea represents a profound constraint on human experience and accounts for many of the world's problems including the diseases that human beings develop.

An entirely different path could have been chosen back in the 17th century when scientists turned down the road of ever increasing reliance on vivisection. Who knows what the state of medicine might be today if they had taken an alternative path that rejected animal research. One fact is certain, which we will explore momentarily. Significant advances are being made today without relying upon animal testing.

In René Descartes' time back in the 17th century, vivisectors justified vivisection because people had gradually lost sight of animals as being conscious, intelligent creatures capable of great emotional depth just because they didn't walk, talk, and think like human beings. In the mechanistic universe envisioned by Descartes, animals were mere mechanical objects. Comments like those made at the time that a kicked dog no more felt pain than a church organ if a key was depressed (discussed in chapter 17) are so strange that they would utterly defy comprehension were it not that some of the most intelligent people today, specifically animal researchers, believe essentially the same thing, that animals are without emotions or consciousness. As difficult as that may seem to believe, it has been an ongoing debate in the scientific community that has bubbled to the surface in recent years in articles appearing in publications like U.S. News and World Report, the Economist, The *New York Times*, the Seattle Times, and many other media sources.

On May 5, 2009, Dr. Doug Melton appeared as a guest on *The Charlie Rose Show* aired by PBS. Melton, the co-director of the Harvard University Stem Cell Institute, was named as one of the world's 100 most influential people in 2007 and 2009 by Time Magazine.[5] He is an Investigator of the Howard Hughes Medical Institute and is the Thomas Dudley Cabot Professor in the Natural Sciences at Harvard University. Rose had invited Melton on the show to discuss his stem cell research work.

Type 1 diabetes is a particularly important area of research for Melton, especially from a personal respect, because he has two children who suffer from the disease. Consequently, learning how to get the pancreas to produce insulin cells — the inability for which is the cause of Type 1 diabetes — is, understandably, one of his top priorities.

Melton is a personable individual, knowledgeable, sophisticated, soft spoken, kind and gentle in his demeanor. He works in three areas: 1) making cells for transplantation, 2) using cells to find drugs that slow disease, and 3) using stem cells to "recapitulate" (as Melton puts it) disease in an animal. He describes this work as "exciting" and though he admits that scientists do not know why success in animals cannot always ["always" was the word Melton used] be transferred to humans, he also points with pride to stem cell researchers who have figured out a way to study human disease by implanting it inside an animal and watching it develop.

In his research with animals, Melton begins with mice because they grow faster and are easier to keep. He says, however, that "in general people like to do large animal studies like a monkey or a pig but those take longer and are more expensive." Melton believes stem cell research will eventually get to the root causes of degenerative diseases like diabetes, cardiovascular disease, and neurodegeneration but admits they are years away.[6] Nevertheless, he finds his work to be "extremely valuable" and says that it is "a huge amount of fun to just go to the lab every day cause there's so many things happening."[7]

Dr. Melton did not discuss or reveal any knowledge on his part about the use of nutrition in preventing and even reversing cardiovascular disease and Type 2 diabetes. He also did not indicate that he had any awareness that nutritional research has already made important strides in understanding Type 1 diabetes, including that it has been linked to dairy products and that a plant-based diet can lower the total cholesterol level of Type 1 diabetic patients to a heart-attack safe level. He might, consequently, be interested in the work of Dr. Joel Fuhrman. As described in chapter 5, Fuhrman has shown that with a nutrition regimen he can control Type 2 diabetes and can help Type 1 diabetic patients reduce their insulin requirements by about half so that they can essentially live, as he describes it, a disease-free life. Dr. Fuhrman is a former world class figure skater and member of the United States World Figure Skating Team. He has appeared on countless radio and television shows including: ABC, CBS, NBC, FOX, CNN, Today, Good Morning America, the Discovery Channel, TV Food Network, and CNBC.

It can be fairly safely assumed that most people will agree that a dog does not like to be kicked and will respond to a kick either by attacking the person who kicked it or by running away and will remember that person in a fearful or very resistive if not aggressive manner in the future.

By inference, the same may be said of any animal that is mistreated in some way. So when mice or pigs or primates in an animal research laboratory experience through their own receptor systems a research person like Dr. Melton, they do not experience a kindly gentleman trying to do good for humanity. They experiences someone or something that is trying to do them harm, and all the self-protective alarms in their systems go off in the same way that would happen with any creature who feels threatened, including humans — unless, of course, the researcher finds some way to prevent those alarms from going off.

It is evident from Dr. Melton's interview with Charlie Rose that to Melton an animal is only a "thing" to be used in whatever way meets his research needs in the laboratory, including implanting human disease in it. As a "thing," a mouse can be used according to a hierarchical system that relegates animals to an inferior status that does not confer on them the right to experience "fear" or other self-protective alarms, or, for that matter, any kind of emotion. This also represents the mechanistic Descartian viewpoint of which more and more scientists, like the renowned biologist Rupert Sheldrake, refuse to accept.

It must be acknowledged from the facts, too, that animal researchers are sometimes less than honest in making their case for animal research. For example, when called upon to justify animal testing when confronted with criticisms of animal cruelty and abuse, the animal research industry ignores the criticisms and trots out a list of medical accomplishments it asserts were made because of animal research. In the year 2005 three Nobel Prize winners and 500 eminent academics including 250 professors signed a collective statement that read "Virtually every medical achievement of the last century has depended directly or indirectly on research with animals."[8] Hyperbole like this is the kind of propaganda the animal research industry relies upon and pushes on the public as a rationale for keeping the animal testing motor running and cranking out the money. Animal testing proponents have often seized upon this particular declaration as proof of the necessity for animal research. Yet none of the signatories who signed the declaration have ever provided any evidence or documentation to back up this claim. Does it really have any basis?

Not according to Robert A.J. Matthews, who occupies the position of visiting reader at the Aston University of Information Engineering in Birmingham, England and who is the author of *25 Big Ideas: The Science that's Changing our World.* He is also a science consultant and writer for the BBC. In an article published in the Journal of the Royal Society of Medicine, Matthews challenged the assertion. In fact, his research exposes the statement that this eminent group of academics signed, including the three Nobel Prize winners, as being as phony as a three dollar bill. Not only does it have no basis, it originated as:

> ...a one page statement by the US Public Health Service, dated February 1994 and published in *The Physiologist* under the title 'The Importance of Animals in Biomedical and Behavioral Research.' It contains no citations to the literature supporting the claim; this is simply asserted. Subsequent reiterations of the claim either cite this original unreferenced source, or merely assert it in turn essentially verbatim.[9],[10]

So this declaration is nothing but a false assertion promoted by an elite group of animal research supporters that gets repeated at will by anyone who wants to speak out in favor of animal research with some appearance of authority. There is, however, an opposite arm of propaganda just as powerful as that flexed by the Nobel Prize winners and their academic colleagues. One such example comes from Dr. Charles Mayo (1898-1968), the son of the founder of the Mayo Clinic, a gifted surgeon. and a member of the Mayo Clinic's Board of Governors. Dr. Mayo, said the following:

> I abhor vivisection. It should at least be curbed. Better, it should be abolished. I know of no achievement through vivisection, no scientific discovery, that could not have

been obtained without such barbarism and cruelty. The whole thing is evil.[11]

Today, many within the scientific community concur and voice their disagreement with Descartes and attitudes such as those evinced by Dr. Melton and his scientific colleagues immersed in the mechanistic school of scientific thinking. As Marc Bekoff, a biologist at the University of Colorado and a leading scientist in the field of animal cognition pointed out, if we begin to regard animals as having emotions then "we can no longer treat them as objects; they're not mere things for us to do with what we please."[12]

Scientists like Bekoff are busy showing just how alike human beings and animals often are. These scientists test and debate animal consciousness in relation to living creatures like primates and various other animal species including birds, insects, and earthworms, and in relation to subjects like anthropomorphism, attention, perception, learning, memory, thinking, consciousness, intentionality, communication, planning, play, aggression, dominance, predation, recognition, assessment of self and others, social knowledge, empathy, conflict resolution, reproduction, ecology, evolution, kin selection, neuroethology, and parent-young interactions and caregiving.[13] In the process they are proving what most people know instinctively, that animals do experience emotions like joy, fear, jealousy, anger, impatience, friendship, and love.

The study of animal cognition is making significant inroads in the debate. Steven Siviy, a behavioral neuroscientist at Gettysburg College in Pennsylvania, asks "if you believe in evolution by natural selection, how can you believe that feelings suddenly appeared, out of the blue, with human beings?"[14] In other words, if humans evolved from apes their emotions evolved also. It makes sense, then, that apes have emotions.

It follows that other species also have emotions. Siviy has

shown that when rats play, their brains release large amounts of dopamine, which is associated with pleasure in humans and which also happens in humans when they play.[15] It seems, therefore, that rats also experience pleasure. This, too, is an emotion. Studies also show how the amygdala, an almond-shaped structure in the brain, is activated in both humans and rats when they are angry.[16] It follows, then, that rats experience anger. This also is an emotion.

Chimpanzees, gorillas, and orangutans have all been proven to recognize themselves in a mirror which suggests consciousness.[17] It appears, consequently, that primates are conscious animals. Food storing by birds also suggests "that animals have conscious forethought."[18] Does this mean that consciousness may extend even to birds with their tiny brains? This may indeed be the case. Crows even have the capacity to distinguish one human being from another by observing the differences in their facial characteristics. This is a remarkable ability. How many human beings are able to distinguish one crow from another by their faces, or any part of their anatomy other than, perhaps, their size? Crows have also been observed hiding their food from other crows.[19] This shows consciousness.

But if doubts persist that animals are sentient beings, it would be difficult to deny the conscious forethought of a male chimpanzee in Sweden's Furuvik Zoo who liked to assemble a collection of rocks in the morning before the zoo opened so that he could have a stash ready to throw at zoo visitors around midday in a fit of rage. Mathias Osvath, who wrote up the incident in a paper for the journal Current Biology, concluded that "These observations convincingly show that our fellow apes do consider the future in a very complex way. It implies that they have a highly developed consciousness, including lifelike mental simulations of potential events."[20]

A primatologist at Emory University's Yerkes National Primate Research Center in Atlanta, Ga., said that substantial evidence exists showing that chimps plan for the future. She noted that she had personally "seen chimps poop in their hand, wait, and then throw it at people."[21]

Some scientists, however, are unwilling to admit that animals are conscious, intelligent creatures with feelings no matter what evidence is offered. They are afraid that such an admission would allow anthropomorphism, the identification of human traits with animals, to creep into their work making it impossible to perform vivisection. And they are right. How does one perform some particularly painful operation on an animal that is looking back at you with terrified eyes that read, "Please don't hurt me. Please be kind. Please don't kill me?" How does one look at a band of 20 or so monkeys in a large cage looking like concentration camp victims and note how they have paired off, the partners in each pair clutching each other in terror awaiting the next horror that will befall them as victims of animal researchers? But then, one would have to believe that animals are capable of experiencing terror and horror to believe that they could look at a human being while reflecting the emotions of terror and horror in their eyes and body language.

Scientists who believe animals have no consciousness fear that a general acceptance by the public at large that animals have emotions, consciousness, and intelligence, would give animals rights similar to those human beings have assigned to themselves, the right not to have their freedom and their lives taken from them without their permission, and the right not to be physically abused and have their lives disrespected. This would be a huge blow to the animal testing industry and to the ambitions of a researcher like Dr. Melton in that without animal research he could not implant disease in an animal and watch it develop. At the same time, it would be a boon to those who think medical research is on the wrong road and needs to start going down the trail that pioneers like Dr. Barnard, Dr. Bekoff , Dr. Campbell, Dr. Esselstyn, Dr. McDougall, Dr. Ornish, Dr. Siviy and many others are forging.

Descartes gave science moral permission to experiment on animals to the degree to which it has developed and science took it and followed his lead. There is no reason why science cannot turn in another direction today, and some scientists are already doing that as we have seen.

Moral imperatives do demand the best possible care for children, as Dr. Young and Dr. Silver tell us, but they also demand the same for other species. There is no reason the two cannot coexist. Dr. Melton can continue to pursue other avenues of inquiry that are important to him like making cells for transplantation [in humans] and using cells to find drugs that slow disease. As for following the path of human disease that has been implanted in an animal, it should not be assumed that the same objective cannot be accomplished by other methods like the following.

From a speculative standpoint, science should soon develop better imaging techniques that will permit scientists to observe human disease develop in humans. After all, we can already observe a baby in the womb. This could conceivably even be accomplished before stem cell research achieves its goals which, as Dr. Melton indicated, seems to be many years away.[22] Observing disease develop in a human would naturally provide better results than observing human disease develop in an animal.

An increasing number of people today, including scientists, no longer want to follow the mechanistic path set by Descartes because it is a route that lacks compassion for animals which most people do have and for which they are thankful. Life would be so much more shallow without it. It is this sense of compassion, more than any other, that is so deeply rooted in the lives of the great humanitarian figures in history. Like a beacon in the night, compassion keeps hope alive, revealing the road ahead that leads to the solution of the world's problems. And like Walt Whitman said, "whoever walks a furlong without sympathy walks to his own funeral drest in his shroud."[23]

The Descartes' mechanistic view of animals is narrow and self-centered, and, more than anything, it lacks compassion.

The wheels on the huge NIH gravy train funded by the tax dollars of the citizenry that the biomedical animal research industry has been riding for decades at the expense of innocent animals are antiquated and beginning to screech. And people are listening. More and more scientists today are shunning animal research, using tools from molecular biology, biochemistry, and analytical pharmacology in combination with human tissue and sophisticated computer technologies in developing drugs and in making other important discoveries that render tests on animals obsolete. In fact, the abandonment of animal testing in favor of alternative methodologies by scientists not married to animal testing has already yielded significant results such as 1) embryonic stem cell tests; 2) human skin testing on leftovers from surgical procedures; 3) cell and tissue culture (in vitro) studies used to screen for anti-cancer, anti-AIDS and other types of drugs as well as for producing and testing pharmaceutical products like vaccines, antibiotics, and therapeutic proteins; and 4) sophisticated scanning technologies (MRI, PET, and CT) that can view internal organs in animals including alligators, snakes, and tarantulas, thus eliminating the need for invasive surgical procedures.

In February of 2008, the National Institutes of Health and the Environmental Protection Agency began a five year collaboration using robotic technology and in vitro testing to reduce the need for animal research in toxicity tests.[24] Further innovations in eliminating drug testing on animals include two biochips (Metachip and Datachip) that can be used to predict drug reactions in humans.[25] At Pharmagene Laboratories in Royston, England, scientists every bit as serious as mainstream scientists are studying how drugs affect human genes and the proteins they make without resorting to animal research. In the United States bioengineers at Brown University are working to create tissue models in place of human organs and have developed "three-dimensional freestanding cellular structures from 'building blocks' of living cells."[26] Progress like this reduces the perception of the need for animal testing.

Other advances continue to be made. Linda Griffith, a bioengineer at MIT, has successfully placed a computer chip in human liver tissue for studying how the liver interacts with various drugs and chemicals.[27] And, in December of 2008, Professor Christine Mummery of Leiden University Medical Center in the Netherlands, speaking before the British Pharmacological Society in Brighton in the United Kingdom, showed how it was possible to cultivate human heart cells from embryonic stem cells. Both these techniques could help eliminate the need for using animals in drug testing.[28] Procedures like these are also safer because drugs safely tested on animals often have devastating and life-threatening consequences when they are used by humans. This is a fact that almost everyone acknowledges, including Dr. Melton, as indicated earlier when he admitted that scientists do not know why success in animals cannot always be transferred to humans.

Last but far from least, epidemiological studies of human populations have led to the discovery of the root causes of human diseases including demonstrating the mechanism of AIDS transmission and how it could be prevented. And, as we have seen, T. Colin Campbell's epidemiological studies have isolated the cause of many forms of cancer, heart disease, diabetes, and other chronic diseases. All that is required to put these discoveries into action is to get the medical establishment to stop ignoring these findings.

Science is a wonderful profession that can explore exciting new directions for humanity and the world. Unfortunately, while some biomedical researchers agree that an exhaustive search for alternatives to animal testing is the future direction for medical research, the profession in general shows little enthusiasm for new methodologies, and animal researchers are dragging their feet. All too many would rather continue down the same tired path, and they do not want to admit that other directions exist.

It seems clear that when human beings venture forth in uncharted waters based on an intuitive sense of the possibilities ahead, only profound discovery and adventure lie in wait. This is the history of humankind and it is so fundamental to human existence that we can surely rely upon it. When it comes to medical research, what alternative do we have — eternal dependency upon weaker species that cannot defend themselves against humankind's callousness and cruelty? Surely humans are capable of much, much more.

It is time we left our 17th century views behind and began reaching for a higher destiny where we do not have to abuse other living creatures in order to find cures for our chronic diseases, many of which we have created ourselves. We are living in the 21st century. As we strive to attain our goals, we can make it a century in which we find a better way than by violating the lives of innocent animals who have done us no harm.

Suffer the Little Children

Chapter 22

How Our Diet Puts Our Children at Risk

Congressional Cave-in to the Junk Food Industry

No one questions that children need protection from abusive adults, school bullies, drug dealers, and pedophiles. But there is another kind of menace that has been preying on the nation's school children for decades, robbing them more and more of one of their most precious gifts: their vitality and health. Its most potent manifestation is childhood obesity.

The leader of the menace is the junk food industry. It sets the children up for nutritional deficiencies and starts them down a road toward a lifetime of disease that can only end in premature death. As matters stand, the food companies are drowning our kids in a sea of hot dogs, hamburgers, pizzas, French fries, milk shakes, sugary and fizzy drinks (soda), and sugar products (candy).

At the same time school administrations have not stood up to the junk food industrialists nor have they guided the children to better health. This does not mean schools should impose all kinds of draconian regulations on the kids. But they can take steps, like including nutrition in the school curriculum that teaches in a progressive and fun way the benefits and joys of a good diet and the dangers of poor nutrition. It can be done, and a few concerned educators and nutritionists are trying to introduce more enlightened nutrition programs into the schools when possible.

The root of the problem begins at home and in the diet the children have inherited from the adult world. The children seldom learn, for example, about the benefits of fruits and vegetables, and advocacy in the homes and in the schools promoting the merits of a plant-based, animal-free diet is almost non-existent.

We are now raising generations of children who will live shorter lives than their parents all because of the food they eat. Adults need to improve their own diets and knowledge about nutrition and pass along better eating habits to their children. Until that happens, the children will continue to be easy targets for predatory food marketers.

The National Center for Health Statistics states that in 2003/2004 17 percent of children and adolescents aged from 2 to 19 were overweight or obese, and that is a conservative estimate. Their excessive weight puts them at risk for asthma, hypertension, and depression.[1] Similarly, the Institute of Medicine of the National Academy of Sciences estimated that nine million children over the age of 6 were considered to be obese with 60 percent of overweight children susceptible to cardiovascular risk and Type 2 diabetes.[2,3] One third of boys and even more girls (39 percent) born in the year 2000 are at lifetime risk of developing diabetes under present diet and lifestyle conditions.[4]

Two major factors are responsible for childhood obesity. They are: 1) increased intake of fat and sugar, and 2) a lack of exercise. Children are now getting more than 50% of their daily calories from fat and added sugar (32% and 20% respectively).[5] This far exceeds the 2005 U.S. dietary guidelines recommending that children and teens aged 4 - 18 get between 25% to 35% of their calories from fat. Physical conditioning has also taken a hit. In the last decade of the 20th century, high-school participation in physical education fell off by one-third. By 1996 only 21 percent of middle and high school students were taking part in physical education even one time a week.[6] Junk foods, TV watching, and video games have created a generation of sedentary youth with decreasing interest in outdoor games and physical exercise.[7]

Obesity in children started gaining momentum in the last decades of the 20th century. From 1970 to 1994 overweight kids increased from 15.2% to 27.2% for children 6 to 11 years of age and from 15.2% to 26.6% for adolescents 12 to 17 years of age. In nearly the same time span, 1960 to 1994, overweight adults increased by 24.3% to 35%.[8] This is a substantial increase, and it suggests that children and adolescents are following the nutritional example set by their parents. That should be obvious enough, but the point is that parents afflicted with obesity themselves are hardly role models for teaching their children about good nutrition. Overweight and obese children are not likely to accept guidance about nutrition from parents and the adult world when the parents and adults themselves are overweight and obese. By 2003/2004 the number of overweight or obese adults in the United States stood at 66 percent.[9]

However much the influence of overweight and obese parents plays a role in children's health, other forces are also at work undermining the children's health such as the aggressive television targeting of children and adolescents by food companies. Of particular interest is that besides the 1200 to 1500 hours of TV viewing annually, children are estimated to watch up to 40,000 television commercials a year, many of them promoting the consumption of sugary foods and soft drinks.[10] Junk food industrialists spend an estimated $10 to $12 billion annually for TV ads for youth marketing such as for sampling, coupons, contests, sweepstakes, youth-targeted public relations, school relations, event marketing, and packaging especially designed for children, all to sell more fast foods, snack foods, candy, soft drinks, and sweetened breakfast cereals that are high in calories and fat, low in fiber, and low in nutrient density.[11] In 2002 the annual sales to America's Youth for food and beverages stood at $27 billion.[12]

Obesity is one of the primary symptoms of diabetes which

tripled in school children from the 1980s to 1990s. The obesity connection to sugar sweetened soda is unmistakable. One study found that drinking just one sugary beverage a day increased the risk of obesity in a child by 60%.[13] From 1985 to 1997, soda purchases in schools increased by 1,100 percent.[14] Researchers at the University of Minnesota have also linked the consumption of large quantities of soda to pancreatic cancer.[15]

Schools provide a major source for junk foods for the kids. According to a 2008 report card on school nutrition issued by the Center for Science in the Public Interest (CSPI), two-thirds of our states have few standards "to limit junk-food and soda sales out of vending machines, school stores, and other venues outside of school meals." Margo Wootan, director of nutrition policy at the CSPI tells us that:

> The majority of states still rely on the U.S. Department of Agriculture's outdated school nutrition standards. Those national standards limit only the sale of jelly beans, lollipops, and other so-called 'foods of minimal nutritional value.' Those standards don't address calories, saturated and trans fat, sodium, or other key nutrition concerns for children today.[16]

The CSPI grade school report on school nutrition standards offers a glimpse at the magnitude of the problem. No states received an A. Two states got an A-. Seven states got B+s. Nine states received a B or B- . Five states and the District of Columbia got a C, seven states got Ds, and twenty states got Fs.

School administrations are also responsible for allowing the sale of junk foods in vending machines in various locations around the school grounds. They are paid off to permit this by food companies through exclusive contracts that bring in money in the form of financial arrangements and a variety of incentives like scoreboards and band uniforms.[17]

American taxpayers spend $10 billion a year for the National School Lunch Program (NSLP) that serves 29 million children lunch every school day and is supposed to provide a nutritional diet for school children.[18],[19] However, the program has been encircled by a range of competing interests trying to regulate its management ever since its inception in 1946. These have included farmers, agribusiness operations, school administrators, nutritionists, children's health advocates, and most importantly, the food industry marketing junk foods.[20]

The school lunch program is undermined by two major factors that prevent it from meeting its objectives of providing school children a solid, nutritional lunch. For one, the USDA nutritional guidelines the schools rely on for government funding of the NSLP program are outdated, as indicated above. These standards even list French fries as a vegetable.

The most significant obstacle leading directly to childhood obesity, however, is the alternate source of food that is available to students and upon which many of them rely. This is the junk food sold in school vending machines, cafeteria à la carte lines, and school stores. [21]

Junk food is called "competitive foods" by health professionals because it competes with the NSLP lunch program.[22]

The "competitive foods" diet in the schools increases fat intake and reduces the consumption of fruits and vegetables on which far too little emphasis is placed. In fact, the concept of a plant-based diet is a stranger on school grounds not only to the school kids but also to most teachers and school administrators. It turns out that almost everyone has gone to school, but practically no one has ever learned much about nutrition. It is just not a priority.

"Competitive foods" also launch lifetime diet patterns of reliance on junk foods and additionally are accompanied by commercialism. Stickers are plastered all over vending machines and students are surrounded by advertising logos and merchandise for sale, like shirts, book covers, sports bags, sunglasses, clocks, cups, coolers, and hats.[23] This kind of crass commercialism defiles the image of schools as a place of learning, creative thinking, intellectual stimulation, social skills interaction, vocation preparation, sports activities, events participation, play, and the joys of youth.

Congress has attempted to rein in competitive foods over the decades, but largely without success. In 1970 Congress directed the USDA to set competitive foods guidelines but at the same time demanded restrictions on only candy and soda sold in the school lunch areas. Meanwhile, candy, and soda could still be sold in other areas of the school along with all the other fast food junk. While the schools themselves had the option of implementing stricter guidelines, few considered it important enough to do so.

Two years later, pressured by industry and schools which were losing profits, Congress rescinded the USDA's authority to regulate soda and candy and returned the power back to the schools. This started another cycle of battles with the public demanding more regulation of fast foods, candy, and sugary drinks, and congressmen and congresswomen trying to get regulatory bills passed. Finally, Congress passed the National School Lunch Act and Child Nutrition Amendments of 1977, yet insisted that the USDA should only limit but not ban "foods of minimal nutritional value (FMNV)." This severely weakened the impact of the amendments.[24] The majority in Congress obviously had yet to catch on to the junk food industry's exploitation of the nation's school children.

The new amendments launched another series of battles over how these regulations were to be interpreted, with the National Soft Drinks Association ultimately winning an appellate court ruling that eviscerated the amendment's intent and permitted the sale of soft drinks at all times and in all school locations except the school lunch areas.[25]A year later the USDA amended its regulations to extend protection against soda limitations to include candy. Apart from the school lunch areas, this made it possible to purchase soda and candy in all other school locations at any time.

Congress was now fully stymied. But rather than face up to its obligations, it was unable to mend the crisis until 1994 when Senator Patrick Leahy introduced legislation to "encourage local school authorities to restrict or ban the sale of soft drinks and other items of 'minimal nutritional value.'" This applied, however, only until the end of the last lunch period.[26] That meant in the afternoons the kids could still go wild stuffing themselves with junk.

Even this weak, watered-down bill was met by an avalanche of protest by the junk food industry with Coca-Cola mounting a letter writing campaign against it. This was more than Congress could withstand. It threw in the towel, finally passing a bill that merely put "the choice of when and whether to offer competitive foods squarely in the hands of State of [sic] local officials."[27]

The food industry for junk had won the battle over Congress which had abandoned the school children to the junk food industrialists. The original trickle of "competitive foods" that by this time had already developed into a stream, now roared uncontested like a mighty river of junk through our nation's schools filling the children with fast foods, candy, and sugary drinks.

Little has been done since Senator Leahy's legislation, though Congress passed the 2004 Child Nutrition and Women, Infants, and Children (WIC) Reauthorization Act in 2004 that required local school districts to establish wellness committees by the beginning of the 2006-2007 school year.[28] A new amendment to be attached to the 2007 Farm Bill was introduced by Senator Tom Harkin [Democrat - Iowa] and Senator Lisa Murkowski [Republican - Alaska] that would have restricted vending machine products and eliminated foods high in fat and sugar from à la carte menus that supplement school lunches. The amendment, which had broad support, was thwarted, unfortunately, by procedural maneuvers. Lawmakers, however, promised to revive the amendment as a stand alone bill or attach it to other legislation at a later date. This did happen, as we shall see in the next chapter.[29]

In the meantime, junk food has been available in the schools with little opposition from school administrations, the government, or the courts. Local and state governments, which should have been helping to protect the children from the unscrupulous practices of the junk food industrialists, have also abdicated their roles as the children's defenders. What is best for the children has all but been forgotten in the ongoing squabble. This is exactly what the junk food industry wanted. It has manipulated the government, the judiciary, and school administrations like they were a company of powerless puppets. In the meantime, the children have been left unprotected and have grown more obese with increasing incidences of diabetes and cardiovascular disease.

The direct and indirect costs of obesity in the United States now amounts to $117,000,000,000 per year according to the Surgeon General.[30] That is a lot of zeros and the "reward" the country gets for letting the high-fat, junk food industry take control of nutrition. This is not a legacy the nation should be proud of bequeathing to its children: disease and huge healthcare costs attributed to poor nutrition incurred by treating diet-related diseases that originated in habits acquired in getting a normal, secondary school education.

As we have seen the problems are significant. The need for education about the role diet plays in disease formation and the creation of good health cannot be emphasized enough. The idea of teaching the children about the dangers of meat and dairy products while promoting a greater reliance on an alternative plant-based diet is the obvious solution. Unfortunately, this is seldom considered by the government or educators.

One independently-minded nutritionist who does think about such matters, however, and actually manages to implement these kinds of programs in some schools is Dr. Antonia Demas. She has won national awards for the Most Creative Implementation of the Dietary Guidelines from the US Department of Agriculture and for Excellence in Nutrition Education from the Society for Nutrition Education. The founder of the Food Studies Institute, Dr. Demas works with schools, non-profit organizations, vegetarian societies, and corporations across the country in developing curricula in the schools for healthy, low-fat meals.[31] Under her guidance, children learn about the dangers of fat and the nutritive benefits of delicious plant-based meals from around the world. She teaches a preference for fruits, vegetables, and whole foods over junk foods in attacking the growing epidemic of obesity, heart disease, Type 2 diabetes, and many forms of cancer in the nation's youth.

Another nutritionist working to improve the health of the nation's children is Dr. Pamela A. Popper. A critic of what goes on in the healthcare profession, she is described as "a straight-talking professional who is not afraid to criticize national health organizations, government agencies, medical professionals, pharmaceutical companies, agricultural organizations and manufacturing companies, many of whom have agendas and priorities that interfere with distributing truthful information and promoting public health."[32]

Other efforts around the country are making some headway. In Baltimore, encouraged by the Johns Hopkins Bloomberg School of Public Health, the schools have instituted a Meatless Monday meal program that has turned out to be immensely popular with the students. In New York City, Manhattan borough President Scott Stringer is pushing a similar program, and nationally, momentum is building to turn Meatless

Mondays in the schools into a national agenda. These kind of efforts are much needed and a step in the right direction.[33]

Other people, too, are not taking the situation lying down. Opposition to the junk food industry's marketing of unhealthy products to the children is growing. Parents, especially, have had enough of poor nutrition in the schools and watching the junk food industrialists ride their children's backs. In the next chapter we will examine how some of these voices are making themselves heard.

Chapter 23

Fight-Back in Paradise!

Executives in the Sandbox

On its website Milk Matters, the Eunice Kennedy Shriver National Institute of Child Health & Human Development of the National Institutes of Health advises that Tweens (kids aged 9 - 12) and Teens should get three cups of low-fat or fat-free milk daily. Few in the adult world question the authority of milk, least of all, our government agencies. However, as noted earlier, scientific evidence has revealed that casein, "the main protein in dairy foods, has been shown to experimentally promote cancer and increase blood cholesterol and atherosclerotic plaque." Milk has also been "linked to Type 1 diabetes, prostate cancer, osteoporosis, multiple sclerosis [and] other autoimmune diseases."[1]

Because of evidence like this, it has become increasingly apparent to many adults that the junk food debate needs to include milk. Its disease-causing potential puts it squarely in the junk foods category that children should be taught to avoid. If we were really concerned about our children's health, we would refuse to allow young innocent bodies to consume dairy and meat products. We would also demand that the Department of Agriculture and the National Institutes of Health pay attention to the scientific evidence that shows irrefutably that these products promote cancer and other diseases.

The dairy industry is using our children to sell their products and make themselves rich. Of that there can be no question, as seen from the 2001 annual report of Dairy Management, Inc., an organization that shares in the management of the American Dairy Association, the National Dairy Council, and the U.S.

Dairy Export Council, and also builds demand for America's dairy producers. It offered this advice for increasing milk demand:

> As the best avenue to increase fluid milk consumption long-term, children are without a doubt the future of dairy consumption. That's why the dairy checkoff continues to implement school milk marketing programs as one way to help increase kids' fluid milk consumption.[2]

[The dairy checkoff is a national fund of contributions from milk producers used to promote dairy products.]

The report also advised that marketing goals should be achieved as follows:

1) ongoing activities in advertising, promotion and public relations efforts targeted to children ages six to twelve and their mothers
2) target students, parents, educators and school food-service professionals
3) guide school-age children to become life-long consumers of dairy products
4) protect and enhance consumer confidence in dairy products and the dairy industry

The National Dairy Council has not been shy about applying this kind of advice and even promotes programs that invade and encroach on the schools. Chef Combo's Fantastic Adventures lessons, in which children play games like tasting hot and cold chocolate milk, "was placed in 76% of pre-school kindergarten sites nationally" while lessons like Pyramid Café and Pyramid Explorations conveyed the message to 12 million students that milk and dairy products are important aspects of a healthy diet.[3] Popular lesson plans the Council has promoted, which teachers could download as free lessons for their pupils, have included making hand puppets of cows and dairy foods. Lesson plans also call for setting up a Dairy Treat Day where the children can taste cheese, pudding, yogurt, cottage cheese, and ice cream.[4],[5] Cute lessons like *A Cheesy Tale* have children listen to the story of two cousin mice with different tastes. The children then are asked to compare orange and yellow cheeses using all five of their senses.[6] No doubt, given the chance, they must like the taste sense the best.

Our dairy executives must be enjoying a second childhood as they invent these games.

Fast foods executives selling high-fat meat products have just as much fun. In Seminole County, Florida, McDonald's recently paid for report cards for schoolchildren from kindergarten through the fifth grade on which was printed pictures of McDonald's red-headed clown and the promise of a free "Happy Meal" to all children receiving good marks for grades, behavior, or attendance.[7] The report card notes that a "Happy Meal" includes French fries, a soft drink, and either a hamburger, cheeseburger, or chicken McNuggets.

Food industry executives from McDonald's have also teamed up with toy companies to produce play-food toys like a McDonald's Barbie "fun time play set" on which is inscribed "Lots of yummy food." It contains miniature French fries, Big Macs, and a Sprite soft drink machine. The Hasbro toy company features a McDonald's Play-Doh set that includes molds for hamburgers and buns, and machines for churning out play milkshakes and soft-serve ice cream.[8]

The Pizza Hut "Book It" program executives are also having a grand time. They reward students with a free Pizza Hut personal pizza when they achieve certain reading goals. The program reaches 22 million school children in 900,000 classrooms.

Many parents are offended that McDonald's is permitted to

supply their children with report cards containing advertising logos, and want to know what food companies are doing in the school classrooms. Free treats like McDonald's "Happy Meals" and Pizza Hut's "Book It" personal pizzas contribute to childhood obesity. Consider that an adult male would have to walk nine miles to burn off the calories from one McDonald's double whopper or that a six-inch Pizza Hut personal pizza contains 630 calories and 27 grams of fat.[9] Add a topping, and you get 770 calories and 39 grams of fat. That's without a soda or any other fast food embellishments.

The total recommended fat intake for lunch for children in grades 7 through 12 (the grades with the highest fat intake requirements for all school children) based on USDA standards is 28 grams. That is 11 grams below the 39 grams of fat provided by one Pizza Hut personal pizza with topping, and, as stated, that is without a soda.[10]

The calorie standards set by the Food and Nutrition Board of the National Academy of Sciences for moderately active children suggest the consumption of 1600 to 2000 calories daily for girls and 1800 to 2200 for boys, aged 9 to 13. From ages 14 to 18, the recommended calorie intake is 2000 for girls and 2400 to 2800 for boys.[11] This means that the 770 calories contained in a six-inch Pizza Hut personal pizza with topping is a sizeable chunk of the daily allowance for calorie intake. For ages 14 to 18 it comes to 38.5% of calories for girls, and ranges from 27.5% to 32% for boys. For children aged 9 to 13, it comes to as much as 38.5% to 48% of calories for girls and 42% for boys. And again, that is without a soda. Add a 12 oz. can of soda, and you get another 150 calories. These percentages leave little room for all the other food (meals and in-betweens) to be eaten during the day. Obviously, many children eating a six-inch Pizza Hut personal pizza with topping will go way over their daily calorie allowance before they go to bed at night. With inducements like this, why obesity in children is on the rise is hardly a mystery.

If there is to be change, much of it will have to come from the public, and a growing number of advocacy groups and civic organizations composed of parents, concerned citizens, and private healthcare professionals are beginning to rise up, though they are still few in number. But more and more parents are becoming outraged by how the junk food industry, the nation's schools, the government regulatory agencies, the Congress, and the courts have worked against the best interests of the nation's children in building the current obesity epidemic. Parents want to know why the government has done so little to protect their children. They would like to know why schools that are supposedly in the business of education and childhood guidance have put the health of their children second and the needs of food companies first.

Food companies marketing junk have grown rich at the expense of the nation's children without embarrassment, shame, or guilt. Even when exposed to the full glare of public light, they battle to continue distributing their cocktail of fat and sugar to the country's youth, unconcerned about the harm they are causing. Opponents have suggested many counteractions to combat their influence including lawsuits. The food companies just argue that lawsuits drive up the price of their foods because they will pass along the legal costs to the consumer.

However that may be, lawsuits have proved effective in causing some companies to revise their advertising and nutritional practices. Under pressure from a suit by the Center for Science in the Public Interest (CSPI), Burger King agreed to stop using trans fats. The Campaign for a Commercial-Free Childhood, the CSPI, and two Massachusetts parents sued Kellogg, forcing the company to agree to adopt nutrition standards for food it advertises to young children and to stop using cartoon characters like SpongeBob unless it meets those standards. CSPI, the Clinton Foundation, and the American Heart Association also negotiated with Coca-Cola, PepsiCo, and

Cadbury Schweppes to phase-out some sugary soft drinks from schools.[12]

Many children's advocates think that in order to stop the food industry from marketing junk to children it will take dozens of lawsuits. They see the same scene playing out that was necessary to force tobacco companies to stop marketing cigarettes to children. These people think it will take years to accomplish their goal and say that the food companies selling junk, as was the case with tobacco, will resist to the end.

Some adversaries propose levying heavy fines on the food companies if they do not participate in obesity-lowering programs. Others want them to pay higher taxes. Still others want the government to step in and order changes in the way food companies market their products. These activists would also like to compel school administrations to control fat and sugar foods they permit on school property.

The obesity crisis is not just an American problem. Food marketers to children have spread across the face of the globe, and wherever they go the obesity problems associated with their activities follow right along.

Food industrialists are more responsive to criticism in Europe where they at least fear whatever government regulations exist enough to comply with them. In the United States it is a different story. Here, where timid government agencies show little inclination to impose regulations, the junk food industry opposes nutritional limitations unrepentantly and often successfully. Bruce Silverglade, legal affairs director for the Center for Science in the Public Interest, describes the picture as follows:

U.S. based food companies are complying with government initiatives in Europe that curb junk food advertising to kids, limit fat and salt content in processed foods, and call for nutrition information on the fronts of food packages, but are opposing such steps in the U.S. — in effect treating European consumers better than Americans.[13]

Silverglade says that the Food and Drug Administration, the Federal Trade Commission, and other U.S. agencies are far from aggressive in cracking down on junk food advertising and points out as an example that the Nestlé company complies with British advertising curbs, but does not even participate in the U.S. self-regulatory initiative to which the food industry agreed. (See below regarding the FTC and corporate self-regulation.) The United Kingdom and France have already set reduction standards for salt content in processed foods, and Denmark has eliminated the use of trans fats. In the United States, however, the FDA requires no restrictions. But even though the FDA and the USDA have proven to be weak defenders of parents' and children's interests when it comes to combating the junk food industry, increasing pressure can get Congress to enact legislation that will, in turn, force these agencies to do a better job.

Many people believe that a total ban on junk food is the only real action that can effect a cure, but until that can be achieved, consumer groups are beginning to network to fight the attempts of the junk food companies to falsely advertise their products.[14] Support groups have formed not only in the United States but around the world where childhood obesity has reached as far as urban China.[15] The Indian Federation of Consumer Organizations in New Delhi, the Consumers Association of Penang in Malaysia, the Swedish Consumers Coalition in Stockholm, and coalitions in Mexico, Australia, Uganda, and Canada have launched campaigns against the obesity menace.[16]

In December of 2007 the Mexican consumer group that calls itself Consumer Power exposed a Coca-Cola elementary school campaign portraying "Coca-Cola as one of several beverages that can be used for thirst after physical activity."[17] In 2008, consumers in 20 countries launched a Center for Science in the Public Interest organized "Global Dump Soft Drinks" campaign aimed directly at Coca-Cola and PepsiCo. The campaign demanded that the companies help curtail childhood obesity. In Japan, where so far obesity is relatively low, but where Coca-Cola is trying to promote sugary teas and other sweetened beverages, the Global Dump Soft Drinks campaign is trying to put a stop to the company's promos before their products can take root. Among its general demands, the campaign is calling on Coca-Cola and PepsiCo to stop marketing sugar and caffeine beverages to children under the age of 16 and to stop selling all sweetened beverages in all private and public elementary schools, middle schools, and high schools.[18]

In England a Scottish member of the Parliament proposed a bill to ban junk food marketing aimed at children that would include a ban on cartoon characters, games, and child friendly competitions printed on food and drink packaging.[19] The Daily Post pointed out, however, that the effort was a mere drop in the ocean. What was needed, the newspaper said, was a total ban of junk food in the schools where vending machines selling sugary drinks and chocolate, and canteens offering chips, burgers, and pizza existed in abundance (just like in America).[20]

According to a poll conducted by the Opinion Research Corporation in April of 2008, 57 percent of Americans, 68 percent of people in Great Britain, 76 percent of Spaniards, and 61 percent of Hungarians want their governments to take stronger action in curbing childhood obesity and other nutritional health problems. As the general public becomes more aware of the harm the children are being exposed to from junk foods, these figures should rise. Presently, only 36 percent think food companies are doing their job in limiting junk food advertising to children.[21]

Opposition to present food standards is growing. Already 82 percent of Americans want food companies to do more to reduce fat, sugar, and salt in all their products, not just for children. And 78 percent stated that they wanted fast-food and chain restaurants to disclose nutrition information on menus and menu boards. In this case, at least, the government seems to have listened. The Obama administration's healthcare legislation of 2010 stipulates that large chains like Burger King, McDonald's, and Starbucks must list the calorie content of their foods. Vending machines must do the same.

As we have seen, The FDA, the USDA, and other industry-favoring government agencies go easy on food companies. It took a barrage of criticism before the FTC finally resigned itself to having to do something, so it accepted a set of nutrition guidelines designed by the food industry itself with which the food industry would voluntarily comply. Weak, self-regulatory initiatives like this are all too typical of the kind of change United States government agencies, subservient to business interests, agree to institute when they are criticized.

Meanwhile, the USDA continues to follow the nutritional guidelines for schools it set in 1966 which do not consider candy bars, snack cakes, or French fries to be junk food.

In the United States Congress a few politicians did finally come forward to make nutrition recommendations for the schools. In 2007, as noted in chapter 22, Senator Tom Harkin and Senator Lisa Murkowski introduced an amendment to the 2007 Farm Bill that would have set new nutritional guidelines according to the "gold-standard" recommendations for school nutrition set by the National Academy of Science's Institute of Medicine, which advises Congress on such matters.[22] When the bill failed due to procedural matters, Senator Harkin reintroduced the amendment in April of 2009 as a companion bill to H.R. 1324 which was introduced by Lynn Woolsley [Democrat – California, 6th District] in the House of Representatives.

Harkin's bill, named the Child Nutrition Promotion and School Lunch Protection Act (S. 934), authorizes the Secretary of

Agriculture to regulate the sale of foods sold outside of the federal school nutrition programs — junk foods, in other words. The bill also amends the Child Nutrition Act of 1966 to require the Secretary of Agriculture to establish science-based nutrition standards for all competitive foods. That means the end of classifying French fries as a vegetable.

The Harkin legislation has 31 co-sponsors including some of the most powerful senators and is supported by the American Dental Association, the American Diabetes Association, the American Dietetic Association, the American Heart Association, the Center for Science in the Public Interest, and the School Nutrition Association. It now sits with the Senate Committee on Agriculture, Nutrition, and Forestry where prospects are high that it will be passed onto the Senate floor for a vote as part of the Healthy, Hungry-Free Kids Act (HHFKA).

It seems fairly certain, unfortunately, that no matter what happens, the dairy industry will escape unscathed and continue to market its products in the schools. And while the consumption of meat products may be reduced to some extent if the HHFKA passes, the dangers of consuming meat will still be hidden from view. That is because the current nutrition guidelines employed by the Institute of Medicine, to which Congress and the USDA will turn for guidance if the HHFKA is passed, are the same ones that all the other government agencies follow which do not fully acknowledge the dangers posed by meat and dairy products.

As should be apparent from the examples offered in this book, once they become adults, many children will eventually pay the price in cancer, heart disease, stroke, diabetes, osteoporosis, and other debilitating conditions if they continue to consume meat and dairy products after they leave school. And, unfortunately, adults often carry forward the dietary patterns they pick up in school for the remainder of their lives. That is why the schools are the perfect place to teach good nutrition, if only we would take advantage of the opportunity.

Kelly Brownell, the Chair of the Psychology Department at Yale University, and co-author with Katherine Battle Horgen of *Food Fight*, describes the childhood obesity epidemic as follows:

> We have failed our children, pure and simple. Nine million just in America are heavy enough to be in immediate health danger. And obesity is but one of many problems brought on by poor diet and lack of physical activity....The nation cannot afford a repeat of the tobacco history, where the federal government was very slow to react because of industry influence. Many other institutional changes are necessary as well, with food marketing to children and foods in schools as prime examples.[23]

Today's children are tomorrow's adults, and we are producing a nation of increasingly obese people prone to diabetes, cardiovascular disease, stroke, cancer, and other life-threatening conditions.

The failure to adequately come to grips with the problem of childhood obesity remains a major challenge. We do everything in our power to keep sexual predators and other criminals away from the children, including enacting legislation that keeps drug dealers at a certain distance from our schools. We should do the same with the junk food industry if we are to protect the children from abuses related to diet and nutrition. At the same time, at home and in the schools we need to begin showing the children the way for a lifetime of healthy living and well-being. But before we can do that, we adults have to learn it ourselves. And there is a considerable distance to travel before we reach that destination.

The Road to a Solution

Chapter 24

Hamburger Heaven

How the Diet of the Western World is Creating Poverty in the Developing Countries and Threatening the Future of the Earth

In his 1964 Nobel Peace Prize acceptance speech, Martin Luther King, Jr. declared: "I have the audacity to believe that peoples everywhere can have three meals a day for their bodies."[1] It is now more than 45 years later and some 1.4 billion people in the world are living in extreme poverty on less than $1.25 a day.[2] With the world's total population presently standing at around 6.7 billion that means that one person out of every five is impoverished.

Today, Martin Luther King would no doubt be very disappointed to learn that his *audacity* still has so far to go before it is realized, especially for children. In impoverished countries more than one-third of the deaths of children under the age of five are due to child or maternal undernutrition.[3] Nearly twenty million children worldwide are severely malnourished, and famine is all too frequently an unwelcome and threatening guest in the developing world.[4]

A closer look at the causes of poverty reveals that the pending storm looming across the world's horizon is stirred in large part by the habits of the Western world where the reliance upon land to grow feed for livestock means not enough land is available to grow food for the developing countries. The connection involving the consumption of animal protein to larger issues such as individual and public health, environmental damage to the earth and the atmosphere, agricultural animal cruelty, and world poverty is unmistakable. Even some nutritionists who take the side of recommending a limited consumption of animal protein recognize the danger. Dr. Andrew Weil, for example, notes that "raising animals for meat wastes precious natural resources, including food and water, and it is a surprisingly important factor in the worsening pollution of soils, water tables, and air all over the planet."[5] Hopefully, the dawning recognition of just how serious the problem really is will give Weil and others, including our healthcare organizations, cause to revise their position on the advisability of consuming animal protein. Even a small amount consumed individually if multiplied by billions of people adds up to an enormous amount of animals being slaughtered for meat or being used in the production of dairy products.

Jeremy Rifkin, President of the Foundation on Economic Trends and author of *Beyond Beef, the Rise and Fall of the Cattle Culture*, reported that in the United States alone, 157 million metric tons of cereal, legumes and vegetable protein is fed to livestock which converts to 28 million metric tons of animal protein for human consumption.[6] While this is an indication that the Protein Gods are presently in control of the American diet, it does not satisfy the meat industrialists who are reaching out to expand the consumption of animal protein in the developing world. There they are busily at work promoting the same process of feedlot production (Confined Animal Feed Operations (CAFOs)) to increase meat output that has been successfully employed in the West.

Food corporations marketing meat can only profit when people eat meat, and so they advertise everywhere to encourage people to eat as much meat as possible. Rifkin points out that sales campaigns equate grain-fed "feedlot" cows (in contradistinction to grass-fed "pasturage" cows) to a country's prestige where consuming animal protein has increasingly become "the mark of success" in the developing countries.[7]

The big difference for the meat executives between grass-fed cows and cows that are grain-fed is that for grass-fed cows, grazing fields can only supply a limited amount of grass to feed a limited number of cows that require a large land space per cow for grazing. With grain-fed cows, a large amount of grain can be brought to a huge number of cows that can be divided up and confined on a limited land space (feedlots). That means more cows on less land where it is far easier to raise large herds of cows economically. This results in much larger profits for the meat executives.

While it goes without saying that CAFOs spell good fortune for agribusiness, they also spell misfortune for the future of the planet. For starters, the process engenders poorer health for feedlot cows, which occurs from feeding on low-nutrient grain. This gets passed onto people who consume the grain-fed beef and then develop various diseases. That occurs as follows.

Feed grain consists of genetically modified grain and soy that may include by-products such as municipal garbage, chicken feathers, stale pastry, candy, and other miscellaneous crud.[8] But it also includes a much more dangerous product. Howard Lyman, author of *Mad Cowboy: Plain Truth from the Cattle Rancher Who Won't Eat Meat*, reports that 80 percent of pesticides used in America is targeted on "four specific crops — corn, soybeans, cotton, and wheat — the major constituents of livestock feed." These pesticides are carcinogenic, and when animals eat feed grain that is contaminated with these poisons they store them in their fat [9] This gets passed onto humans if they eat the meat of cows because this meat is infused with the contaminated fat. The meat industry proudly calls this fat "marbling" because the more marbling in the meat, the juicier and more flavorful the meat is held to be. The USDA uses the amount of marbling in beef to determine quality grades. Meat with the highest concentration of marbling is awarded the highest grade, Prime. Next comes Choice followed by Select, Standard, Commercial, Utility,

Cutter, and Canner.

Cud-chewing animals are born to roam freely in wide-open pastures. Grazing is natural and good for the welfare of cows. They are destined by nature to eat high-fiber content grass and shrubs, not to be confined in small pens to be fed low-nutrient, starchy, low-fiber modified grains contaminated with pesticides and filled with by-products which increase their fat content.

The feed grain when consumed by cows also results in unhealthy but common conditions like subacute acidosis that cause cows to kick at their stomachs and to eat dirt. To prevent negative reactions like this, cows are given chemical additives and a continuous diet of low-level antibiotics to which bacteria become resistant. No medications have been developed to treat these disease-resistant bacteria which also get passed onto humans when they consume beef. In addition, grain-fed cows have less vitamin E, beta-carotene, vitamin C, and omega-3 fatty acids in their systems.[10]

Beef, as we have seen, is one of the chief causes of nutritionally-related diseases in humans. It is an unhealthy and dangerous product because of the saturated fat and cholesterol it contains. Eating the high-calorie fat that has materialized in the cows from the carcinogenic feed grain just adds to the danger, especially for developing cancer. Consuming meat that contains drug-resistant bacteria is not exactly healthy either. The USDA seems not to have caught on yet even though the healthcare industry now uniformly recommends meat consumption only in the form of lean (low-fat) meat precisely because of the linkage of fat to cancer and heart disease. It is time for the USDA to reappraise its grading system for beef so that the most marbling gets the lowest grade, not the highest.

Dairy cows that are grain fed, like beef cows, require antibiotics too, because they need protection from diseases caused by excessive milking. These antibiotics get into the milk the cows produce and are also suspects as disease-producing agents. The same applies to bovine growth hormone which is injected into the cows to increase their milk production and, as noted earlier, is suspected as a cause of breast cancer, colon cancer, and prostate cancer.

A major problem caused by cows living on feedlots also occurs because cows dump an enormous quantity of manure on the ground which farmers are unable to dispose of in an economically feasible and ecologically safe manner. The farmers either have to move the manure out of the feedlot pens to a vacant area where it collects in huge "mountains," haul it off their property and deposit it elsewhere, create water lagoons to contain it, or dispose of it through a combination of these methods. But however they manage the manure, a sizeable portion ends up seeping into the soil as groundwater where it contaminates streams and rivers. Groundwater is an important source for drinking water and is used by more than 50% of the people in the United States. It is important to keep it pristine clear and as free from contaminants and pesticides as possible.

Just how much waste is involved? Howard Lyman reports that on a typical feedlot containing 10,000 cows, the cows produce half a million pounds of dung every day. Larger feedlots containing 100,000 cows "have a waste problem equal to that of the largest American cities." Lyman further notes that it has been "estimated that animal wastes are responsible for ten times as much water pollution in America as the human population....Moreover, every year thousands of cattle carcasses are left to rot in streams and rivers, polluting them further."[11]

With an estimated 27 billion animals being slaughtered in the United Sates alone every year for food, and countless billions more waiting until their time comes to be slaughtered, the many problems that are present in relation to animal waste disposal are staggering to contemplate.

Developing nations that want to emulate Western countries are too desperate to adequately assess the problems associated with their ambitions, and so set about increasing their meat supply. The first step in fulfilling the rags to riches saga is to install affordable chicken and egg production facilities. Next in the sequence comes the production of pork along with milk and dairy products produced by *grass-fed* cows. The penultimate step is to produce cows that are *grain-fed*. The final goal is to become a country where the mainstay of the diet is grain-fed beef and dairy products.[12]

The grain required to feed the livestock that rich countries consume is a key ingredient in the creation of poverty in the developing countries. That is because much of the developing world's land is being converted from grain or crop-bearing fields, which could be used to feed the poor, into grain-growing fields which are used to feed livestock to be slaughtered for the wealthy to consume.[13] This model of growing grain to feed livestock for human consumption has become the worldwide trend as agribusiness corporations promote the conversion of land that is used to grow crops for food, to land that is used to grow feed for animals.

The process started in the 1970s after green revolution technologies of the mid-20th century enabled farmers to increase food production in Mexico, India, and Pakistan by employing fertilizers, pesticides, and improved irrigation technologies, and by planting high-yielding crops. The new technology was welcomed and spared an estimated billion people from starvation. It was a brilliant success.

During this period the Food and Agriculture Organization (FAO) of the United Nations urged developing countries to grow coarse grains that could be used to feed livestock. The United States government stepped in and tied food-aid to countries that were willing to develop feed grain markets. At the same time agriculture companies were procuring low-interest government loans to set up livestock operations in these developing countries.[14] All was well so long as the food surpluses created by the green revolution held out. But when food supplies dwindled, the FAO still advised the developing countries to continue on the same path of converting croplands for people to grainlands for livestock.[15] This was not such a brilliant success.

Many nations have now switched from being food producers for people to being feed producers for livestock. Without surpluses to back up this kind of policy, as was the case in the "green revolution," however, the results can be devastating. For countries without enough food, land needs to be used to grow crops for people, not grain for livestock. In 1984, for example, Ethiopia was using a sizeable portion of its land to produce linseed cake, cottonseed cake, and grapeseed meal for export to the United Kingdom and other European nations as feed for livestock.[16] At the same time thousands of Ethiopians were dying from famine. This land used to grow feed for livestock could have been used to grow crops for the people who were starving.

A huge environmental problem also occurs when it comes to feeding livestock because of the worldwide emission of greenhouse gasses that emanate from the mammoth herds of billions of animals used for food. According to a major report by the FAO called *Livestock's Long Shadow*, livestock is responsible for 18 percent of greenhouse gasses, the three most potent being carbon dioxide, methane, and nitrous oxide.[17] Animals contribute 9% of total carbon dioxide, 37% of methane, and 65% of nitrous oxide emissions globally with the percentages increasing yearly. Agricultural emissions of greenhouse gasses are even higher than the entire transportation sector (automobiles, trucks, etc.). In fact, manure alone is said to produce a global-warming effect equal to 33 million automobiles.

Many people connect livestock emissions to global warming, and citizens have begun to mount international campaigns to combat climate change such as Meatless Mondays, and Less Meat = Less Heat. Beatle Paul McCartney has lent his name in support of the latter. A few scientists, however, like University of

California at Davis Professor Frank Mitloehner, claim that cattle emissions have little to do with climate change. Among scientists, this is a minority view.

Added to the environmental woes described above is the fact that 8% of the water that should be for human use goes to irrigate the crops that are used to feed the world's livestock.[18]

As seen in the foregoing narrative, the world is facing a growing crisis. It's cause is the consumption of animal-protein.

U.S. Census figures reveal that the world population presently stands at 6.7 billion. It will reach 9 billion by the year 2045. How much land will then be required to house and feed the billions of livestock the world depends upon for animal protein, and how many more animals will need to be slaughtered to produce it? How will the manure even be disposed of that all these animals will generate? At present, annual methane emissions from manure decomposition is estimated at 17.5 million tons. [20]And, according to a USDA report made in 1986, already only one-sixth of the manure from hog-raising operations was usable in any way. The rest ended up as groundwater that flowed into streams and rivers where it contributed to nitrogen, phosphorus, and nitrate pollution.[19]

Agribusiness corporations, however, operating in poorer countries tend not to be overly concerned about problems like these. They are focused primarily on profit which they acquire in a variety of ways like the sale of seed, farm chemicals, and cattle; the purchase and ownership of land; the production of livestock; and the manufacture of food.

An example of corporate, industrial expansion into foreign lands is Virginia-based Smithfield Farms, the world's largest producer of pork. In the year 2000 Smithfield killed 27 million pigs. Pigs produce three times more excrement than humans do, and the waste at Smithfield Farms comes to an estimated 26 million tons a year. Much of the waste is allowed to run out into the fields where it sits until the elements break it down and it becomes groundwater that eventually finds its way into rivers and streams.[21]

Smithfield has expanded into a 7.75 billion Euro multinational conglomerate operating in 13 countries on three continents. It buys up farms and converts them into Smithfield operations that are politically connected to the governance of local economies in ways that often have devastating consequences to local residents.[22] Using its political muscle, for example, the Smithfield operation in Romania, where Smithfield owns 25 pig farms, managed to sidestep environmental laws so that it was allowed to pollute as a heavy industry. In Northern Poland, Smithfield's political allies managed to get liquid manure reclassified as an agricultural product which weakened the local laws on waste.

Smithfield now owns several farms in Poland where the company operates behind a front company, Prima Foods, because the Polish laws prohibit foreign companies from purchasing farms. Smithfield has also acquired a controlling interest in Animex, one of the country's largest meat processors. Besides their farms containing 55,000 pigs, Smithfield operations in Poland also involve cows, turkeys, chickens, geese, and feed grain.

Wherever Smithfield locates, the area's residents live with foul odors, headaches, and falling property values. Local populations have suffered eye infections and rashes emanating from lagoons on Smithfield properties containing pig waste.[23] The stench from Smithfield farms also affects the tourist industry, and small farms that cannot compete are forced into bankruptcy. In Wiezkowice, Poland in 2002, pigs died by the hundreds in overstocked storage buildings, and their bodies laid for days sickening the local population with the stench.

Adding to Smithfield's tarnished reputation, in Starachowice, Poland, workers at a Smithfield-run Constar plant were discovered scraping the mold off of old sausage meat and sending it to stores with new expiration dates.[24] After they got to know what Smithfield was all about by contending with three of their farms, residents in the Goldap region of Poland picketed and protested Smithfield plans to build four new farms in the area which would have contained over 4,000 pigs on each. The locals were victorious.

According to the Helsinki Commission, Smithfield is damaging the ecosystem with its pollution. The manure on the company's fields is contaminating water systems around the Baltic sea, and ammonia and nitrogen waste from Smithfield farms is seeping into the soil.[25]

Filthy conditions on farms like Smithfield also increase the possibility of animals spreading diseases like avian flu, pig fever, and Nipah that can be transmitted to nearby communities. Nipah is a central nervous system and respiratory virus contracted from fruit bats that infect pigs and can be transmitted to humans. It can be fatal. Swine fever (a different disease) struck a Smithfield farm in Romania in 2007. As in Poland, the bodies of pigs laid for days before being carted away. Thirty-nine thousand pigs in the surrounding region had to be killed to stop the spread of this highly infectious disease.[26]

The kind of name a company like Smithfield builds hardly recommends the United States to the rest of the world. Yet Congress continues to tolerate companies like Smithfield whose activities damage the country's reputation abroad.

An important question worth asking is how long will the planet survive the voracious and insatiable appetites of agribusiness corporations like Smithfield farms? Land space has already become an issue of global proportions. Stephen Leckie of the International Development Research Center lays out the problem in very clear terms in a report titled *How Meat-Centered Eating Patterns Affect Food Security and the Environment*. Leckie points out the startling possibility that "as the human population expands to close to 9 billion hungry people in the coming decades, it is not hard to imagine every last forest, wetland, and grassland being leveled for agriculture."[27]

Already 70% of global freshwater consumption and 38 percent of the entire ice-free land surface is used for livestock, as stated in a report by the United Nations Environment Program (UNEP).[28] In addition, the *Livestock's Long Shadow* FAO United Nations' report referred to earlier tells us that:

> ...the livestock sector is a major stressor on many ecosystems and on the planet as a whole. Globally, it is one of the largest sources of greenhouse gasses and one of the leading causal factors in the loss of biodiversity.... Livestock is a sector of striking contrasts.... It causes considerable environmental damage in terms of climate change and air pollution, water supply and quality, and biodiversity. This is in stark contrast to the positive effects in waste recycling and conservation of non-renewable resources that characterized most mixed farming following the Agricultural Revolution. At the same time livestock-dependent livelihoods of people living in, or at the margins of poverty, are threatened....Given the planet's finite resources, and the additional demands on the environment from a growing and wealthier world population, it is imperative for the livestock sector to move rapidly toward far-reaching change.[29]

As our study has revealed, vast areas of land in the developing world are being used for producing feed for livestock that could be used to raise plant-based foods for the impoverished people of the world. According to the UNEP report cited above "more than half of the world's crops are used to feed animals, not people."[30] Paul Roberts, author of *The End of Food*, says that "every time an American bites down on a steak or hamburger, they're contributing to global hunger....If the rest of the world were to eat like we do, the planet would collapse."

More and more people in the developing world, however, are copying Western habits and biting into that hamburger, one of the great symbols of Western prosperity. And as the developing countries turn increasingly toward the West for ways to achieve wealth, they also are inheriting the consequences of Western success which includes assimilating the diseases associated with the affluent nations. Rifkin sums up the dilemma as follows:

> The irony of the present system is that millions of wealthy consumers in the first world are dying from diseases of affluence (heart attacks, strokes, diabetes, cancer) brought on by gorging on fatty grain-fed meats, while the poor in the third world are dying of diseases of poverty brought on by the denial of access to land to grow food grain for their families. We are long overdue for a global discussion on how best to promote a diversified, high-protein, vegetarian diet for the human race.[31]

Worldwatch Institute, an independent interdisciplinary research organization on environmental issues since 1974, informs us that 56 billion animals are already raised and slaughtered for food each year, a conservative approximation.[32] As we have also seen, an estimated 27 billion animals are slaughtered in the United States alone.[33] Present world demand for meat of 280 million tons is expected to increase by twice as much by the year 2050. Milk production is also expected to almost double to 1043 million tons in the same time frame.[34] Most of this increase will happen in the developing world. This presents a very large problem because the environmental damage caused by livestock is already significant, and, according to the FAO, "the environmental impact per unit of livestock production must be cut by half, just to avoid increasing the level of damage beyond its present level"[35]

The Western world's obsession with eating animal protein has brought cancer, heart disease, stroke, diabetes, and many other chronic diseases to our relatives and friends. The air we breathe is poisoned and our streams and rivers are contaminated. And now big money industrialists have exported this obsession to the developing countries where the people eagerly grasp for the next rung up the economic ladder of success. This means they want more meat and diary products like their wealthy friends to the West. Fast food restaurants are everywhere, and the people living in the developing world are falling victim to the affluent killer diseases of the Western world.

There is no escaping that considerable blame for the enormous problems facing the people of the earth today must be laid at the doorstep of animal consumption. And, it is happening to an extent that is beginning to threaten the future of the earth.

T. Colin Campbell says "it turns out that if we eat the way that promotes the best health for ourselves, we promote the best health for the planet. By eating a whole foods, plant-based diet, we use less water, less land, fewer resources and produce less pollution and less suffering for our farm animals."[36]

If this earth is to survive far into the future without cataclysmic disruption and intense global suffering that is directly connected to the eating habits of the world's citizens, the consumption of animal protein must be looked at in the hardest and most objective terms. All of the problems that are inherent in consuming animal protein can be avoided. All we have to do is to stop eating animals and dairy foods. When we do, many of our diseases will fade away, much of the pollution of our rivers will stop, a significant percentage of the poisoning of our atmosphere will disappear, a major percentage of the exploitation and abuse of animals on factory farms and in research laboratories will end, and we will have taken an enormous step toward eliminating poverty everywhere in the world.

Chapter 25

The World is Waiting for the Sunrise

The Divorce of Ethics and Profit

In 1953 newly elected President Dwight D. Eisenhower named General Motors President Charles E. Wilson to be his Secretary of Defense. At the confirmation hearing before Congress, Wilson was asked if he was capable of making a decision contrary to the interests of General Motors. He replied that he could, but that it was difficult to imagine a situation that would require him to do so because he had assumed for years that "what was good for the country was good for General Motors and vice versa." General Motors was the largest corporation in the United States at the time, and Wilson's comment was soon fashioned into one of the most famous misquoted quips: "What is good for General Motors is good for the country!" It quickly became the watchword for describing hard-nosed, cynical businesses and business people.

Misquoted or not, all too often this is the model that businesses pursue in their relentless pursuit of profit. In February of 2009 the president of a peanut butter company was subpoenaed before Congress to investigate charges he had knowingly shipped salmonella contaminated products to customers with a false certificate certifying they were satisfactory. Upon receipt of a positive laboratory reading for salmonella, he had also reportedly sent the peanut butter to another lab to try to get a negative reading and complained in an e-mail to his plant manager that "the time lapse, besides the cost is costing us huge $$$$$."[1]

Some people would call this man's actions criminal. Others

would say he was just following "business as usual" procedures in the tough-minded business world where the normal range of ethics need not apply. In this kind of world "what is good for [fill in the name of the company] is good for the country" is the only ethical standard worth pursuing. If you are a business person and you want to play with the big boys and girls, come in as hard as nails, and come in prepared to win at any cost. If you don't like the way the game is played and you're still in love with business, go open a Ma and Pa shop on Main Street someplace. But if that's the case, don't call us. We'll call you.

On a financial advice television program that aired several years ago, the host regularly invited stock brokers specializing in tobacco products to appear on his show to be interviewed by himself and a panel of other stock brokers.[2] The host and his panel would sit around discussing market forecasts, past performance charts, and future profit expectations with the guest in relation to tobacco, indifferent to the fact that the very nature of their conversation was an endorsement of a known promoter of lung cancer and heart disease. It almost seemed like they were intentionally saying, "See! We are a special brand of business people. Ethics have no place in guiding our decisions. All that matters in this kind of world is profit."

In this book we have seen how profit as the bottom line has prevented healthcare information from reaching the public that could eliminate suffering and save the lives of many people. We have seen how it has destroyed the lives of many of our children and is continuing to do so. We have seen how profit motive undeterred by ethical considerations has reached out across the world to exploit and use land for profit without consideration of the poverty left behind. We have seen how it has imposed cruelty and brutality upon innocent, defenseless animals in university laboratories and on factory farms, and we have seen how it damages our forests, fields, rivers, and streams and the atmosphere upon which the population of the world depends for survival.

In 2009, National Public Radio reported that the Japanese national economy had declined 12% because of its dependency on the U.S. economy which itself was in crisis. In the United States, institutional, private, and foreign investors lured on by huge profit potential inflated by bankers and mortgage lenders with phony mortgage derivatives, all came tumbling to earth in a great humpty dumpty fall, sending the economy into a downward spiral that carried the world economy along with it. This caused immense suffering for the world in the loss of jobs, the loss of homes, the disappearance of life-fulfilling opportunities, the splitting up of families, and increased poverty around the world where in some instances even peasants in China had their wages cut in half. To some it was just another game the finance boys and girls played that turned sour, like with the dot-com companies that soared into the stratosphere in the late 1990s before that balloon burst and also came crashing to earth.

The reality is that the world is surrounded by profit that is strangling it, and the world is being called upon to decide what to do about it.

Today tobacco has such a bad name that financial experts and stock brokers specializing in pushing tobacco stocks would hardly dare appear on a major network television show to openly admit they were promoting tobacco. One would hope in hindsight that those who played that game might recognize that their endorsement of tobacco made them players in selling a product that caused people to develop lung cancer and heart disease.

Yet not much has changed. Today's current economic mess always gets cleaned up and then the game begins again. The lure of profit divorced from ethics continues, as in the examples of drug companies which create nonexistent diseases to get the public to buy their drugs. They will never admit that fact until they too take the great fall and all their victims along with them.

In the meantime, it's "just good business," as in the same manner in which some of our major nonprofit health organizations and government healthcare agencies have recommended drugs not because they legitimately solved a healthcare problem, but because some of their officials were tied to the drug industry through personal connections that padded their wallets or created wealth for their institutions.

Now that cardiac disease arrest and reversal treatment is available, expensive and invasive surgical procedures for cardio-vascular disease should be phasing out. But surgery and drug treatment for heart disease and cancer earns enormous sums of money for those who practice and promote this approach, and it connects to an enormous animal research network upon which university and medical center research facilities rely for huge grants of tax money in the billions of dollars handed over by the NIH and other government funding agencies. Animal researchers and their university sponsors have been living off of curiosity testing, repetitive research projects, and unethical substance abuse testing for decades indifferent to the harm their work causes innocent animals and, ultimately, the public. But never mind. What is good for university medical centers and other animal research laboratories is good for America. And that applies equally to the meat and dairy industries with their factory farms, though they are not eager to discuss all the diseases associated with the products they deliver to the public.

The linkage between meat and dairy products to cancer, heart disease, stroke, and diabetes has now been well enough estab-lished to warrant the strongest warnings to the public, but if these diseases were eliminated, profit to the healthcare organiza-tions might diminish significantly. "So why would anyone in their right mind want to do that?" asks the savvy business entre-preneur. "That would not be good for business."

The answer, of course, is that they should do it because the healthcare industry is obligated by virtue of the ethics of the profession to ignore considerations of profit that are harmful to the public's best interests.

Scientists like Dr. Campbell have now provided overwhelming evidence of the cause of the killer diseases, but the healthcare establishment will neither refute nor admit this claim. The nutrition programs developed by Dr. Esselstyn and Dr. Ornish for cardiac disease arrest and reversal treatment have made a bit more headway, peripherally speaking, and a few glimmers of hope sparkle through, though these treatment options also are essentially ignored by mainstream medicine. Certainly, it is difficult not to notice that to date not one healthcare organization has been willing to unequivocally acknowledge that animal protein is the major cause of our healthcare crisis and that this epidemic could be stopped and reversed.

Just as the Royal College of Physicians in England made the announcement in 1962 that tobacco was a direct cause of lung cancer and heart disease, and just as the American Cancer Society seconded that announcement followed by the U.S. Surgeon General's report on smoking, some agency needs to step forward today to make the new announcement. The message is simple enough. "Meat and dairy products cause cancer, heart disease, stroke, and diabetes and pose significant risks for other chronic diseases. Many of these risks can be eliminated and many of these diseases reversed by eliminating animal protein from the diet."

Institutions are capable of change over time. Enlightened leadership can take the helm of a ship in trouble and guide it to safe shores, or the forces of ignorance can do their best to prevent new stewardship from taking its place at the helm, leaving the ship foundering in high seas that threaten to drive it onto rocky shores. Ignorance can be overcome through teaching. But when ignorance is fostered by agents lurking in the shadows who have something personal to gain by continuing that ignorance, this is the real danger as we see by studying the tobacco, animal research, and factory farm industries.

It will be up to citizens individually and together to set a new course for the future by insisting that the healthcare establishment take the findings of healthcare pioneers like Dr. Barnard, Dr. Campbell, Dr. Esselstyn, Dr. McDougall, Dr. Ornish, and a few others seriously. The public has the capacity to press the healthcare industry into validating the new nutritional guidelines for the protection of their children and their families as well as for friends and associates. It took complaints to Congress by the public to force the NCI to start spending some of its money to investigate the link of nutrition to cancer, and it took citizens groups to force the FTC into putting warning labels on cigarette packages. Now it is time for the good people of the earth to make their voices heard once again.

Government healthcare agencies and nonprofit healthcare organizations, hospitals and health facilities, and physicians, nurses, and medical practitioners are already nearly unanimous in recommending that people limit their intake of meat and dairy products. These organizations and medical personnel have just one final step to take. They know what it is. Start revealing the facts. The consumption of animal protein and dairy products is dangerous to the health of the citizens of the world.

Facts like these cannot be repeated often enough until they have fully penetrated our consciousness so let us state it just once again. We now know scientifically and unambiguously that to consume animal foods is to put us within closer range of being struck by one of the killer diseases. As individuals we have the personal power to keep that from happening. All we have to do is to stop consuming animal products, whether it is beef, pork, lamb, poultry, fowl, or fish. In the process we will have taken a step toward restoring the eco balance of the planet and ending the poverty that continues to plague all countries, but especially those in the developing world. When we do, we will have rediscovered a communion with life itself, and we will have joined hands in unity with our neighbors all around the world. Every person who has done this already, and there are many, can attest to this fact. They are forming a new kind of planetary community where respect and appreciation for all forms of life is the guiding principal that determines their actions.

It is not just meaningless chatter when Titus in Shakespeare's *Titus and Andronicus* chides Marcus for having killed a fly.

> Poor harmless fly,
> That with his pretty buzzing melody,
> Came here to make us merry! And thou hast killed him.

Winston Churchill understood when he said to his butler, "Please put the ladybug outside without harming her." It is the same message of respect for other life forms and species that Albert Schweitzer conveyed when he spoke these words: [3]

> What is this recognition, this knowledge within the reach of the most scientific and the most childlike? It is reverence for life, reverence for the unfathomable mystery we confront in our universe, an existence different in its outward appearance and yet inwardly of the same character as our own, terribly similar, awesomely related. The strangeness between us and other creatures is here removed....

The comprehension of nature as it exists from the absurdly grotesque to the implausibly sublime and the recognition that as human beings we are equally a part of it all, transforms our egocentric aspirations into a contemplation of the unity of life where we become more at one with nature and the universe.

When human beings stop killing animals because their compassion leads them to stop, they will stop killing their neighbors. This will open new channels for funneling human energies, and those energies lead toward a world able to function without slavery, genocide, and war. The key to this level of integration is to cease the abuse and exploitation of animals. In this state of mind we can build a new and better world and find a fuller life enriched by love and compassion. At the same time we will be protecting our own health and the health of our families and those we love and cherish.

Animal Research Funded by Charities

Personal Use and Toxicity Testing on Animals Not Related to Medical Research by Government and Private Sector Companies

A few of the hundreds of charities that either fund or conduct animal research are the Alzheimer's Association, American Cancer Society, American Diabetes Association, American Federation for Aging Research, American Foundation for AIDS Research, American Heart Association, American Lung Association, American Red Cross, Cystic Fibrosis Foundation, Epilepsy Foundation of America, March of Dimes, Muscular Dystrophy Foundation, National Osteoporosis Foundation, St. Jude Children's Research Hospital, Susan G. Komen Breast Cancer Foundation, United Cerebral Palsy, and the United Muscular Dystrophy Association.

Many people are surprised to learn that charities use the donations people give them to fund animal research. But that is the case, though the charities are not out broadcasting the news. The March of Dimes, for example, has funded research in visual development tests in which the eyelids of kittens were sewn shut for an entire year before killing them. The visual development this research claimed to have studied occurs in cats after birth while it occurs in humans before birth so that the tests were meaningless. This organization has spent millions of charity dollars for laboratory studies on primates, rats, mice, cats, dogs, rabbits, pigs, sheep, guinea pigs, opossums, and other species. The research includes experiments such as giving cocaine and nicotine to pregnant animals, freezing newborn ferrets, tethering pregnant monkeys to cages by cables running through the mothers' uteruses and into their fetuses' bodies, subjecting pregnant sheep to severe dehydration, and deliberately injuring the lungs of newborn lambs. None of these experiments have led to better healthcare for children.[1]

Besides charities, the animal research industry also includes private sector companies and government agencies which engage in a wide range of personal use and toxicity testing on animals. The private sector includes cosmetic companies, industrial chemical companies, and pharmaceutical companies with names like Arm & Hammer, BIC, Clairol, Dial, IAMS, Johnson & Johnson, Max Factor, Oil of Olay, Platex, Procter and Gamble, Right Guard, Unilever, and many others.

Some of the government agencies that require or conduct nonmedical animal research include the Consumer Product Safety Commission, the Department of Defense, the Department of Energy, The Department of Transportation, the Environmental Protection Agency, the Food and Drug Administration, the National Aeronautics and Space Administration (NASA), the National Institute of Environmental Health Sciences, the National Institute for Occupational Safety and Health, the National Toxicology Program, and the Occupational Health and Safety Administration.[2]

The Occupational Health and Safety Administration, for example, runs toxicity tests for chemicals in the workplace. The Environmental Protection Agency (EPA) tests insecticides, fungicides, rodenticides, pesticides, and herbicides The Consumer Product Safety Commission uses animal in tests on household cleaners, laundry detergents, fabric softeners, office products, and toys.

Many experiments are cruel beyond belief. The EPA confines dogs in inhalation chambers where they are forced to inhale pesticides.[3] They struggle in vain to escape. The programs run by the Department of Defense shoot, blast, burn, scald, and poison animals. They have subjected animals to irradiation, nerve gas, mustard gas, breaking their bones, decompression, and torture in ways that included attaching cartons of mosquitoes to restrained monkeys and pinning down rabbits so that mosquitoes could feed on them in mosquito virus tests.[4]

Animals don't make war, but they are made to suffer the consequences of the brutal wars human beings wage.

Cosmetic companies have their own range of projects. Procter and Gamble scientists test cosmetics for irritancy by locking rabbits, guinea pigs, hamsters, ferrets, and other animals into restraining devices and then applying burning chemicals to the animals' eyes and shaved portions of their skin. This is done without sedation or pain killers and causes excruciating pain. Some of the animals strain so forcefully against their restraints that they break their backs trying to escape, causing them even more needless suffering. Those that survive are put through additional tests until they are finally killed.

Animal research, whether it is conducted by university and medical facilities, charities, the private sector, or government agencies, exploits defenseless animals supposedly to better the welfare of human beings. But does it make the human condition better or worse when researchers torture animals in order to produce a better lipstick or shaving cream? What does it do to the spiritual and intellectual development of the human mind when it relies on cruelty toward animals to achieve its materialistic goals? Mark Twain, the iconic literary genius whose centennial death anniversary America celebrated on April 21, 2010, answered the question for the ages when he said:

> I believe I am not interested to know whether vivisection produces results that are profitable to the human race or doesn't. To know that the results are profitable to the race would not remove my hostility to it. The pains which it inflicts upon unconsenting animals is the basis of my

enmity toward it, and it is to me sufficient justification of enmity without looking further.

How to Get an NIH Grant (Satire)

Animal researchers are adept at disguising their work and connecting it in some way to human physiological processes in order to make it look like legitimate animal research. It is not difficult to do, and anyone with even the most primitive comprehension of human and animal anatomy can do the same. For example, if researchers wanted to get funding of a few hundred thousand dollars, they could file an application with the NIH to explore neuroplasticity in schizophrenia. Neuroplasticity is the ability of the brain to reorganize neural pathways based on new experiences.

In their research proposal, they would advise that they intended to induce schizophrenia in animals by injecting them with dissociative drugs, like phencyclidine (PCP), methamphetamine, or lysergic acid diethylamide (LSD), and then study the resulting correlations with human schizophrenia by conducting MRI and CT brain scan imaging of the cortical and subcortical subtypes. This would be followed by dissecting the brains of the animals in postmortem exams. From that point forward the researchers would have an open book into which they could pour their research findings on schizophrenia.

A study like this could last decades with no end in sight. Whenever additional funding was needed, all the researchers would have to do would be to write an impressive sounding progress report on how the subjects (primates) reacted to disorientation and hallucination-producing drugs and make the report sound like it had human applicability.

It is easy to do. How about, for example, a paper titled "Discordant Neuroplasticity Variants of Genomic Modifications through Recurrent Schizophrenic Applications in Non-human Animal Populations."

How many hundred thousand dollars would a title like that be worth annually adding up to a few million tax dollars?

If this sounds like a joke, it is presented only to emphasize that animal researchers are joking their way through billions of tax dollars that belong to the public. The example above, excluding the fictitious title of the paper for additional funding, actually does resemble somewhat the work of a researcher at UCLA who addicts monkeys to PCP and methamphetamine ostensibly to create human schizophrenia, after which he kills some of them to measure their dopamine levels. Do scientists actually think that schizophrenia, a human condition, can be created in animals by injecting them with hallucinogens when science has yet to understand what schizophrenia is in humans?

Cruel animal research like this is not a joke to innocent animals, and it should not be a joke to taxpayers who, without their authorization, end up funding this very non-funny, meaningless animal research.

Additional Examples of Unnecessary Cruel Animal Research

The cruelty and abuse of animals in animal research laboratories in unnecessary experiments that are funded by the NIH and other government agencies is occurring in laboratories across the country every day. Some of this cruelty and abuse stems from the design of the research project itself, and some of it results from the way animals are handled.

In 2005 the United States Department of Justice awarded a University of Wisconsin professor $500,000 to electrocute pigs with Taser guns to try to determine if stun guns are safe. This was an unnecessary project that could have been done using follow-up medical studies of Taser victims instead — as many previous studies had already done — so this was a total waste of taxpayer money, and it was exceedingly cruel.

At the University of North Carolina 59 undercover videotapes revealed that in tests for alcohol, dopamine, and nicotine, rodents were infected with oversized tumors so large the animals could hardly carry them around and some of the tumors ulcerated and burst; a researcher broke the necks of rats to get rid of those for whom she had no need; rodents were packed together under such crowded conditions that they resorted to cannibalism and suffocated to death; mice with untended teeth grew so long that they could not eat and some of them starved to death; researchers amputated the toes of rodents for identification purposes; rats screamed when being beheaded with scissors without anesthesia or numbing agents; and a researcher jokingly held up a tiny white mouse and said, "Say Bye, bye," and then beheaded the mouse with a pair of scissors.[1,2]

None of the other researchers at the University of North Carolina said a word about the abuses going on all around them, and this cruelty would have gone unreported if an undercover investigator had not been present to document the events.

At Rockefeller University in New York City cats have had their brains severed from their spinal cords after which anesthesia was discontinued while they were locked in frames and experimented upon for hours. In other experiments at this university cats were forced to vomit 97 times in the space of three and one-half minutes.

At New York University, chimpanzees were locked in old refrigerators filled with cocaine smoke. In other experiments at NYU, monkeys were subjected to a continuous three hour-long studio-generated sound that was 10 decibels louder than a shotgun blast. One NYU researcher took baby monkeys from their mothers by force, then drilled holes in the baby monkeys' heads for the purpose of studying artificially created vision abnormalities that had no practical use.[3] This researcher did this for fourteen years while collecting $1,500,000 from the NIH. The babies were either killed and dissected instantly after being experimented upon or were subjected to years of continuing experimentation. The mothers in these experiments were left bereft of their babies and suffered wretchedly because of their loss.

Taking infant animals from their mothers by force is a favored technique among animal researchers. See below for an instance of the same technique employed at Emory University and chapter 20 where an animal researcher does this at the Oregon Health and Science University.

New York University has been one of the most notorious protectors of institutional animal abuse in the nation. It has been charged with more than 400 violations of the Animal Welfare Act and has been fined $450,000, the largest fine ever leveled by the USDA. Reports indicate that New York University and the New

York University Medical Center experiment on 50,000 animals annually and collect $100,000,000 of the people's money in federal funding.[4]

Researchers forced monkeys to endure heart attacks and seizures at the University of Connecticut Health Center. (That it is unethical to do cardiovascular experiments on animals, especially when heart disease can be prevented and reversed through nutrition, is discussed in chapter 10.) Not to be outdone, at the University of Washington researchers cut open the skulls of monkeys and implanted electrodes into their brains. The research done at these universities was so extreme that the NIH forced them to return their grant money following documented complaints by PETA.[5]

Many other examples exist. Not yet discussed is a professor at Emory University in Atlanta, Georgia who pulls infant monkeys from their frantic mothers so that he can strap them into body chairs inside of wooden boxes in order to repeatedly subject the babies to noises up to 120 decibels (a sound equivalent to thunder, pneumatic drills, and airplane engines) just so that he can measure their heart rates.[6] Strapping animals into chairs that rotate and taking babies from their mothers are the kinds of techniques researchers copy from each other in repetitive projects. They have learned that these are the kinds of techniques that impress the NIH funders.

Cocaine and heroin addiction animal tests are being done at Harvard University, the world's most elite university, where a researcher addicts monkeys at an expense of $1,250,000 to the tax payers and then forces them to endure drug withdrawal. (That it is unethical to conduct drug addiction testing on animals is discussed in chapter 20.) At Johns Hopkins University at Baltimore a researcher studies drugs on monkeys and baboons at a cost of $1,000,000 annually. The university also employs a researcher who implants metal coils into primates' eyes and puts steel poles into their skulls. He then locks them into a chair that spins rapidly just to study different spin reactions to brain damage.

This researcher also cuts out pieces of the primates' brains to see if this causes a different reaction. His work costs the public $500,000. He conducts the same research on chinchillas.

Another researcher at the University of California San Francisco claims that he measures the neurological activity of monkeys.[7] If they behave nicely during the experiments, he rewards them with some juice. If they don't perform to his expectations they get nothing until the next day. But before he does that he slices the monkeys' eyes open so that he can place a wire coil inside. (This is another of those techniques animal researchers copy from one another.) Next he drills screws into their heads and places a metal plate under the scalp. After that he drills into the brain and removes part of it by suction after which the monkeys cannot move or stand for several days. (Removing a portion of primates' brains is another technique researchers copy from each other.) This is followed by drilling more holes into the monkeys' heads into which the researcher inserts stainless steel recording cylinders (yet another copy technique). Then he drives electrodes through the cylinders directly into the brain and uses the bolts that protrude through the scalp to screw the monkeys by the head into rotating, restraining chairs so that they cannot move for eight hour stretches. (More rotating chairs. More confining experiments.)

This researcher claims he is doing Alzheimer's research, but another University of California neuroscientist, Lawrence Hansen, M.D., said "I have never previously encountered experiments which would deliver quite so much suffering for so comparatively little scientific gain." He stated that the neural pathway this researcher claimed to be studying "is one of the few neural pathways not involved in AD [Alzheimer's Disease]!" Hansen, an NIH-funded neuroscientist and Alzheimer's researcher who has authored or co-authored 86 peer-reviewed scientific articles on Alzheimer's and has published 131 articles in the world's foremost scientific journals, added that "this cynical attempt to justify animal cruelty by linking it with a treatment for devastating human disease is disingenuous at best, and can more fairly be viewed as deceptive."[8]

The examples of institutional animal abuse presented in this book like the foregoing examples of needless, useless, curiosity research represent only a snapshot of what goes on behind the closed doors of animal research laboratories all across the country. This is barely the tip of the iceberg of this nether world of animal research that is routinely rubber-stamped by the NIH and other government funding agencies every year.

It should be evident that some serious restraints need to be placed on the NIH and other government agencies to prevent them from funding cruel animal research. It is an enormous waste of the public's money and it is acquiescence to unscrupulous individuals who unconstrained by ethics invent animal research projects that are so patently cruel and fantastically bizarre that they can only be termed nightmarish.

References

Prelude to Health

1. Colin T. Campbell and Thomas M. Campbell II, *The China Study*, (Dallas: BenBella Books, 2005), pp. 6, 7.
2. Ibid., p. 75.
3. *Foundation for Responsible Medicine*, "Mission Statement," http://www.frtv.org/about-foundation.html

Chapter I

1. *American Cancer Society*, "Estimated New Cancer Cases and Deaths by Sex," 2008.
   http://www.cancer.org/docroot/NWS/content/NWS_1_1x_Cancer_Facts_and_Figures_2008_Released.asp
2. *American Heart Association*, "AHA Statistical Update: Heart Disease and Stroke Statistics - 2009 Update," p. e22, http://circ.ahajournals.org/cgi/reprint/CIRCULATIONAHA.108.191261
3. Ibid, p. e51.
4. *Department of Health and Human Services, Center for Disease Control*, "National Diabetes Fact Sheet 2007," http://www.cdc.gov/diabete s/pubs/pdf/ndfs_2007.pdf
5. Ibid.
6. *Nationmaster.com*, "Health Statistics: Life expectancy at birth, Total population by country, 2008," http://www.nationmaster.com/graph/hea_lif_exp_at_bir_tot_pop-life-expectancy-birth-total-population&date=2008
7. *Kaiseredu.org*, "U.S. Healthcare Costs: Background Brief." http://www.kaiseredu.org/topics_im.asp?imID=1&parentID=61&id=358#1b

Chapter 2

1. Marion Nestle, *Food Politics: How the Food Industry Influences Nutrition and Health,* (Berkeley and Los Angeles: University of California Press, 2003), p. 39, digitized at http://books.google.com/books?id=yD_RCqOE5goC&dq= Marion+Nestle,+Food+Politics:+How+the+Food+Industry+I nfluences+Nutrition+and+Health&printsec=frontcover&so urce=bn&hl=en&ei=wasxSrjFCIHcM7GpwPsJ&sa=X&oi=bo ok_result&ct=result&resnum=4

2. Campbell, p. 252.

3. Ibid., pp. 308, 309.

4. The Atkins Diet is a high protein, high fat, low carbohydrate diet.

5. Campbell, p. 308.

6. Ibid., p. 327.

7. Ibid.

8. Roberrt N. Proctor , *Cancer Wars: How Politics Shapes What We know & Don't Know,* (New York: Basic Books, 1995), 1-8, 16.

9. Ibid.

10. Beginning with Hippocrates, Greek, Roman, and Islamic physicians followed a medical theory which believed disease was caused by an imbalance of bodily humors. The humors were black bile, yellow bile, phlegm, and blood. The correct balance of the humors was dependent on factors like diet and the kind of life activity in which one was involved. This theory was followed for centuries right into the Renaissance and only began to give way in the 16th and 17th centuries. See Proctor, pp. 16 and 26.

11. Ibid., p. 26

12. Ibid., p. 27.

13. Ibid., p. 18.

14. Ibid., p. 32.

15. Ibid., pp. 1-8.
16. Ibid.
17. The top ranked metropolitan hospitals and university teaching hospitals are Johns Hopkins, the Mayo Clinic, Ronald Reagan UCLA Medical Center, the Cleveland Clinic, Massachusetts General Hospital, New York Presbyterian University Hospital of Columbia and Cornell, University of California San Francisco Medical Center, Brigham and Women's Hospital of Boston, Duke University Medical Center, Hospital of the University of Pennsylvania, and the University of Washington Medical Center Seattle. See "Best Hospitals Honor Roll," *U.S. News and World Report* (July 10, 2008) http://health.usnews.com/articles/health/best-hospitals/2008/07/10/best-hospitals-honor-roll.html
18. Campbell, p. 23

Chapter 3

1. Campbell, p. 21.
2. Ibid., p. 294.
3. Ibid., p. 4.
4. Ibid., p. 5.
5. Ibid.
6. Ibid., p. 5.
7. Ibid., p. 6.
8. Ibid.
9. Samuel S. Epstein, *The Politics of Cancer Revisited*, (New York: East Ridge Press, 1998), 39.
10. Campbell, p. 70.
11. Ibid.
12. Ibid., pp. 69-72.
13. Ibid.
14. Ibid., p. 21.
15. Ibid., p. 76.

16. Ibid., p. 12.

17. Ibid., p. 76

18. Ibid.

19. Mark Gold, "The Global Benefits of Eating Less Meat," *Compassion in World Farming Trust*, (2004), 16, http://www. wellfedworld.org/PDF/CIWF%20Eat%20Less%20Meat.pdf

20. Paul N. Appleby et al., "The Oxford Vegetarian Study: an Overview," *American Journal of Clinical Nutrition*, (September 1999), vol. 70, No. 3, 525S-531S, digitized at http://www.ajcn.org/cgi/content/abstract/70/3/525S?maxtos how=&HITS=10&hits=10&RESULTFORMAT=&fulltext=veg etarian+heart&andorexactfulltext=and&searchid=11323679 86572_14818&stored_search=&FIRSTINDEX=0&sortspec=r elevance&resourcetype=1&journalcode=ajcn

21. Gary E. Fraser, "Associations between diet and cancer, ischemic heart disease, and all-cause mortality in non-Hispanic white California Seventh-day Adventists," The American Journal of Clinical Nutrition, (September 1999), Vol. 70, No. 3, 532S-538S, http://www.ajcn.org/cgi/content /full/70/3/532S

22. J. Chang-Claude, R. Frentzel-Beyme, U. Eilber, "Mortality pattern of German vegetarians after 11 years of follow-up," *Epidemiology*, 1992 Sept.; 3(5):395-401

23. Patricia R. Betron, R.D. et al (Nutrition Panel), "Vegetarian Diets : Advantages for Children," *Physicians Committee for Responsible Medicine*, See footnotes 18 and 19, http:// www.pcrm.org/health/veginfo/vegetarian_kids.html See also Thorogood M, "Risk of death from cancer and ischemic heart disease in meat and non-meat eaters," Brit Med J 1994; 308:1667-70 http://www.ncbi.nlm.nih.gov/ pubmed/8025458

24. John H. Cummings and Sheila A. Bingham, "Diet and the Prevention of Cancer," (December 12, 1998), *BMJ*, 317(7173): 1636-1640,

http://www.ncbi.nlm.nih.gov/pmc/articles/PMC1114436/

25. *goveg.com*, "Cancer: Killing Animals is Killing Us."

26. Animal Aid, "Pancreatic Cancer Linked to Animal Products," (June 30, 2009) http://www.animalaid.org.uk/h/n/NEWS/news_veggie/ALL/2157//

27. Cummings and Bingham, "Diet and the Prevention of Cancer," http://www.ncbi.nlm.nih.gov/pmc/articles/PMC1114436/

28. Animal Aid, "Pancreatic Cancer Linked to Animal Products."

29. *CA: A Cancer Journal for Clinicians*, "American Cancer Society Guidelines on Nutrition and Physical Activity for Cancer Prevention," (Oct 2006) 56(5):254-81, quiz 313-4, http://caonline.amcancersoc.org/cgi/content/full/56/5/254

Chapter 4

1. Epstein, pp. 286, 287.

2. Devra Davis, *The Secret History of the War on Cancer*, (New York: Basic Books, 2007), p. 161.

3. *U.S. National Libraries of Medicine, NIH*, "The Reports of the Surgeon General: The 1964 Report on Smoking and Health," http://profiles.nlm.nih.gov/NN/Views/Exhibit/narrative/smoking.html

4. Epstein, p. 114.

5. Davis, p. 161.

6. *The New York Times*, "Ernst Wynder, 77, A Cancer Researcher Dies," (July 16, 1999) http://www.nytimes.com/1999/07/16/us/ernst-wynder-77-a-cancer-researcher-dies.html?pagewanted=1

7. Ibid., pp. 13, 14.

8. Ibid.

9. Ibid., p. 166.

10. *World Health Organization*, "Launch of the Chronic Disease

Report," (2006).
http://www.oxha.org/knowledge/publications/mauritius-launch-of-the-who-chronic-disease-report.pdf

11. Ibid., p. 166

12. *American Cancer Society*, "Prevention and Early Detection: Cigarette Smoking," http://www.cancer.org/docroot/PED/content/PED_10_2X_Cigarette_Smoking.asp

13. *World Health Organization*, "Launch of the Chronic Disease Report."

14. Mike Stobbe, "Smoking ban leads to major drop in heart attacks," newsvine.co, http://www.newsvine.com/_news/2008/12/31/2262215-smoking

15. Dr. Samuel Epstein interviewed by Amy Goodman, "Most Censored Story: Does the American Cancer Society Work to Prevent Cancer?" *Democracy Now, daily TV/radio news program*, (April 13, 2000), http://www.democracynow.org/2000/4/13/most_censored_story_does_the_american

16. *American Institute of Philanthropy*, "Top 25 Compensation Packages," http://www.charitywatch.org/hottopics/Top25.html

17. *CA: A Cancer Journal for Clinicians*, "American Cancer Society Guidelines on Nutrition and Physical Activity for Cancer Prevention," http://caonline.amcancersoc.org/cgi/content/full/56/5/254

18. Ibid.

19. Procter, p. 26.

20. Campbell, p. 88.

21. Ibid., pp. 160 - 161.

22. *Senior Journal.com*, "Cancer to Replace Heart Disease as Leading Killer in World by 2010, Says International Study," Health and Medicine for Senior Citizens, http://senior-journal.com/NEWS/Health/2008/20081209-Cancer ToRepleaceHeart.htm

23. Campbell, p. 168.

24. Ibid., p. 170
25. Ibid., p. 172
26. Ibid., p. 174.
27. *CA: A Cancer Journal for Clinicians*, "American Cancer Society Guidelines."
28. *CA: A Cancer Journal for Clinicians*, "More Details On Red Meat, Colon Cancer Link," (2005); 55:143-144, doi: 10.3322/ canjclin.55.3.143, http://caonline.amcancersoc.org/cgi/cont ent/full/55/3/143, See also *JAMA* (2005, 293, No. 2: 172-182).
29. Ibid.
30. Campbell, p. 177.
31. *CA: A Cancer Journal for Clinicians*, "American Cancer Society Guidelines."
32. Campbell, p 178. See p. 386 footnote 97, Giovannucci E, "Dietary influences of 1,25 (OH)2 vitamin D in relation to prostate cancer: a hypothesis." *Cancer Causes and Control* 9 (1998): 567-582.
33. Ibid., See p. 386 footnote 96, Chan, JM, and Giovannucci, EL. "Dairy products, calcium, and vitamin D and risk of prostate cancer." Epidemiol, Revs. 23 (2001): 87-92
34. *CA: A Cancer Journal for Clinicians*, "American Cancer Society Guidelines."
35. *University of Michigan Health System,* "Calcium and Vitamin D," http://www.med.umich.edu/1libr/guides/calcium.htm
36. *The American Institute for Cancer Research, Stories,* "Summertime Tales: NW: Questions about calcium needs, crab and clams, grapefruit and weight loss," (July 27, 2009) http://www.aicr.org/feed/rss2_0/stories.rss
37. *CA: A Cancer Journal for Clinicians*, "American Cancer Society Guidelines."
38. Leo Galland, "Four Patterns of Dysbiosis" in Comprehensive Digestive Stool Analysis Application Guide, *Genova Diagnostic,* http://www.genovadiagnostics .com /files/profile_assets/referenced_materials/CDSA-App

Guide.pdf

39. Leo Galland, *Power Healing*, (New York: Random House, 1997), back cover.

40. Dr. Dean Ornish is also the director of the Preventive Medicine Research Center in Sausalito, California.

41. Campbell, p. 7.

Chapter 5

1. *American Heart Association*, "Calcium, Dietary," http://www.americanheart.org/presenter.jhtml?identifier=4453

2. *American Cancer Society*, "Shopping List: Basic Ingredients for a Healthy Kitchen," http://www.cancer.org/docroot/subsite/greatamericans/content/Shopping_List_Basic_Ingredients_for_a_Healthy_Kitchen.asp

3. Ibid.,

4. Rob McLean, "Calcium and Osteoporosis," *Cyberparent*. http://www.cyberparent.com/nutrition/osteoporosis-causemilk.htm

5. Hegsted, Mark D., "Fractures, calcium, and the modern diet," American Journal of Clinical Nutrition, (November 2001), Vol. 74, No. 5, 571-573; "Reply to H.B. McDonald," American Journal of Clinical Nutrition, (May 2002), Vol. 75, No. 5, 951; http://www.ajcn.org/cgi/search?pubdate_year=&volume=&firstpage=&DOI=&author1=Mark+Hegsted&author2=&title=&andorexacttitle=and&titleabstract=&andorexacttitleabs=and&fulltext=&andorexactfulltext=and&journalcode=ajcn&fmonth=Sep&fyear=1952&tmonth=Aug&tyear=2010&fdatedef=1+September+1952&tdatedef=1+August+2010&flag=&RESULTFORMAT=1&hits=50&hitsbrief=50&sortspec=relevance&sortspecbrief=relevance&sendit=Search

6. Rob McLean

7. Campbell, pp. 204 - 208.
8. Rob McLean.
9. Gold, p. 19.
10. Ibid.
11. Ibid.
12. Campbell, p. 219.
13. Ibid., p. 221.
14. Ibid.
15. Fran Lowry, "Dietary Pattern Associated with Reduced Alzheimer's Disease Risk," Medscape Medical News, http://www.medscape.com/viewarticle/720517
16. Campbell, pp. 215, 216.
17. Ibid., p. 195.
18. Ibid., p. 196.
19. Ibid, p. 146.
20. Ibid., p. 187.
21. Ibid.
22. Ibid., p. 151, 152. The "veggie" diet consisted of "whole plant foods and the equivalent of ...a cold cut or two of meat a day."
23. Ibid., p. 152.
24. *Diabetes Care*, "A Low-Fat Vegan Diet Improves Glycemic Control and Cardiovascular Risk Factors in a Randomized Clinical Trial in Individuals With Type 2 Diabetes," (August 2006), Volume 29, No. 8, http://www.nealbarnard.org/pdfs/Diabetes-Care.pdf
25. *femail.com.au*, "The Reverse Diabetes Diet," http://www.femail.com.au/the-reverse-diabetes-diet.htm
26. Campbell, p. 152.
27. Ibid., pp. 212 - 214.
28. Ibid., p. 214.
29. John McDougall, "Diet: Only Hope for Arthritis," *Dr. McDougall's Health and Medical Center*, http://www.drmcdougall.com/res_arthritis.html

30. *Johns Hopkins Health Alert,* "Going Vegan with RA," http://www.johnshopkinshealthalerts.com/alerts/arthritis/JohnsHopkinsArthritisHealthAlert_3353-1.html?type=pf
31. John McDougall, "Diet: Only Hope for Arthritis."
32. *Vegetarians in Paradise,* "24 Carrot Award," http://www.vegparadise.com/24carrot73.html
33. Ibid.

Chapter 6

1. But note that most large health organizations, including the National Cancer Institute (NCI), recommend that cancer patients undergoing treatment try to eat high-calorie diets that emphasize protein. In its publication, "Eating Hints for Cancer Patients," the NCI stresses foods like milk, cream, eggs, and cheese and recommends cooking with butter or oil. Salynn Boyles, "Confusion Over Dietary Recommendations," *Annieappleseed Project,* http://annieappleseedproject.stores.yahoo.net/conovdietrec.html
2. *USDA website,* "Nutrition and Your Health: Dietary Guidelines, Choose a diet that is low in fats, saturated fats, and cholesterol," http://www.nal.usda.gov/fnic/dga/dguide95.html
3. Bernard J. Gersh, M.D., ed., *Mayo Clinic Heart Book,* 2nd ed., (New York: William Morrow, 2000), pp. 190-196.
4. *American Heart Association,* "Diet and Lifestyle Recommendations," http://www.americanheart.org/presenter.jhtml?identifier=851
5. *The American Cancer Society,* "The Complete Guide, Nutrition and Physical Activity," http://www.cancer.org/docroot/PED/content/PED_3_2X_Diet_and_Activity_Factors_That_Affect_Risks.asp?sitearea=PED
6. *National Institutes of Health, National Heart, Lung, and Blood*

Institute, "Dash Eating Plan:
Your Guide to Lowering Your Blood Pressure with Dash,"
http://www.nhlbi.nih.gov/health/public/heart/hbp/dash/new_dash.pdf

7. *American Institute for Cancer Research*, "Second Expert Report: Food, Nutrition, Physical Activity, and the Prevention of Cancer: a Global Perspective," see Read the Recommendations for Cancer Prevention, http://www.aicr.org /site/PageServer?pagename=res_report_second

8. *American Institute for Cancer Newsletter*, "Getting Back in Balance With Your Meals," (Spring 2009), Issue 103, p. 6, http://www.aicr.org/site/DocServer/NL103-Spring09.pdf?docID=2821

9. *American Institute for Cancer Research*, "For Red Meat, Another Red Light," (May 2007), http://www.aicr.org/site /News2?page=NewsArticle&id=11809. See also T. Colin Campbell, PhD, "Critique of Report on 'Food, Nutrition and the Prevention of Cancer: A Global Perspective,'" (March/April 2001), *Nutrition Today*, vol. 36(2), pp. 80-84.

10. *American Institute for Cancer Research*, "Eggplant Lasagna," (November 10, 2008), http://www.aicr.org/site/News2?page =NewsArticle&id=14059&news_iv_ctrl=0&abbr=pr_hf_

11. *Human Ecology Forum*, "China study shows diet-disease connection," 22.n3 (Fall 1994): 9(1), http://www.accessmylibrary.com/article-1G1-16642776/china-study-shows-diet.html.

Chapter 7

1. *Prevention Magazine*, "Take This Letter To Your Doctor," (Reader Service Report), (November 1996), pp. 61-64,

2. *The National Cancer Institute*, "Breast Cancer Prevention, Estrogen (Endogenous)," http://www.cancer.gov/cancer-topics/pdq/prevention/breast/Patient/page3#Keypoint5

3. Ibid.
4. Campbell, p. 161.
5. *The National Cancer Institute*, "Breast Cancer Prevention, Estrogen (Endogenous)."
6. *Nutrition Action Healthletter*, "Breast Cancer," (Jan/Feb 1996). See also Steve Lustgarden with Debra Holton, "Women on the Verge of Health: The Vital Role of Food," *EarthSave: Healthy People Healthy Planet*, http://www.earthsave.org/health/women_verge_health.htm
7. *The National Cancer Institute*, "The National Cancer Institute: More Than 70 Years of Excellence in Cancer Research," http://www.cancer.gov/aboutnci/excellence-in-research
8. Ornish, *Eat More, Weigh Less*, (New York: Harper Perennial, 1994), p. 28.
9. Ibid., p. 35.

Chapter 8

1. Campbell, p. 271.
2. Campbell, p. 315.
3. *Harvard School of Public Health*, "The Nutrtition Source, Low-Fat Diet Not a Cure -All," http://www.hsph.harvard.edu/nutritionsource/nutrition-news/low-fat/
4. R. L. Prentice, B. Caan, RT Chlebowski, "Low-fat dietary pattern and risk of invasive breast cancer: the Women's Health Initiative Randomized Controlled Dietary Modification Trial," *JAMA*, (February 8, 2006), 295:6, 629-42, http://jama.ama-assn.org/cgi/content/full/295/6/629)
5. S.A. Beresford et al., "Low-fat dietary pattern and risk of colorectal cancer: the Women's Health Initiative Randomized Controlled Dietary Modification Trial," *JAMA*, (2006), 295:6, 643-54, http://www.jama.ama-assn.org/cgi/content/full/295/6/643

6. B.V. Howard, L. Van Horn, J. Hsia et al., "Low-fat dietary pattern and risk of cardiovascular disease: the Women's Health Initiative Randomized Controlled Dietary Modification Trial," *JAMA*, (2006); 295:6, 655-66, http://jama.ama-assn.org/cgi/content/full/295/6/655

7. *Harvard School of Public Heatlh*, "Fats and Cholesterol: Out with the Bad, In with the good," http://www.hsph.harvard.edu/nutritionsource/what-should-you-eat/fats-full-story/index.html

8. *Harvard School of Public Health*, "Low-Fat Diet Not a Cure-All."

9. Campbell, pp. 275-277.

10. *The McDougall Newsletter*, (February 2006), Vol 5, No. 2. http://www.drmcdougall.com/misc/2006nl/february/response.htm

11. Campbell, p. 329.

12. *The McDougall Newsletter*, (February 2006), Vol. 5, No. 2.

13. Ibid.

14. Campbell, 272.

15. Ibid., pp. 273, 274

16. Ibid.

17. Ibid., p. 277

18. Ibid., p. 281

19. Ibid., p. 272

20. *Harvard School of Public Health*, http://www.hsph.harvard.edu/nutritionsource/what-should-you-eat/fats-full-story/index.html

21. David Irving, "Reply to Dr. Andrew Weil's Article on Saturated Fats," *all-creatures.org*, http://www.all-creatures.org/health/weil.html

22. Campbell, p. 287.

23. The McDougall Newsletter, (February 2006), Vol. 5, No. 2.

Chapter 9

1. *National Cholesterol Education Program*, "High Blood Cholesterol, What You Need to Know," http://www.n hlbi.nih.gov/health/public/heart/chol/wyntk.htm#numbers
2. Martin S. Lipsky, MD, Marla Mendelson, MD, Stephen Havas, MD, MPH, and Michael Miller, MD, *American Medical Association Guide to Preventing and Treating Heart Disease*, (Hoboken, NJ: John Wiley & Sons, Inc., 2008), pp. 26, 27, digitized at http://books.google.com/books?id=4iSo MzkwStMC&printsec=frontcover&dq=American+Medical+ Association+Guide+to+Preventing+and+Treating+Heart+Di sease&source=bl&ots=Wu7XOW-5le&sig=yOOT2N6ljFl_R 11wUOyWzfuLQD8&hl=en&ei=KXxETKvYFsL6lwfCvIDj DQ&sa=X&oi=book_result&ct=result&resnum=2&ved=0C CEQ6AEwAQ#v=onepage&q&f=false
3. Campbell, p. 131.
4. Caldwell B. Esselstyn, Jr., MD, *Prevent and Reverse Heart Disease*, (New York: Penguin Group, 2007), pp. 57-58, digitized at http://books.google.com/books?id=hihHaBi KKU8C&dq=Caldwell+Esselstyn,+B.+Jr.,+MD,+Prevent+an d+Reverse+Heart+Disease&printsec=frontcover&source=b n&hl=en&ei=OrIxSsqTA4zyMpDhqYcK&sa=X&oi=book_re sult&ct=result&resnum=4
5. Campbell, p. 132.
6. Esselstyn, p. 58.
7. Karen Iaccobo and Michael Iaccobo, *Vegetarian America*, (Westport, CT.: Greenwood Publishing Group, Inc., 2004), p. 210, http://books.google.com/books?id=0AiAz62C_jcC &printsec=copyright&dg=had+a+heart+attack+in+Framing ham+in+35+years+in+anyone+who+had+a+cholesterol+und er+150#PPA210,M1
8. *Scientific American Frontiers*, "Frontiers Profile: Bill Castelli," panel 4, http://www.pbs.org/saf/1104/features/ castelli4.htm

9. *WebMD*, "What is Atherosclerosis?" http://www.webmd.com/heart-disease/what-is-atherosclerosis

10. *Merck Source*, "For Your Heart's Sake, Lower Your Cholesterol," http://www.mercksource.com/pp/us/cns/cns_healthink_template.jspzQzpgzEzzSzppdocszSzuszSzcnszSzcontentzSzhealthinkzSzlowercholesterolzPzhtml

11. *goveg.com*, "Meat and Strokes," http://www.goveg.com/strokes-meat.asp

12. Jill Bolte Taylor, Ph.D., *My Stroke of Insight* (New York: Viking Penguin, 2008).

13. Esselstyn, fig. 17 after p. 116

14. goveg.com, "Meat and Strokes."

15. Ibid.

16. Ibid.

17. Ibid.

18. Campbell, p. 220, 221.

19. Maggie Mahar, "The Bad Science that Created the Cholesterol Con," (March 3, 2008), Alternet, http://wwwalternet.org/healthwellness/78554/the_bad_science_that_created_the_cholesterol_con/ See also http://www.alternet.org/health/78554?page=entire

20. Ibid.

21. Ibid.

22. *UniSci*, "Lower Cholesterol Reading Can Mask Heart Attack Risk," (March 2001), http://www.unisci.com/stories/20011/0321013.htm

23. Mahar.

24. John Carey, "Do Cholesterol Drugs Do Any Good?" (January 17, 2008,), *Business Week*, p. 1 http://www.businessweek.com/magazine/content/08_04/b4068052092994.htm?chan=search

25. Mahar.

26. Ibid.

27. Ibid.

28. Campbell, p. 81.

29. Lipsky, p. 89.

30. Gersh, pp. 195, 196.

31. Peter O. Kwiterovich, Jr., M.D., *The Johns Hopkins Complete Guide for Preventing and Reversing Heart Disease,*(Rocklin, California: Prima Publishing, 1993), pp. 197, 198.

32. A preponderance of evidence linking high animal protein (including fish) and high-fat intake to heart disease, high blood cholesterol, and cancer is available for consideration and study from many sources.

33. Barnard, Neal, Contributor, Physicians Committee for Responsible Medicine, *Healthy Eating for Life for Women*, (New York: John Wiley and Sons, 2002), http://books. google.com/books?id=yrT1-yPg7PIC&dq=Healthy+ Eating+for+Life+for+Women&printsec=frontcover&source= bn&hl=en&ei=ZoFETIbnJoP7lwfVooXOAg&sa=X&oi=book _result&ct=result&resnum=5&ved=0CDEQ6AEwBA#v=on epage&q&f=false

34. Gold, p. 18.

35. *American Cancer Society*, "Making Treatment Decisions," see Are there any possible problems or complications, http://www.cancer.org/docroot/ETO/content/ETO_5_ 3X_Omega-3_Fatty_Acids.asp

36. *Oceans Alert*, "PCB Information," http://www.oceansalert. org/pcbinfo.html

37. *Raysahelian.com*, "Alpha Linolenic Acid, ALA," http://www. raysahelian.com/linolenic.html

38. Esselstyn, pp. 83, 84.

39. Ingeborg A. Brouwer et al., "Dietary Linolenic Acid Is Associated with Reduced Risk of Fatal Coronary Heart Disease, but Increased Prostate Cancer Risk: A Meta-Analysis," *The American Society for Nutritional Sciences*, J. Nutr (April 2004), 134:919-922. ALA is the only omega 3 fatty acid found in vegetable sources. The studies were

unable to determine if this alpha-linolenic acid came from meat consumption or flax seed consumption. Another investigation revealed that five studies which examined alpha linolenic acid and found a prostate cancer connection were "extremely inconsistent." With advanced prostate cancer this report suggested an "association with total and saturated fat with advanced prostate cancer, but showed no associations with linoleic acid, alpha-linolenic acid, polyunsaturated fat, eicosapentaenoic acid, or docosahexaenoic acid fatty acids." It concluded that the "associations between dietary fatty acids and prostate cancer remain unclear." See Leslie K. Dennis et al., "Problems with the Assessment of Dietary Fat in Prostate Cancer Studies," *American Journal of Epidemiology* (2004), 160(5):436-444; doi:10.1093/aje/kwh243. http://aje.oxfordjournals.org/cgi/content/full/160/5/436. Another study showed that flax seed reduced prostate cancer risk. See Wendy Demark-Wahnefried, et al., "Flaxseed Supplementation (Not Dietary Fat Restriction) Reduces Prostate Cancer Proliferation Rates in Men," *Presurgery, Cancer Epidemiology Biomarkers & Prevention* (December 1, 2008), 17, 3577-3587,. Doi 10.1158/1055-9965.EPI-08-0008, http://cebp.aacrjournals.org/cgi content/abstract/17/12/3577 http://jn.nutrition.org/cgi/content/full/134/4/919

40. Karen Iaccobo and Michael Iaccobo, *Vegetarian America.*
41. Campbell, p. 119.
42. Ibid., p. 79.
43. *goveg.com*, "Cholesterol and Atherosclerosis," http://www.goveg.com/heartdisease_cholather.asp

Chapter 10

1. *American Heart Association*, "Cardiovascular disease death rates decline, but risk factors still exact heavy toll,"

(12/1/2007), http://www.americanheart.org/presenter.jhtml?
identifier=3052670 2. Esselstyn, pp. 89 - 91.

3.   Ibid., see Chapter 5.

4.   Gersh, p. 190.

5.   Ibid.

6.   Campbell, p. 126

7.   Ibid., p. 23.

8 . Ibid., pp. 125, 323.

9.   Ibid., pp. 338 - 341.

10. Ibid.

11. Ibid., pp. 339, 340.

12. Ibid.

13. Ibid.

14. Ibid.

15. Richard Horton, *Health Wars: On the Global Front Lines of
     Modern Medicine*, (New York: The New York Review of
     Books , 2003), p. 436.

16. Ibid.

17. Esselstyn, p. 55.

18. Jerome Groopman, *How Doctors Think*, (New York: First
     Mariner Books, 2007), p. 155.

19. Esselstyn, pp. 11, 108.

20. PBS interview of Dr. John Young, "Animal Testing Ethics,"
     Religious & Ethics Newsweekly, (August 15, 2008), Episode
     no. 1150, contains interview transcription and video,
     http://www.pbs.org/wnet/religionandethics/week1150/cov
     er.html

21. Esselstyn, p. 4.

22. *American Heart Association*, "AHA Statistical Update, Heart
     Disease and Stroke Statistics - 2009 Update," p. e22,
     http://circ.ahajournals.org/cgi/reprint/CIRCULA-
     TIONAHA.108.191261

23. Campbell, pp. 111 - 123.

24. Ibid., p. 124.

25. Ibid.

26. *Annieappleseed Project*, "Dean Ornish, Nutrition and Prostate Cancer," from Dr. Gregor Newsletter, (Fall 2005), http://www.annieappleseedproject.org/deanornutpro.html See also Washington Post, Rob Stein, "Study Shows Diet, Exercise, and Reduced Stress Slow Prostate Cancer," (August 11, 2005), http://www.washingtonpost.com/wp-dyn/content/article/2005/08/10/AR2005081001882.html

27. Robert Winston and Lori Oliwenstein, *Superhuman*, (New York: Dorling Kindersly, 2000).

28. Ibid., p. 165.

Chapter 11

1. Compared to the difficulties of those facing the challenges of tobacco addiction, meat eaters are far more fortunate. A potent narcotic addiction like nicotine can take decades to break. Its most serious lethal effects may not even be fully felt until years into the dependency, and by then the habit is extremely difficult to overcome. But animal protein is not physically addicting and no deprivation is involved in giving it up. It is really just a matter of switching from an animal-based protein source to a plant-based protein source with the addition of trace amounts of vitamin B12 (a vitamin not found in non-meat foods) and becoming accustomed to new tastes and new habits. Unlike smoking, where people who give it up have to stop smoking, people who stop consuming animal products still get to continue eating food. In fact, once the custom of eating animal food fades away, most people think non-animal food is far better tasting than animal products. Getting completely over tobacco addiction can take weeks and months before the urge to smoke subsides. People can become reacclimatized to food without animal protein, on the other hand, the same

340

day they give it up if they wish.

2. *The American Cancer Society,* "The Complete Guide, Nutrition and Physical Activity," http://www.cancer.org /docroot/PED/content/PED_3_2X_Diet_and_Activity_Facto rs_That_Affect_Risks.asp?sitearea=PED

3. *Craines Detroit Business,* "Western Chic at the sixth-annual Cattle Baron's Ball," (September 30, 2008), http://www. crainsdetroit.com/article/20080930/GIVERS/809309985

4. *My Fox Detroit, WJBK Web Team,* "2008 American Cancer Society Cattle Barron's Ball," (Sept. 7, 2008), http://www. myfoxdetroit.com/myfox/pages/InsideFox/Detail?contentI d=7377482&version=2&locale=EN-US&layoutCode=TSTY &pageId=5.7.1

5. *American Cancer Society,* "American Cancer Society to Host Cattle Barron's Ball in Youngstown," (September 7, 2007), http://www.cancer.org/docroot/COM/content/div_OH/CO M_1_1x_AS_2007_American_Cancer Society_to_Host_ Cattle_Barons_Ball.asp

6. Kwiterovich, Appendix B.

7. *Craine's Detroit Businss,* "Western Chic at the sixth-annual Cattle Baron's Ball: See more photos from this event," http://www.crainsdetroit.com/apps/pbcs.dll/gallery?Avis= CD&Dato=20080929&Kategori=GIVERS&Lopenr=92900999 8&Ref=PH

8. Ibid., main text. *Craines Detroit Business,* "Western Chic at the sixth-annual Cattle Baron's Ball," (September 30, 2008)

9. Ibid.

10. *The Candle Café,* "Candle Café Valentine's Day 2009," http://www.candlecafe.com/

11. *CA: A Cancer Journal for Clinicians.*

Chapter 12

1. Campbell, pp. 262-264.

2. Ibid.

3. Marian Burros, "Prudent Diet and Cancer Rise," *The New York Times*, (June 23, 1982), http://query.nytimes.com/gst/fullpage.html?sec=health&res=9807EFD7143BF930A15755C0A964948260

4. Ibid.

5. Campbell, p. 261.

6. Ralph W. Moss, *The Cancer Industry*, (New York: Paragon House, 1991), p. 231.

7. Mishio Kushi, *The Macrobiotic Approach to Cancer*, (New York: Avery, 1991), p. 72, digitized at http://books.google.com/books?id=H_DSJn3DCeYC&pg=PA7&lpg=PA7&dq=Mishio+Kushi,+The+Macrobiotic+Approach+to+Cancer&source=bl&ots=DeoVWPMiau&sig=8o0emRnqzN7hXdCyUQkvDrpiKKo&hl=en&ei=dkp8StiyNJHONej0teUC&sa=X&oi=book_result&ct=result&resnum=1#v=onepage&q=&f=false

8. Moss, *The Cancer Industry*, p. 216.

9. Ralph W. Moss, *Cancer Therapy*, (Brooklyn: Equinox Press, 2001), pp. 187, 188.

10. Moss, *The Cancer Industry*, p. 216.

11. *AMA website*, "AMA History," http://www.ama-assn.org/ama/pub/category/1854.html

12. John Robbins, *Reclaiming Our Health*, (Tiburon, CA: HJ Kramer, Inc., 1996), p. 187.

13. Ibid., p. 193

14. Ibid., p. 279

15. Ibid., p. 280

16. Moss, *The Cancer Industry*, p. 217.

17. Robbins, p. 280.

18. Ibid.

19. Moss, *The Cancer Industry*, p. 217.

20. Ibid.

21. At first the AMA promoted the idea of finding a safe cigarette (as did the American Cancer Society), and then

supported cigarette filters. When the hazards of cigarette smoking could no longer be denied, the AMA advised the public to "smoke if you feel you should, but be moderate." The AMA's retirement fund owned stock to the tune of $1.8 million in tobacco securities, which at the time was an enormous sum. When challenged, they defended the investment saying the purpose was "'to make the biggest buck,' not to make a social statement." This brought an uproar of criticism. When the Federal Trade Commission first agreed to put health warnings on cigarette packages, the AMA blocked the way. Outraged, Dr. Alton Ochsner, an eminent chest surgeon at Tulane University School of Medicine, accused the AMA of being "derelict" in its health responsibilities. The President of the AMA, F.J.L. Blasingame, responded as follows: "It seems to me that Dr. Ochsner and those who share his opinion are really advocating that an agency of the federal government be granted the power to destroy an $8 billion industry on the extreme theory that the American people need to be protected from themselves in the matter of smoking." The AMA continued to support the tobacco industry well into the 1990s as indicated by its backing of pro-tobacco congress people like J. Roy Rowland, M.D. and others. In 1994 the New England Journal of Medicine stated that the AMA "gave significantly larger average contributions to House members who favored tobacco-export promotion than to those who opposed it." See Robbins, John, *Reclaiming Our Health*, (HJ Kramer, Inc., Tiburon, CA, 1996), p. 209.

Chapter 13

1.   Kenny Ausubel, *When Healing Becomes a Crime: The Amazing Story of the Hoxsey Cancer Clinics and the Return of Alternative*

Therapies, (Rochester, Vermont: Healing Arts Press, 2001), p. 13.

2. Ibid.

3. Moss, *Cancer Therapy,* p. 160.

4. *American Botanical Council,* "Herbs in the Hoxsey Cancer Tonic," Herb Clip TM, ed. Mark Blumenthal, http://74.125.47.132/search?q=cache:9JBXjVatgbsJ:content.herbalgram.org/tomsofmaine/HerbClip/pdfs/070217211.pdf+%E2%80%9CHerbs+in+the+Hoxsey+Cancer+Tonic,%E2%80%9D+American+Botanical+Council&cd=1&hl=en&ct=clnk&gl=us, or http://content.herbalgram.org/tomsofmaine/HerbClip/pdfs/070217-211.pdf

5. *The Products, Tools & Info that you need to choose Health over Disease,* "The Hoxsey Formula," https://www.illnessisoptional.com/cms/index2.php?option=com_content&do_pdf=1&id=104

6. If the AMA, the NCI, the FDA, and others like Sloan-Kettering Hospital, which has also voiced opposition to the Hoxsey treatment, have reason to disagree with the chemical tests already conducted on the Hoxsey tonic by the USDA that showed it had "very significant chemical and biological anticancer activity," is it too much to ask them to conduct their own chemical tests — hopefully, with a nonaffiliated, independent referee? Surely the Hoxsey tonic has accumulated enough anecdotal evidence for success to merit that kind of testing. Until full and convincing testing on the Hoxsey treatment is done, people will continue to go to Mexico to get the tonic for better or worse.

7. Max Gerson used coffee enemas in his cancer treatment.

8. Moss, *The Cancer Industry,* pp. 267.

9. Ibid., pp. 288 - 297.

10. Ibid., pp. 290 - 297.

11. Ibid.

12. Ibid.
13. Ibid., p. 307.
14. Ibid., p. 308.
15. Ibid., p. 328.
16. Ibid., p. 329.
17. Ibid., p. 326.

Chapter 14

1. Campbell, p. 346.
2. *Daily News Central*, "US Turning Blind Eye to Rx Drug-Abuse Epidemic," http://health.dailynewscentral.com/content/view/1232/0
3. Howard Wolinsky, "Disease Mongering and Drug Marketing," *EMBO* (European Molecular Biology Organization), (July 6 (7) 2002), Report 612-614; doi: 10.1038/sj.embor.7400476, http://www.pubmedcentral.nih.gov/articlerender.fcgi?artid=1369125
4. Lynn Payer, *Disease-Mongers: How Doctors, Drug Companies, and Insurers Are Making You Feel Sick*, (New York: Wiley & Sons, 1992), p. 136.
5. Ibid.
6. Ibid.
7. Ray Moynihan, "Disease-Mongers: How Doctors, Drug Companies, and Insurers Are Making You Feel Sick," Review, *BMJ* 2002;324(7342):923, see http://ukpmc.ac.uk/articlerender.cgi?artid=477342
8. Ray Moynihan and Alan Cassels, *Selling Sickness: How the World's Biggest Pharmaceutical Companies are Turning us All Into Patients*, (New York: Nation Books, 2006), p. 140, digitized at http://books.google.com/books?id=fftKR4y2NMIC&dq=Ray+Moynihan+and+Alan+Cassels,+Selling+Sickness:+How+the+World%E2%80%99s+Biggest+Pharmaceutical+Companies+are&printsec=frontcover&source=bl&ots=

4yKwHKtMch&sig=DYvqecWKTd120JpENJAfHfCEcgA&h
l=en&ei=x8QxSpqpHY7KtgeG-ZG4CQ&sa=X&oi=book
_result&ct=result&resnum=2

9. Wolinsky, "Disease Mongering."

10. Ibid.

11. Ibid.

12. Moynihan, *Selling Sickness*, p. 63.

13. Ibid., Ch. 4.

14. *Frontline*, "ADHD - An Update," http://www.pbs.org/wgbh/
pages/frontline/shows/medicating/etc/adhdupdate.html

15. Ibid., p. 62.

16. Ibid., pp. 69, 72.

17. Ibid., p. 69.

18. Moynihan, *Selling Sicknes*, pp. 65, 66. See also footnote 20.

19. *Friends of Narconnon*, "History of Methamphetamine,"
http://www.friendsofnarconon.org/drug_education/drug_i
nformation/meth_%10_speed/history_of_methamphet-
amine/

20. *WebMD Health*, "Sudden Death in 12 Kids on ADHD Drug
Adderall," http://www.medscape.com/viewarticle/511400

21. Ibid., p. 80.

22. *Physicians Committee for Responsible Medicine*, "PCRM Sues
Glickman and Shalala: Dietary Guidelines For 2000, the
Politics of Food: A Brief History of the U.S. Dietary
Guidelines," http://www.pcrm.org/news/lawsuit_history
.html

23. The Beef Industry Council consists of a federation of 44
state beef councils. See http://findarticles.com/p/articles/mi
_m3190/is_n16_v26/ai_12093138/

24. William T. Jarvis, Ph.D., "PCRM, National Council Against
Heatlh Fraud," *The Physicians Committee for Responsible
Medicine*, http://www.ncahf.org/articles/o-r/pcrm.html

25. Christopher Lee, "Doctors, Legislators Resist Drugmakers'
Prying Eyes," *The Washington Post*, (May 22, 2007), see

http://www.washingtonpost.com/wp-dyn/content/article/2007/05/21/AR2007052101701.html

26. Mike Adams, ed., "Scientific medical journals like JAMA fail basic credibility standards; medical journals become increasingly irrelevant," *Natural News.com*, (Aug. 19, 2004), http://www.naturalnews.com/001890.html

27. *Natural News.com*, "JAMA refuses to exclude authors who hide financial ties to drug companies," (Aug. 6, 2006), http://www.naturalnews.com/019914.html

28. Ibid.

29. Ibid.

30. Dr. Samuel Epstein interviewed by Amy Goodman.

31. *Forbes.com*, "David R. Bethune," http://people.forbes.com/profile/david-r-bethune/14859

On March 31, 2008, the Board of Directors of the Company named David R. Bethune interim chief executive officer in addition to his role as Chairman. Mr. Bethune has been a member of the board since 2005, its Chairman since May 2007 and Executive Chairman since August 2007. Mr. Bethune is a member of the boards of directors of Cambrex Corporation and the Female Health Company. From 1999 until his retirement in 2004, he was Chairman and Chief Executive Officer of Atrix Laboratories, Inc., a drug delivery and product development company. Prior to his work at Atrix Laboratories, Mr. Bethune was President and Chief Operating Officer of IVAX Corporation, a pharmaceutical company. Before joining IVAX, Mr. Bethune began a start-up pharmaceutical company venture formed by Mayo Medical Ventures, a business unit of Mayo Clinics of Rochester. Mr. Bethune previously served as group vice president of American Cyanamid Company and a member of the Executive Committee where he had executive authority for human biologicals, consumer health products, pharmaceuticals and ophthalmics as well as global medical research. He was also President of the Lederle Laboratories Division of American Cyanamid Company.

32. *Surfwax Health News*, "Zila sees revenue leap, continued loss as operations refocus," (Oct. 16, 2007). "With this strategic re-direction of the company, we now possess the operational capabilities to realize the market opportunity for ViziLite Plus in oral cancer screening," said Executive Chairman David R.Bethune, http://news.surfwax.com /health/archives/Oral_Cancer.html

33. Forbes.com, "Essex Dental Benefits to Cover Zila's ViziLite Plus for Oral Cancer Screenings," (Nov. 4, 2008), http://www.forbes.com/businesswire/feeds/businesswire/2 008/11/04/businesswire20081104005228r1.html, "ViziLite Plus is being adopted by dentists in the U.S. and other parts of the world," said David Bethune, Zila's chairman and chief executive officer. "We are delighted to have Essex Dental Benefits join the insurance industry movement to cover ViziLite Plus exams and help improve the overall care of patients."... Zila manufactures and markets ViziLite(R) Plus with TBlue(R) ("ViziLite(R) Plus"), the company's flagship product for the early detection of oral abnormalities that could lead to cancer. ViziLite(R) Plus is an adjunctive medical device cleared by the FDA for use in a population at increased risk for oral cancer. In addition, Zila designs, manufactures and markets a suite of proprietary products sold exclusively and directly to dental professionals for periodontal disease, including the Rotadent(R) Professional Powered Brush, the Pro-Select Platinum(R) ultrasonic scaler and a portfolio of oral pharmaceutical products for both in-office and home-care use.

34. Integrity in Science, "American Cancer Society, Tied to Drug companies, von Eschenbach," *Center for Science in the*

Public Interest, (March 3, 2006), http://www.cspinet.org /integrity/watch/200603241.html

35. Dani Veracity, "Is the American Cancer Center more interested in cancer profit than cancer prevention?" (July 31, 2005), http://www.naturalnews.com/010244.html

36. The Corporate Social Responsibility Newswire, "Corporate Impact Awards Recognize Companies' $1 Million-Plus Annual Gifts to American Cancer Society," (November 19, 2009), http://www.csrwire.com/press_releases/28220-Corp orate-Impact-Awards-Recognize-Companies-1-Million-Plus-Annual-Gifts-to-American-Cancer-Society

Chapter 15

1. Howard Wolinsky, "Disease Mongering."
2. Jamie Holguin, "Statins' Side Effects Under Fire," *CBS Evening News,* (October 11, 2004), http://www.cbsnews. com/stories/2004/10/11/eveningnews/ main648685.shtml
3. David Tuller, "Seeking a Fuller Picture of Statins," *The New York Times,* (July 20, 2004), http://www.nytimes.com/2004/ 07/20/health/seeking-a-fuller-picture-of-statins.html? sec=health&&fta=y
4. Ibid.
5. Ibid.
6. *Spacedoc.net,* "Statin Drugs Side Effects," (Duane Graveline website), http://www.spacedoc.net/index.php
7. Tuller, "Seeking a Fuller Picture of Statins."
8. John Carey, "Do Cholesterol Drugs Do Any Good?"
9. Ibid.
10. Moynihan, *Selling Sickness,* p. 7.
11. *Center for Science in the Public Interest,* "FDA Web Site on Drug Ads Developed by Drug Industry PR Firm," (Sept. 15, 2008), http://www.cspinet.org/new/200809152.html
12. Ibid., pp. 110, 111.

13. Ibid.

14. Dani Veracity.

15. Jerome P. Kassirer, *On the Take, How Medicine's Complicity with Big Business Can Endanger Your Health*, (New York: Oxford University Press, 2005), p. 106, digitized at http://books.google.com/books?id=5jsiffLtnm8C&dq=Jerome+P.+Kassirer,+On+the+Take,+How+Medicine%E2%80%99s +Complicity+with+Big+Business+Can+Endanger+Your+Health&printsec=frontcover&source=bl&ots=NCo-gfZ-pj&sig=WJ4Mb79aF8z7XijQEvPkKSCwa7s&hl=en&ei=d8Ux StLtN-CLtgfVu5SwCQ&sa=X&oi=book_result&ct=result& resnum=3

16. Maggie Mahar, "The Bad Science that Created the Cholesterol Con."

17. *Physicians Committee for Responsible Medicine*, "PCRM Sues Glickman and Shalala," http://www.pcrm.org/news/ lawsuit_summary.html

18. Mike Stobbe, "Cancer to be Top Killer by 2010, WHO says," *newsvine.com* http://www.newsvine.com/_news/2008/12/09/ 2194410-cancer-to-be-worlds-top-killer-by-2010-who-says

19. Ibid.

Chapter 16

1. *USDA Agricultural Research Service*, "ARS Timeline: Founding American Nutrition Science," http://www.ars. usda.gov/is/timeline/nutrition.htm

2. Justus von Liebig was the chemist who developed a method of determining the amount of protein in plant and animal tissue. See Chapter 7.

3. Frank L. Katch, "History Makers, Wilbur Olin Atwater (1844-1907)," http://www.sportsci.org/news/history/atwat er/atwater.html

4. USDA Agriculture Research Service.

5. Katch.

6. Ibid.

7. USDA Agriculture Research Service.

8. Carole Davis and Etta Saltos, "Dietary Recommendations and How They Have Changed Over Time," *USDA publication*, AIB-750, USDA/ERS, p. 33, http://www.ers.usda.gov /publications/aib750/aib750b.pdf

9. Katch.

10. USDA Agriculture Research Service.

11. Ibid.

12. Katch.

13. Davis and Saltos, p. 34

14. Carpenter, "The Life and Times of W.O. Atwater."

15. Ibid..

16. Davis and Saltos, p. 34.

17. Ibid., p. 35.

18. Ibid., p. 36.

19. *NutritionCancer.com*, "History of the Link Between Nutrition and Cancer," http://www.nutritioncancer.com/hi story.html

20. Nestle, *Food Politics*, p. 38.

21. Nestle, p. 39. See also The George S. McGovern Page, http://www.smokershistory.com/McGovern.htm

22. Ibid., p. 40.

23. Ibid.

24. Ibid., p. 41.

25. Ibid., p. 42.

26. Senator McGovern personally told T. Colin Campbell that "he and five other powerful senators from agricultural states lost their respective elections in 1980 in part because they had dared to take on the animal foods industry." Campbell, p. 252.

27. Davis and Saltos, p. 36.

28. Campbell, p. 83.

29. *NutritionCancer.com*, "History of the Link Between Nutrition and Cancer." http://www.nutritioncancer.com /history.html

30. Ibid.

31. Ibid.

32. Ibid.

33. T. Colin Campbell, PhD, "Critique of Report on 'Food, Nutrition and the Prevention of Cancer: A Global Perspective,'" (March/April 2001), *Nutrition Today*, vol. 36(2), pp. 80-84.

34. Campbell, p. 23.

35. Paul R. Thomas and Robert Earl, *Opportunities in the Nutrition and Food Sciences: Research Challenges and the Next Generation of Investigators*, (Washington, D.C.: National Academy Press, 1994), p. 28, http://books.nap.edu/open book.php?record_id=2133&page=R1

36. See Campbell, p. 258. "I turned on a morning TV news show and Tom Brokaw appeared on the screen and started talking about nutrition with Bob Olson...They were discussing a recent report that Olson and friends had produced at the National Academy of Sciences called "Toward Healthful Diets." This report, which was one of the briefest, most superficial reports on health ever produced by the NAS, extolled the virtues of the high-fat, high-meat American diet and basically confirmed that all was well with how America was eating."

37. Ibid.

38. Eric Schlosser, *Fast Food Nation*, (New York: Houghton Mifflin, 2001), p. 204, digitized at http://books.google.com

39. Davis and Saltos, Table 1, p. 38.

40. Campbell, p. 255.

41. Ibid.

Chapter 17

1. Campbell., p. 30.
2. Ibid.
3. Ibid., p. 31.
4. Ibid., p. 102-103.
5. Ibid., p. 101.
6. John McDougall, Dr., "A Brief History of Protein: Passion, Social Bigotry, Rats, and Enlightenment," http://www.all-creatures.org/mfz/health-protein-jm.html
7. Campbell, p. 308.
8. McDougall, "A Brief History of Protein."
9. Campbell, p. 58, 80.
10. Stephen F. Mason, *A History of the Sciences*, (New York: Colier Books, 1977), p. 75.
11. Ibid., pp. 76-78.
12. Kenneth Carpenter, *Protein and Energy: A Study of Changing Ideas in Nutrition*, (Cambridge, New York: Cambridge University Press, 1994), p. 1, digitized at http://books. google.com/books?id=GtQThfnhKLsC&dq=Kenneth+Carp enter,+Protein+and+Energy:+A+Study+of+Changing+Ideas +in+Nutritio&printsec=frontcover&source=bn&hl=en&ei=L q 8 x S u K 7 A 5 - a M q 3 A h J M K & s a = X & o i = b o o k _ result&ct=result&resnum=5
13. Cynthia M. Piccolo, "Timeline: Ibn al-Nafis, c. 1210-1288," *Medhunters*, http://www.medhunters.com/articles/timeline IbnAlNafis.html
14. Mohamad S. M. Takrouri, MB. ChB. FFARCS, "Medical aspects of Ala al-Din Abu'l-Hasan Ali Ibn Abi'l-Haram `al-Qurashi (Ibn al-Nafis)'s contributions to science," http:// www.angelfire.com/md/Takrouri/Ibn_alNafis.htm
15. Dr. Abu Shadi Al-Roubi, "Ibnul-Nafees as a Philosopher," Islamic Organization for Islamic Scientists, http://web .archive.org/web/20080206072116/http://www.islamset.co

m/isc/nafis/drroubi.html

16. Ibid., p. 3.
17. Mason, p. 490.
18. E. Brouwer, "Gerritt Jan Mulder: Biography," *The Journal of Nutrition*, (The Wistar Institute of Anatomy and Biology, 1952), http://jn.nutrition.org/cgi/reprint/46/1/1.pdf
   Mulder's discovery about protein chemistry won him fame and with the backing of Jöns Jacob Berzelius, Michael Faraday, and Justus von Liebig, secured him the position of Professor of Chemistry at the University of Utrecht in 1840.
19. Carpenter, *Protein and Energy*, p. 43.
20. Ibid., pp. 50, 54.
21. Mervyn G. Hardinge, "The Protein Myth: when too much of a good thing is a bad thing," *BNET*, http://findarticles.com/p/articles/mi_m0826/is_n1_v6/ai_8174479
22. Carpenter, *Protein and Energy*, p. 78.
23. Ibid., p. 77.
24. Ibid., p. 79.
25. McDougall, "A Brief History of Protein."
26. Hardinge.
27. McDougall, "A Brief History of Protein."
28. Campbell, p. 28
29. Rupert Sheldrake, *The Rebirth of Nature: The Greening of Science and God*, (Rochester, Vermont: Park Street Press, 1994), pp. 49-53.
30. Mason., p. 58.
31. Sheldrake, pp. 44-53.
32. Ibid.
33. Laurel Robertson et al, *The New Laurel's Kitchen: A Handbook for Vegetarian Cookery & Nutrition*, 2nd ed., (Berkeley, CA: Ten Speed Press, 1986), p. 412, digitized at http://books.google.com/books?id=TsChEsPHL5cC&pg=PA407&lpg=PA407&dq=Laurel+Robertson+et+al,+The+New+Laurel%E2%80%99s+Kitchen:+A+Handbook+for+Vegetarian+Coo

kery+%26+Nutrition&source=bl&ots=yPaYQ8GbCb&sig=S
X3MEQajgpIN_omACcf_Ir3X9CQ&hl=en&ei=oK8xSqyyO
YSoM4Sr5Z4K&sa=X&oi=book_result&ct=result&resnum=
5

34. Ibid.

35. McDougall, "A Brief History of Protein."

36. Bradford L. Nichols, Jr. and Peter J. Reeds, "History of Nutrition: History and Current Status of *Research in Human Energy Metabolism*," (USDA Symposium, Baylor College of Medicine and Texas Children's Hospital, Houston, TX), *American Institute of Nutrition, (Journal of Nutrition*, (April 1991), 121: 1889-1890), http://jn.nutrition.org/cgi/reprint/121/11/1889.pdf.

37. McDougall, "A Brief History of Protein."

38. Ibid..

39. Ibid.

40. Ibid.

41. Dean Ornish, M.D., *Eat More, Weigh Less*.

42. McDougall, "A Brief History of Protein."

43. Ibid.

44. Ibid.

45. Ibid.

46. Ibid.

47. Michael Bluejay, "A History of Vegetarianism with an emphasis on the U.S. from 1970 +," http://michaelbluejay.com/veg/history.html, see reference to McDougall, John A. M.D., *The McDougall Program*, 1990, p. 45.

48. It might also be noted that Quinoa, a grain, is another complete plant-based protein providing as many essential amino acids as meat or fish. It is also a significant source of iron, fiber and B vitamins. (Rinsing it in cold water before cooking, removes what has been called a bitter taste.) See Selene Yeager et al, *Complete Book of Alternative Nutrition*, (Emmaus, PA: Rodale Press, 1997), p. 127.

49. T. St. Jeor Sachiko, RD PhD; Barbara V. Howard, PhD; T. Elaine Prewitt, RD DrPH; Vicki Bovee, RD MS; Terry Bazzarre, PhD; Robert H. Eckel, MD; "Dietary Protein and Weight Reduction," *The American Heart Association*," http://circ.ahajournals.org/cgi/content/full/104/15/1869 ?ijkey=02c8fa98ff287d30167717c3ee0f126da3311fa5

50. *American Heart Association*, "Correspondence, Plant Foods Have a Complete Amino Acid Composition," Letter from John McDougall, M.D. (2002), 105:e197. http://www.circ. ahajournals.org/cgi/content/full/105/25/e197

51. Ibid.

52. Francis Moore Lappé, *Diet for a Small Planet Revisited*, (New York: Random House, Inc. 1982), p. 162, digitized at http://books.google.com/books?id=djAaUJlny0cC&pg=PA1 15&lpg=PA115&dq=Francis+Moore+Lapp%C3%A9,+Diet+f or+a+Small+Planet+Revisited,&source=bl&ots=FsOcs5YR1 V&sig=QtyF5uZM3Jv7XCHNG3Hst8x1Qgo&hl=en&ei=Y7 AxSur-M4-oM-iFgZcK&sa=X&oi=book_result&c t=result&resnum=2

53. Ibid.

54. Ornish, *Eat More, Weigh Less*, p. 22.

55. Angela Roysten, *Proteins for a Healthy Body*, (Chicago: Heinemann Library, 2003), p. 29.

56. *CA: A Cancer Journal for Clinicians*.

57. Campbell, p. 31.

Chapter 18

1. Charles Patterson, *Eternal Treblinka: Our Treatment of Animals and the Holocaust*, (New York: Lantern Books, 2002), pp. 7, 8, http://books.google.com/books?id=zkvY1-t3VxMC &dq=Charles+Patterson,+Eternal+Treblinka&printsec=front cover&source=bn&hl=en&ei=pqhcTIHYCoP78Abu5Nz1Ag &sa=X&oi=book_result&ct=result&resnum=4&ved=0CCUQ

6AEwAw#v=onepage&q&f=false

2. Sheldrake, pp. 44-49.

3. Patterson, p. 3.

4. Gretel H. Pelto and Pertti J. Pelto, *The Human Adventure: An Introduction to Anthropology*, (New York: Macmillan Publishing Co., 1976), p. 460

5. Ibid., p. 27.

6. Ibid., p. 48.

7. Pelto, p. 203.

8. Howard F. Lyman and Glen Merzer, *Mad Cowboy: Plain Truth from the Cattle Rancher Who Won't Eat Meat*, (New York: Touchstone, 1998), pp. 11, 12, http://books.google.com/books?id=_L-N1DsKjZcC&dq=Howard+Lyman,+Mad+Cowboy&printsec=frontcover&source=bn&hl=en&ei=MKhcTNieBML58Aby2-GBAw&sa=X&oi=book_result&ct=result&resnum=7&ved=0CDoQ6AEwBg#v=onepage&q&f=false

9. Ibid.

10. *International Vegetarian Union*, "Ancient Greece and Rome: Socrates (470-399 BCE)," http://www.ivu.org/history/greece_rome/socrates.html

11. Paul Blum, "The Moral Life of Babies," *The New York Times*, (3 May 2010), http://www.nytimes.com/2010/05/09/magazine/09babies-t.html?_r=1&ref=magazine

12. *Sea Shepherd Conservation Society*, "United States Senate Condemns the Canadian Seal Slaughter," (May 11, 2009), http://www.seashepherd.org/news-and-media/news-090511-1.html

Chapter 19

1. Davis, pp. 61 - 63.

2. Epstein, p. 112, 113.

3. *Reuters*, "Humane Society Says Video Shows Abused

Livestock," (May 7, 2008), http://www.reuters.com/article/domesticNews/idUSN0716185920080507

4. *PETA.com*, "Undercover Investigation Reveals Hormel Supplier's Abuse of Mother Pigs and Piglets," http://getactive.peta.org/campaign/iowa_pigfarm_abuse2   See video, http://www.petatv.com/tvpopup/video.asp?video=iowa_sow_farm_investigation_9-08_web_edit_peta&Player=wm

5. Donald G. McNeil, Jr., "Group Documents Cruelty to Turkeys," *The New York Times*, (November 18, 2008), http://www.nytimes.com/2008/11/19/dining/19peta.html?_r=1&scp=1&sq=Aviagen%20Turkey%20Plant&st=cse

6. See, for example, www.all-creatures.org

7. *goveg.com*, "Peta Undercover: Sacred and Federal Laws Violated at Iowa Slaughterhouse," http://www.goveg.com/feat/agriprocessors/

8. Ibid.

9. Jaime Chamber, "The Pig on Your Plate: The Injustice of Factory Farming," *The Humanist*, Essay, Kirksville, MO, http://www.thehumanist.org/humanist/articles/essay.chambers.doc

10. Brian Halweil, "Meat Production Continues to Rise," *Worldwatch Institute*, (August 20, 2008), http://www.worldwatch.org/node/5443

11. *Simplot*, "Feedlots," http://www.simplot.com/land/cattle_feeding/feedlots.cfm

12. Lloyd Alter, "Cows Can Be Transported For 52 Hours Without Food or Water," *treehugger.com* (September 8, 2008), http://www.treehugger.com/files/2008/09/cows-can-be-transported-52-hours.php

13. *Farm Sanctuary*, "Factory Farming.com: Factory Beef Production," (April 2006), http://farmsanctuary.org/issues/factoryfarming/beef/

14. See chapter 24 for more on CAFOs and feedlots.

15. *Farm Sanctuary*.

16. *goveg.com*, "Cows Used for Their Milk," http://www.goveg.com/factoryFarming_Cows_Dairy.asp

17. Samuel S. Epstein, *What's In Your Milk*? (Bloomington, IN: Trafford Publishing, 2006).

18. Schlosser, p. 204.

19. *United Poultry Concerns, Inc.*, "Forced Molting of "Laying" Hens — Fact Sheet," http://www.fda.gov/ohrms/dockets/dailys/00/may00/050300/c000019.pdf

20. *goveg.com*, "The Egg Industry," http://www.goveg.com/factoryFarming_chickens_egg.asp

21. Ibid.

22. Ibid.

23. *PETA TV*, "45 Days in Hell: The Life and Death of a Broiler Chicken," http://www.petatv.com/tvpopup/video.asp?video=45_days&Player=wm

24. *PETA*, "Undercover Investigations: Thousands of Chickens Tortured by KFC Supplier," http://www.kentuckyfriedcruelty.com/u-pilgrimspride.asp

25. Schlosser, Ch. 7,"*Cogs in the Great Machine*," p. 149.

26. Schlosser, p. 156.

27. Ibid.

28. Julia Preston, "Meatpacker Is Fined Nearly $10 Million," *The New York Times*, October 29, 2008, http://www.nytimes.com/2008/10/30/us/30fine.html

29. Schlosser, p. 197.

30. Ibid., p. 195.

31. Ibid., p. 138.

32. Ibid., p. 158.

33. Matthew Green, "Udder Confusion: Difficult Choices in the Dairy Aisle," *Edible East Bay* (Spring 2008), http://www.edibleeastbay.com/content/pages/articles/spring08/udder.pdf

34. Schlosser, p. 158.

35. Ibid., p. 155.

Chapter 20

1. *PETA Media Center*, "Animal Experiments: Overview, Funding and Accountability," http://www.peta.org/mc /factsheet_display.asp?ID=126
2. Ibid.
3. *Humane Society International, HSUS*, "Scientific Research," http://www.hsus.org/hsi/animal_experiments/scientific _research/
4. *Physicians Committee for Responsible Medicine*, "Good Medicine, Illegal Experiments: Physicians File Lawsuit Against USCF for Violating Animal Welfare Law," (Autumn, 2007), Volume XVI, Number 4, http://www. pcrm.org/magazine/gm07autumn/illegal_experiments.html See also http://www.pcrm.org/newsletter/sep07/physi- cians_sue.html
5. *PETA Media Center*, "Animal Experiments: Overview, Funding and Accountability," http://www.peta.org/mc/ factsheet_display.asp?ID=126
6. Jim Giles and Meredith Wadman, "Grants Fall Victim to NIH Success," Nature (October 26, 2006), 443, 894-895, http://www.nature.com/nature/journal/v443/n7114/full/443 894a.html
7. Dana Yarri, *The Ethics of Animal Experimentation: A Critical Analysis and Constructive Christian Proposal,* (New York: Oxford University Press, 2005), p. 14.
8. "Number of Active Research Facilities," Laboratory Primate Advocacy Group, http://www.lpag.org/lay person/lay person.html#labsnumber
9. The North Carolina Associates for Biomedical Research, for example, relies upon this data. See *North Carolina Associates for Biomedical Research*, "How Many and What Kinds of

Animals are Used in Biomedical Research," http://www. ncabr.org/biomzed/FAQ_animal/faq_animal_13.html

10. Yarri, p. 14.

11. Tzachi Zamir, *Ethics and the Beast*, (Princeton, NJ: Princeton University Press, 2007), p. 80, digitized at http://books.google.com/books?id=3oEKodnhg48C&dq=Tzachi+Zamir,+Ethics+and+the+Beast&printsec=frontcover&source=bn&hl=en&ei=2LwxSovNN56qtgePz_yqCQ&sa=X&oi=book_result&ct=result&resnum=4.

12. Campbell, p. 316.

13. *Stop Animal Exploitation Now* (S.A.E.N.), "Animal Experimentation in the United States (2007)," http://www.all-creatures.org/saen/fact-anex-2007.html

14. *World Laboratory Animal Liberation Week*, "The Animal Experimentation Scandal: An Audit of the National Institutes of Health Funding of Animal Experimentation," http://www.all-creatures.org/wlalw/report-anexp-audit.html

15. *Humane Society of the United States*, "USDA Animal Welfare Act Enforcement Report," http://www.hsus.org/animals_in_research/animals_in_research_news/usda_report_on_animal_welfare.html

16. *Stop Animal Exploitation Now* (S.A.E.N), "Animal Experimentation in the United States."

17. The movement for the divestiture of university stocks and bonds in South African investments started at Stanford, Michigan State University, Ohio University, the University of Wisconsin at Madison, and Columbia University but quickly spread across the country to other campuses like UCLA, UC Berkeley, Ohio State University, Harvard/Radcliffe, SUNY Albany, and many, many others.

18. Daniela Derson, "Just Like South Africa," *New Voices, National Jewish Student Magazine,* (November 17, 2002), http://newvoices.org/features/just-like-south-africa.html

19. *In Defense of Animals,* "Help End Nicotine Experiments on Monkeys at OHSU," http://www.vivisectioninfo.org/campaigns/spindel/

20. Ibid.

21. *Oregon Health and Science University,* "Eliot Spindel," http://www.ohsu.edu/xd/research/centers-institutes/onprc/scientific-discovery/scientists/eliot-spindel.cfm

22. *Animal Rights History,* "Cicero: Cicero Marcus Tullius 106 - 43 BCE," http://www.animalrightshistory.org/timeline-antiquity/cicero.htm

23. *International Vegetarian Union,* "Herodotus (484 - 425 B.C.)," http://www.ivu.org/history/greece_rome/herodotus .html

24. Animal research as a branch of science has a well-deserved bad name, no matter how much university prestige and the award of the Nobel Prize to some scientists who have practiced vivisection may try to ennoble it. All justifications for what is going on in animal research laboratories pale in comparison to the criticisms of some of the greatest artists, philosophers, poets, scientists, theologists, thinkers, and writers in the history of the world. How do these animal research scientists hold their heads high and answer to people like Jeremy Bentham, William Blake, Robert Browning, Lord Byron, Rachel Carson, Margaret Cavendish, Winston Churchill, Cicero, Thomas Edison, Albert Einstein, St. Francis of Assisi, Sigmund Freud, Mahatma Gandhi, Thomas Hardy, Herodotus, Hippocrates, Victor Hugo, C.W. Hume, William Ralph Inge, Immanuel Kant, Pope John Paul II, Carl Jung, Jiddu Krishnamurti, C.S. Lewis, Abraham Lincoln, John Locke, Ashley Montague, John Muir, Ovid, Thomas Paine, Plutarch, Pythagoras, Alexander Pope, Romaine Rolland, Eleanor Roosevelt, George Bernard Shaw, Arthur Schopenhauer, Albert Schweitzer, Isaac Bashevis Singer, Socrates, Robert Louis Stevenson, Harriet Beecher Stowe, Henry David Thoreau,

Leo Tolstoy, Mark Twain, Leonardo da Vinci, Francois Voltaire, Alice Walker, and Emile Zola.

25. *Animal Rights History*, "Voltaire [Francois Marie Arouet] 1694 - 1778." http://www.animalrightshistory.org/animal-rights-enlightenment/voltaire.htm

26. *Poetwilll.org*, "Running for Their Lives," http://www.poetwill.org/billman_dogs.htm

27. Ibid.

28. *Rush PR News*, "Meet Dog 3017 — Ohio State University's Latest Lab Casualty," (April 22, 2009), http://www.rushprnews.com/2009/04/22/meet-dog-3017-ohio-state-universitys-latest-lab-casualty/

29. Dana Yarri, p. 69.

30. *Physicians Committee for Responsible Medicine*, "Good Medicine, Illegal Experiments: Physicians File Lawsuit Against USCF for Violating Animal Welfare Law."

31. *Stop Animal Exploitation Now* (S.A.E.N.), "Government Grants Promoting Cruelty to Animals, University of Minnesota, Minneapolis, MN, Marilyn E. Carroll, Primate Testing, 2005 - 2007," http://www.all-creatures.org/saen/res-fr-mn-um-grant-carroll-2005.html

32. *Columbia University*, "Department of Psychiatry," http://ps-handbook.com/2008/node/289

33. *University of California San Francisco*, "UCSF Institutional Animal Care and Use Committee," http://www.iacuc.ucsf.edu/

34. Ibid.

35. *Sourcewatch Encyclopedia*, "Ten Worst Laboratories," http://www.sourcewatch.org/index.php?title=Ten_Worst_Laboratories

36. *Physicians Committee for Responsible Medicine (PCRM)*, "Good Medicine, Illegal Experiments: Physicians Sue California University for Violating Animal Welfare Law."

37. *Physicians Committee for Responsible Medicine*, "March of

Dimes-Funded Animal Experiments: An Overview," reviewed by Peggy Carlson, M.D., and Kristie Stoick, M.P.H., http://www.pcrm.org/resch/charities/mod_over view.html See also http://www.pcrm.org/newsletter/apr07 /mod.html

38. *Sourcewatch Encyclopedia*, "Ten Worst Laboratories."

39. Ann Stauble, "Cats and NEAVS don't fancy this Cat Fancy Article," *New England Anti-Vivisection Society*, (June 29, 2001), http://www.neavs.org/programs/avoiceforanimals /lte_catfancy_06292001.htm

40. PCRM, "Physicians File Lawsuit Against USCF."

41. Jane Goodall, "A Plea for the Chimps," *NY Times Magazine*, May 17, 1987.

42. Ibid.

Chapter 21

1. *Columbia University*, "Medical Research with Animals," http://cumc.columbia.edu/research/animal/standards.html

2. Ibid.

3. Madhusree Mukerjee, "Trends in Animal Research," *Scientific American Magazine*, (February 1997).

4. John Young interviewed by Saul Gonzalez, Tim O'Brien, anchor, "Animal Testing Ethics," *Religious & Ethics Newsweekly*, (August 15, 2008), Episode no. 1150, http://www.pbs.org/wnet/religionandethics/week1150/cove r.html Contains interview transcription and video.

5. Doug Melton interviewed by Charlie Rose in "Stem Cells with Dr. Doug Melton," *Charlie Rose Show*, http://www. charlierose.com/view/interview/10274

6. Ibid.

7. Ibid.

8. Robert A.J. Matthews, "Medical progress depends on animals, doesn't it," *Podium*, (2008), J R Soc Med, 101: 95-98.

DOI 10.1258/jrsm.2007.070164, http://www.animalexperi
ments.info/assets/studies/Human%20relevance%20Contrib
utions%20to%20medical%20progress%20Matthews%20200
8%20JRSM.pdf

9.   Ibid.

10. See also Animal Information Center Newsletter, (Summer
     1994), Vol. 5, No. 2, ISSN. 1050-561X, http://www.nal
     .usda.gov/awic/newsletters/v5n2/5n2toc.htm

11. *Animal Rights Quotes*, http://www.animalliberationfront
     .com/Saints/Authors/Quotes/SortQuotesVivis.htm

12. Marc Bekoff, "In Conversation," *Bark Magazine*, No. 10,
     (2000), http://www.sheldrake.org/interviews/bark_inter
     view;:.html

13. Marc Bekoff et al., *The Cognitive Animal: Empirical and
     Theoretical Perspectives on Animal Cognition*, (Cambridge,
     MA: MIT Press, 2002), digitized at http://books.google.com
     /books?id=TztyW8eTnIC&pg=PA105&lpg=PA105&dq=Mar
     c+Bekoff+et+al.,+The+Cognitive+Animal:+Empirical+and+T
     heoretical+Perspectives+on+Animal+Cognition&source=bl
     &ots=uHmbTAnmCk&sig=r8KsoLR5fNJi4ut1jyvUQermZx
     k&hl=en&ei=gL4xSrvAGYSGtgfuyIyCQ&sa=X&oi=book_r
     esult&ct=result&resnum=2

14. Jeremy Rifkin, "Our Fellow Creatures Have Feelings — So
     We Should Give Them Rights Too," Common Dreams.Org
     (August 16, 2006), http://www.commondreams.org/views
     03/0816-05.htm

15. Laura Tangley, "Animal Emotions, " *U.S. News and World
     Report*, (October 22, 2000), http://www.usnews.com/usnews
     /culture/articles/001030/archive_010364_3.htm See also
     Connie Garfalk, "Help, My Cat Loves Me, " Offbeat Cats,
     http://www.offbeat-cats.com/feature_feelings_e.html

16. Ibid.

17. Robert W. Shumaker and Karyl B. Schwartz, "When
     Traditional Methodologies Fail, Cognitive Studies of Great

Apes," in Bekoff, *The Cognitive Animal*, p. 337.

18. Sara J. Shettleworth, "Spatial Behavior, Food Storing, and the Modular Mind," in Bekoff, *The Cognitive Animal*, p. 126.

19. *World Science*, "Rock-throwing zoo chimp stocked ammo in advance: study," (March 10, 2009), http://www.world-science.net/othernews/090310_chimp

20. Coco Ballantyne, "Planning of the Apes: Zoo Chimp Plots Rock Attacks on Visitors," *Scientific American*, (March 9, 2009), http://www.scientificamerican.com/article.cfm?id=chimpanzee-plans-throws-stones-zoo

21. *World Science*, "Rock-throwing chimp."

22. Charlie Rose Interview with Doug Melton.

23. Walt Whitman, "Song of Myself" from *Leaves of Grass*.

24. *Scientific American*, "Feds Agree to Toxicity Tests That Cut Animal Testing," http://www.scientificamerican.com/article.cfm?id=feds-agree-to-toxicity-test&page=2

25. Ibid.

26. *boston.com*, "Are the lab rat's days numbered?" http://www.boston.com/business/healthcare/articles/2009/03/30/are_the_lab_rats_days_numbered/?page=1

27. Ibid.

28. Matthew Knight, "Scientist: stem cells could end animal testing," (Dec. 22, 2008), Animals and Animal Rights in the Media Worldwide, http://animals-in-the-news.blogspot.com/2008/12/professor-christine-mummery-van-leids.html

Chapter 22

1. John Cawley, "Markets and Childhood Obesity Policy," *The Future of Children*, (2006), 16, no. 1, http://www.futureofchildren.org/information2826/information_show.htm?doc_id=355339

2. Jeffrey P. Koplan, Catharyn T. Liverman, Vivica I. Kraak, Eds., *Preventing Childhood Obesity, Health in The Balance*,

Institute of Medicine of the National Academies, (Washington, D.C.: The National Academies Press), p.1, http://www.nap. edu/openbook.php?isbn=0309091969&page=1

3. Mary Story and Simone French, "Food Advertising and Marketing Directed at Children and Adolescents in the U.S.," *International Journal of Behavioral Nutrition and Physical Activity,* (2004), **1**:3doi:10.1186/1479-5868-1-3, http://www.ijbnpa.org/content/1/1/3

4. Ellen Fried and Michele Simon, "The Competitive Food Conundrum: Can Government Regulations Improve School Food?" *Duke Law Journal,* (2007), 56, no. 6, p. 1492. See www.law.duke.edu/shell/cite.pl?56+Duke+L.+J.+1491 +pdf

5. Ibid.

6. *The Journal of Physical Education, Recreation & Dance,* "Child Obesity-What Can Schools Do?" (2001), vol. 72, Issue: 2.

7. Koplan, *Preventing Childhood Obesity, Health in the Balance,* p. 172.

8. Smith, J. Clinton, M.D., M.P.H., *Understanding Childhood Obesity,* (Jackson, MS: University Press of Mississippi, 1999), pp. 26, 27.

9. National Center for Health Statistics, http://www.cdc.gov/ nchs/products/pubs/pubd/hestats/overweight/overwght_a dult_03.htm

10. Ibid.

11. Story and French.

12. Koplan, *Preventing Childhood Obesity, Health in the Balance,* p. 172.

13. Fried and Simon, p. 1498.

14. Ibid.

15. *Care2,* "Soft Drinks & Cancer, Chocolate & Strokes," http://www.care2.com/greenliving/soft-drinks-cancer-chocolate-strokes.html. The researchers theorize that stressing the pancreas repeatedly with high doses of sugar leads to inflammation, which in turn sets up a vulnerability

to pancreatic cancer.

16. *Center for Science in the Public Interest*, "Two-thirds of States Get Poor Grades on School Food Report Card," (Feb. 7, 2008), Newsroom, http://www.cspinet.org/new/200711281.html

17. Fried and Simon, p. 1498.

18. Ibid., p. 1492.

19. *Tom Harkin, Iowa's Senator*, "It's Time For Better Nutrition In Our Schools," (May 14, 2007), http://harkin.senate.gov/pr/col.cfm?id=274213

20. Fried and Simon, p. 1502.

21. Ibid., p. 1493.

22. Ibid., p. 1502.

23. Ibid., p. 1500.

24. Ibid., p. 1507.

25. Ibid., p. 1508.

26. Ibid., p. 1509.

27. Ibid.

28. Ibid., p. 1510.

29. Kim Severson, "National Briefing/Education; Trying Anew To Rein In School Foods," *The New York Times*, (December 18, 2007), http://query.nytimes.com/gst/fullpage.html?res=9C07E6DD1F3AF93BA25751C1A9619C8B6

30. *Text of H.R. 1363*, "Child Nutrition Promotion and School Lunch Protection Act of 2007," http://www.open congress.org /bill/110-h1363/text -

31. *The Food Studies Institute*, http://www.foodstudies.org/Curriculum/LessonSummaries.htm

32. *Wellness Forum*, http://www.wellnessforum.com/

33. Bao Ong, "A Push to Start the School Week Without Meat," *The New York Times: City Room*, (February 22, 2010), http://cityroom.blogs.nytimes.com/2010/02/22/a-push-for-students-to-start-their-week-without-meat/

Chapter 23

1. Campbell, p. 294
2. Ibid., p. 292.
3. Ibid., p. 293.
4. Ibid.
5. *National Dairy Council*, "Educators Journey Into Nutrition Educeation," Nutrition Explorations," (March 2009), http://www.nutritionexplorations.com/educators/lessons/chef-combo/chef-combo.asp?tab=1
6. Ibid.
7. *Campaign for Commercial-free Childhood*, "Guest Opinion: Schools should ditch partnerships with McDonald's," (January 2, 2008), http://www.commercialexploitation.org/news/schoolsshould.htm
8. Susan Linn and Diane E. Levin, "Stop marketing 'yummy' food to children," Commentary, *The Christian Science Monitor*, (June 20, 2002), http://www.csmonitor.com/2002/0620/p09s01-coop.html.
9. *Sustainweb.org.*, "Children's food campaigners complain about ads for 'manly' burgers," Children's food campaign, news, http://www.sustainweb.org/news.php?id=165
10. Darlene Martin, "NF97-315 Overview of the USDA School Meals Initiative for Healthy Children," Historical Materials from University of Nebraska - Lincoln Extension, (January 1997), http://digitalcommons.unl.edu/cgi/viewcontent.cgi?article=1416&context=extensionhist
11. *azcentral.com*, "How do school menus jibe with kids' calorie needs," (January 8, 2005), http://www.azcentral.com/health/kids/articles/0108ob26schoolfoodgraphic.html
12. *Center for Science in the Public Interet*, Litigation Project: Current Docket, http://www.cspinet.org/litigation/
13. *CSPI Newsroom*, "Americans and Europeans Want Tougher Action on Childhood Obesity and Diet-Related Disease," (April 2, 2008), http://www.cspinet.org/new/200804022

.html

14. Ibid.

15. Patricia M. Anderson and Kristin F. Butcher, "Childhood Obesity: Trends and Potential Causes," *The Future of Children*, (2006), 16, no. 1, p. 21. See http://www.future-ofchildren.org/usr_doc/02_obesity_anderson-butcher.pdf

16. *CSPI Newsroom*, "Consumer Groups in 20 Countries Urge Coke, Pepsi to Limit Soft Drink Marketing to Children," (January 3, 2008), http://www.cspinet.org/new/200801031 .html

17. Ibid.

18. Ibid.

19. Helen Rae, "Healthy Start to the War on Junk Foods: in Association with the NHS. A North East MP Is Keen to See an End to Junk Food Advertising," Report, *Evening Chronicle* (Newcastle, England), (May 19, 2008), http://www .entrepreneur.com/tradejournals/article/179162632.html

20. *Daily Post Comment*, "Junk Food Ad Ban Is a Drop in the Ocean," (Liverpool, England), (November 15, 2004), http:// www.highbeam.com/Search.aspx?q=Daily+Post+Comment +%e2%80%9cJunk+Food+Ad+Ban+Is+a+Drop+in+the+Ocea n%e2%80%9d+

21. *CSPI Newsroom*, "Americans and Europeans Want Tougher Action."

22. *Tom Harkin, Iowa's Senator.*

23. Kelly D., Brownell, "Childhood Obesity," Issues in Science and Technology, *Forum*, (Summer 2005), http://www. issues.org/21.4/forum.html

Chapter 24

1. John Blake, "As Children Starve, World Struggles for Solutions," *CNN.com*, (November 18, 2008), http://www. cnn.com/2008/US/11/17/hunger.week/index.html

2. Shaohua Chen and Martin Ravallion, "The developing world is poorer than we thought, but no less successful in the fight against poverty," Policy Research Working Paper, *World Bank*, (August 1, 2008), http://econ.worldbank. org/external/default/main?pagePK=64165259&theSitePK=4 69372&piPK=64165421&menuPK=64166093&entityID=0001 58349_20080826113239. See also http://siteresources. worldbank.org/DEC/Resources/Poverty-Brief-in-English.pdf

3. *World Health Organization, The Lancet: The Lancet's Series on Maternal and Child Undernutrition, Executive Summary*, p. 2, http://www.who.int/nutrition/topics/Lancetseries_ ExecutiveSummary.pdf

4. *World Health Organization*, "Under-nutrition is the underlying cause of death for at least 30% of all Children under age five," *Fact File*, http://www.who.int/features/factfiles /global_burden/facts/en/index9.html

5. Andrew Weil, *Eating Well for Optimal Health*, (New York: Random House, 2001), p. 112

6. Jeremy Rifkin, "The World's Problem on a Plate, 2002," *News Center, CommonDreams.org* Originally published in The Guardian of London, http://www.commondreams. org/views02/0517-03.htm

7. Ibid.

8. *Northwestern Health Sciences University*, "Grain-Fed Versus Grass-Fed Animal Products," Healthy U, Sources, J Animal Sci 80(5): 1202-11, 2002, http://www.nwhealth.edu/healthy U/eatWell/grassfed.html See also *Eat Wild*, http://www. eatwild.com/

9. Lyman and Merzer, p. 127.

10. *Northwestern Health Sciences University*, "Grain-Fed Versus Grass-Fed Animal Products."

11. Lyman and Merzer, p. 127.

12. Rifkin, *The World's Problem on a Plate*.

13. Stephen Leckie, "How Meat-Centered Eating Patterns Affect Food Security and the Environment," *International Development Research Center*, http://www.idrc.ca/en/ev-30610-201-1-DO_TOPIC.html

14. Rifkin, *The World's Problem on a Plate.*

15. Ibid.

16. Ibid.

17. *Food and Agriculture Organization of the United Nations*, "Livestock's Long Shadow," Summary and Conclusions, p. 272, (Rome 2007), http://www.fao.org/docrep/010/a0701e /a0701e00.HTM

18. Ibid.

19. Leckie.

20. *Food and Agriculture Organization of the United Nations*, "Livestock's Long Shadow," Section V, Livestock's role in water depletion and pollution, p. 98, (Rome 2007).

21. Jeff Tietz, "Boss Hog," *Rolling Stone*, (December 14, 2006), http://www.rollingstone.com/politics/story/12840743/porks _dirty_secret_the_nations_top_hog_producer_is_also_one_ of_americas_worst_polluters

22. *Food & Water Europe*, "A Factory Farm Force: US Multinational Smithfield Moves into Europe," (2008), See Scribd, http://www.scribd.com/doc/6303027/A-Factory-Farm-Force-US-Multinational-Smithfield-Moves-into-Europe

23. Ibid.

24. Ibid.

25. Ibid.

26. Ibid.

27. Leckie.

28. UNEP, E. Hertwich, E. van der Voet, S. Suh, A. Tukker, M. Huijbregts, P. Kazmierczyk, M. Lenzen, J. McNeely, Y. Moriguchi, "Assessing the Environmental Impacts of Consumption and Production: Priority Products and

Materials, A Report of the Working Group on the Environmental Impacts of Products and Materials to the International Panel for Sustainable Resource Management," (2010), p. 80. See also Warren McLaren, "Half of World Crop is Feeding Animals, Not People," *Treehugger.com* June 22, 2010. http://www.treehugger.com/files/2010/06/half-of-world-crop-feeding-animals-not-people.php http://www.unep.org/resourcepanel/documents/pdf/PriorityProducts AndMaterials_Report_Full.pdf

29. *Food and Agriculture Organization of the United Nations,* "Livestock's Long Shadow," pp. 267-284

30. E. Hertwich et al

31. Rifkin, *The World's Problem on a Plate*

32. Brian Halweil, "Meat Production Continues to Rise."

33. *Peta2 Free For All*, "Take Charge: Stop School Slaughter," http://www.peta2.com/takecharge/t-stoptheslaughter.asp

34. *Food and Agriculture Organization of the United Nations,* "Livestock's Long Shadow," Livestock a major Threat to environment, *Executive Summary, p. xx.*

35. Ibid.

36. Campbell, pp. 239, 240.

Chapter 25

1. Lindsay Layton, "Peanut Executive Takes The Fifth," *Washington Post,* (February 12, 2009), http://www.washingtonpost.com/wp-dyn/content/article/2009/02/11/AR2009 021104174.html

2. Amy Kover, "Wall Street Week: Unhip, Unabashed, Unbeaten Louis Rukeyser, Superstar," *Fortune,* (Aug 3, 1998), http://money.cnn.com/magazines/fortune/fortune_ archive /1998/08/03/246302/index.htm

3. Albert Schweitzer, *Reverence for Life,* (Irvington Publishers, Second Printing, 1993), p. 115, http://books.google. com/

books?id=FHRAVQYFDlYC&printsec=frontcover&dq=Albe
rt+Schweitzer,+Reverence+for+Life&source=bl&ots=5YUsH
wZ7Dc&sig=H_Hk8CUDTFNSc-SKNTD2gGAA_6E&hl=
en&ei=YmNcTIDgO8H8Aaxw9nXAg&sa=X&oi=book_resul
t&c t=result&resnum =8&ved=0CDkQ6AEwBw#v=onepage
&q&f=false

Appendix I

1. *Physicians Committee for Responsible Medicine*, "March of Dimes-Funded Animal Experiments: An Overview."
2. *The National Humane Education Society*, "Research Issues, U.S. Agencies and Animal Testing," http://www.nhes.org/articles/view/750
3. *StopAnimalTests.com*, "U.S. Government Testing Programs," http://www.stopanimaltests.com/us-gov.asp
4. Sourcewatch.org, "U.S. Government's War on Animals," http://www.sourcewatch.org/index.php?title=U.S._Govern ment's_War_on_Animals#DoD_animal_testing_programs

Appendix III

1. *Animal Times Summer 2002*, "Special Undercover Investigation," www.peta.org/Living/at-summer2002/UN Clab/
2. *Stop AnimalTests.com*, "Peta's '10 Worst Laboratories' List," http://www.stopanimaltests.com/f-worstlabs_09.asp
3. *In Defense of Animals*, "The Horrific Monkey Experiments of New York University," http://www.vivisectioninfo.org/nyu.html
4. Ibid.
5. *Rush PR News*, "Meet Dog 3017."
6. *Sourcewatch Encyclopedia*, "Ten Worst Laboratories."
7. *In Defense of Animals*, "The Truth About Vivisection," http://www.vivisectioninfo.org/lisberger.html

8. *In Defense of Animals*, "IDA's Response to NIH Defense of Lisberger," http://www.vivisectioninfo.org/uscf/nihre-sponse.html

Bibliography

Adams, Mike, ed., "Scientific medical journals like JAMA fail basic credibility standards; medical journals become increasingly irrelevant," *Natural News.com* (Aug. 19, 2004), http://www.naturalnews.com/001890.htm

Agatston, Arthur, M.D., *The South Beach Diet*, (New York: St. Martin's Press, 2003), http://books.google.com/books?id=HGOqFd5ALhsC&dq=Arthur+Agatston,+M.D.,+The+South+Beach+Diet&printsec=frontcover&source=bn&hl=en&ei=qL8xSovMBcKltgfWncjACQ&sa=X&oi=book_result&ct=result&resnum=4

Allegheny General Hospital, "Dean Ornish Program for Reversing Heart Disease,"
http://www.wpahs.org/agh/services/index.cfm?mode=view&medicalspecialty=547

"Alpha Linolenic Acid, ALA," *Raysahelian.com*, http://www.raysahelian.com/linolenic.html

Al-Roubi, Dr. Abu Shadi, "Ibnul-Nafees as a Philosopher," Islamic Organization for Islamic Scientists, http://web.archive.org/web/20080206072116/
http://www.islamset.com/isc/nafis/drroubi.html

Alter, Lloyd, "Cows Can Be Transported For 52 Hours Without Food or Water," *treehugger.com* (September 8, 2008),
http://www.treehugger.com/files/2008/09/cows-can-be-transported-52-hours.php

AMA website, "AMA History," http://www.ama-assn.org/ama/pub/category/1854.html

American Botanical Council, "Herbs in the Hoxsey Cancer Tonic," Herb Clip TM, ed. Mark Blumenthal,
http://74.125.47.132/search?q=cache:9JBXjVatgbsJ:content.herbalgram.org/tomsofmaine/HerbClip/pdfs/070217211.pdf+%E2%80%9CHerbs+in+the+Hoxsey+Cancer+Tonic,%E2%80%9D+A

merican+Botanical+Council&cd=1&hl=en&ct=clnk&gl=us, or
http://content.herbalgram.org/tomsofmaine/HerbClip/pdfs/0
70217-211.pdf

American Cancer Society, "American Cancer Society to Host
Cattle Barron's Ball in Youngstown," (September 7, 2007),
http://www.cancer.org/docroot/COM/content/div_OH/COM
_1_1x_AS_2007_American_Cancer_Society_to_Host_Cattle_
Barons_Ball.asp

American Cancer Society Foundation, "Board of Trustees,"
American Cancer Society.

http://foundation.cancer.org/foundation/content/Board_of_Trus
tees.asp

American Cancer Society, "Estimated New Cancer Cases and
Deaths by Sex," (2008), http://www.cancer.org/docroot/NWS/
content/NWS_1_1x_Cancer_Facts_and_Figures_2008_Releas
ed.asp

American Cancer Society, Eating Lots of Red Meat Linked to
Colon Cancer, *see JAMA* (Vol. 293, No. 2: 172-182) http://
www.cancer.org/docroot/NWS/content/NWS_1_1x_Eating_L
ots_of_Red_Meat_Linked_to_Colon_Cancer.asp

American Cancer Society, "The Complete Guide, Nutrition and
Physical Activity," http://www.cancer.org/docroot/PED/
content/PED_3_2X_Diet_and_Activity_Factors_That_Affect_
Risks.asp?sitearea=PED

American Cancer Society, "Making Treatment Decisions," see Are
there any possible problems or complications, http://www.
cancer.org/docroot/ETO/content/ETO_5_3X_Omega-
3_Fatty_Acids.asp

American Cancer Society, "Prevention and Early Detection:
Cigarette Smoking," http://www.cancer.org/docroot/PED/
content/PED_10_2X_Cigarette_Smoking.asp

American Cancer Society, "Shopping List:Basic Ingredients for a
Healthy Kitchen," http://www.cancer.org/docroot/subsite/
greatamericans/content/Shopping_List_Basic_Ingredients_fo

r_a_Healthy_Kitchen.asp

American Heart Association, "AHA Statistical Update: Heart Disease and Stroke Statistics — 2009 Update," p. e22, http://circ.ahajournals.org/cgi/reprint/CIRCULATIONAHA.108.191261

American Heart Association, "Calcium, Dietary," http://www.americanheart.org/presenter.jhtml?identifier=4453

American Heart Association, "Cardiovascular disease death rates decline, but risk factors still exact heavy toll," (December 1, 2007), http://www.americanheart.org/presenter.jhtml?identifier=3052670

American Heart Association, "Correspondence, Plant Foods Have a Complete Amino Acid Composition," letter from John McDougall, M.D. (2002), 105:e197, http://www.circ.ahajournals.org/cgi/content/full/105/25/e197

American Institute for Cancer Newsletter, "Getting Back in Balance With Your Meals," (Spring 2009), Issue 103, http://www.aicr.org/site/DocServer/NL103-Spring09.pdf?docID=2821

American Institute for Cancer Research," Second Expert Report: Food, Nutrition, Physical Activity, and the Prevention of Cancer: a Global Perspective," see Read the Recommendations for Cancer Prevention., http://www.aicr. org/site/PageServer?pagename=res_report_second

American Institute for Cancer Research, Stories, "Summertime Tales: NW: Questions about calcium needs, crab and clams, grapefruit and weight loss," (July 27, 2009), http://www.aicr.org/feed/rss2_0/stories.rss

American Institute of Philanthropy, "Top 25 Compensation Packages," http://www.charitywatch.org/hottopics/Top25.html

American Physiological Society Policy Action Center, "Opponents of Research Target Charities." http://www.the-aps.org/pa/resources/bionews/charities.htm

Anderson, Patricia M. and Kristin F. Butcher, "Childhood

Obesity: Trends and Potential Causes," *The Future of Children* (2006), 16, no. 1, p. 21. See http://www.futureofchildren.org/usr_doc/02_obesity_anderson-butcher.pdf

Animal Rights History, "Cicero Marcus Tullius 106-43 BCE," http://www.animalrightshistory.org/timeline-antiquity/cicero.htm

Animal Rights Quotes, http://www.animalliberationfront.com/Saints/Authors/Quotes/SortQuotesVivis.htm

Annieappleseed Project, "Dean Ornish, Nutrition and Prostate Cancer," from Dr. Gregor Newsletter, (Fall 2005), http://www.annieappleseedproject.org/deanornutpro.html

Appleby, Paul N., Timothy JA Key, Jim I. Mann, and Margaret Thorogood, "The Oxford Vegetarian Study: an Overview," American Journal of Clinical Nutrition, Vol. 70, No. 3, 525S-531S, (September 1999), http://www.ajcn.org/cgi/content/abstract/70/3/525S? maxtoshow=&HITS=10&hits=10&RESULTFORMAT=&fulltext=vegetarian+heart&andorexact-fulltext=and&searchid=1132367986572_14818&stored_search=&FIRSTINDEX=0&sortspec=relevance&resourcetype=1&journalcode=ajcn

Ausubel, Kenny, *When Healing Becomes a Crime: The Amazing Story of the Hoxsey Cancer Clinics and the Return of Alternative Therapies,* (Rochester, Vermont: Healing Arts Press, 2001).

azcentral.com, "How do school menus jibe with kids' calorie needs," (January 8, 2005).

Balzer, Ben, M.D., "Introduction to the Paleolithic Diet," *Earth 360.com,* http://www.earth360.com/diet_paleodiet_balzer.html

Barnard, Neal, Contributor, Physicians Committee for Responsible Medicine, *Healthy Eating for Life for Women,* (New York: John Wiley and Sons, 2002), see at http://books.google.com/books?id=yrT1-yPg7PIC&dq=Healthy+Eating+for+Life+for+Women&printsec=frontcover&source=bn&hl=en&ei=ZoFETIbnJoP7lwfVooXOAg&sa=X&oi=book_result&ct

=result&resnum=5&ved=0CDEQ6AEwBA#v=onepage&q&f=f
alse

Bekoff, Marc, "In Conversation," *Bark Magazine*, No. 10, (2000), http://www.sheldrake.org/interviews/bark_interview.html

Bekoff, Marc, Allen Colin and Gordon M. Burghardt, *The Cognitive Animal: Empirical and Theoretical Perspectives on Animal Cognition*, (Cambridge, MA: MIT Press, 2002), http:// books.google.com/books?id=T-ztyW8eTnIC&pg=PA105& lpg=PA105&dq=Marc+Bekoff+et+al.,+The+Cognitive+Animal: +Empirical+and+Theoretical+Perspectives+on+Animal+Cogni tion&source=bl&ots=uHmbTAnmCk&sig=r8KsoLR5fNJi4ut1j yvUQermZxk&hl=en&ei=gL4xSrvAGYSGtgfuyIyCQ&sa=X& oi=book_result&ct=result&resnum=2

Beresford, SA, et al. "Low-fat dietary pattern and risk of colorectal cancer: the Women's Health Initiative Randomized Controlled Dietary Modification Trial," *JAMA*, (2006), 295:64354, http://www.jama.ama-assn.org/cgi/content/full /295/6/643

Biomed.com, "The Protein Connection," http://biomedx.com/zeta /page6.html

Blake, John, "As Children Starve, World Struggles for Solutions," *CNN.com*, (November 18, 2008), http://www.cnn.com/2008/ US/11/17/hunger.week/index.html

Bluejay, Michael, "A History of Vegetarianism with an emphasis on the U.S. from 1970 +," http://michaelbluejay.com/veg/ history.html see reference to McDougall, John A. M.D., The McDougall Program, (1990).

boston.com, "Are the lab rat's days numbered?" http://www. boston.com/business/healthcare/articles/2009/03/30/are_the_l ab_rats_days_numbered/?page=1

Brouwer, E., "Gerritt Jan Mulder: Biography," *The Journal of Nutrition*, (The Wistar Institute of Anatomy and Biology, 1952), http://jn.nutrition.org/cgi/reprint/46/1/1.pdf

Brouwer, Ingeborg A., Martin B. Katan and Peter L. Zock,

"Dietary -Linolenic Acid Is Associated with Reduced Risk of Fatal Coronary Heart Disease, but Increased Prostate Cancer Risk: A Meta-Analysis," The American Society for Nutritional Sciences J. Nutr. 134:919-922, (April 2004), http://jn.nutrition.org/cgi/content/full/134/4/919

Brownell, Kelly D., "Childhood Obesity," *Issues in Science and Technology, Forum*, (Summer 2005), http://www.issues.org/21.4/forum.html

Burros, Marian, "Prudent Diet and Cancer Rise," *The New York Times*, (June 23, 1982), http://query.nytimes.com/gst/fullpage.html?sec=health&res=9807EFD7143BF930A15755C0A964948260

CA: A Cancer Journal for Clinicians, "American Cancer Society Guidelines on Nutrition and Physical Activity for Cancer Prevention," (Oct 2006) 56(5):254-81, quiz 313-4, http://caonline.amcancersoc.org/cgi/content/full/56/5/254

The Candle Café, "Candle Café Valentine's Day 2009," http://www.candlecafe.com/

Campaign for Commercial-free Childhood, "Guest Opinion: Schools should ditch partnerships with McDonald's," (January 2, 2008), http://www.commercialexploitation.org/news/schools should.htm

Campbell, Colin T., and Thomas M. Campbell II, *The China Study*, (Dallas: BenBella Books, 2005).

Campbell, T. Colin, PhD., "Critique of Report on 'Food, Nutrition and the Prevention of Cancer: A Global Perspective,'" (March/April 2001), *Nutrition Today*, vol. 36(2).

Carpenter, Kenneth J., "The Life and Times of W.O. Atwater: The 1993 W.O. Atwater Centennial Memorial Lecture," *Department of Nutritional Sciences, University of California, Berkeley*. http://jn.nutrition.org/cgi/reprint/124/9_Suppl/1707S.pdf

Carpenter, Kenneth, *Protein and Energy: A Study of Changing Ideas in Nutrition*, (Cambridge, New York: Cambridge University Press, 1994), http://books.google.com/books?id=GtQThfnh

KLsC&dq=Kenneth+Carpenter,+Protein+and+Energy:+A+Stu dy+of+Changing+Ideas+in+Nutritio&printsec=frontcover&so urce=bn&hl=en&ei=Lq8xSuK7A5-aMq3AhJMK&sa=X&oi =book_result&ct=result&resnum=5

Carey, John, "Do Cholesterol Drugs Do Any Good?" (January 17, 2008), *Business Week,* http://www.businessweek.com/ magazine/content/08_04/b4068052092994.htm?chan=search

Cawley, John, "Markets and Childhood Obesity Policy," *The Future of Children,* (2006), 16, no. 1, http://www.future-ofchildren.org/information2826/information_show.htm?doc_ id=355339

Center for Science in the Public Interest, "FDA Web Site on Drug Ads Developed by Drug Industry PR Firm," (Sept. 15, 2008), http://www.cspinet.org/new/200809152.html

Center for Science in the Public Interest, Litigation Project: Current Docket, http://www.cspinet.org/litigation/

Center for Science in the Public Interest, "Two-thirds of States Get Poor Grades on School Food Report Card," (Feb. 7, 2008), Newsroom, http://www.cspinet.org/new/200711281.html

Chamber, Jaime, "The Pig on Your Plate: The Injustice of Factory Farming," *The Humanist,* Essay, Kirksville, MO, http://www. thehumanist.org/humanist/articles/essay. chambers.doc

Chan, JM, and EL Giovannucci, "Dairy products, calcium, and vitamin D and risk of prostate cancer," Epidemiol, Revs. 23 (2001): 87-92.

Chen, Shaohua and Martin Ravallion, "The developing world is poorer than we thought, but no less successful in the fight against poverty," Policy Research Working Paper, *World Bank* (August 1, 2008) http://econ.worldbank.org/external/default/ main?pagePK=64165259&theSitePK=469372&piPK=64165421 &menuPK=64166093&entityID=000158349_20080826113239. See also http://siteresources.worldbank.org/DEC/Resources /Poverty-Brief-in-English.pdf

Chinese scripted title, http://www.yozemi.ac.jp/les/bb-tvnet/

jissen/tomita/tomita10.pdf

Columbia University, "Department of Psychiatry," http://ps-handbook.com/2008/node/289

Columbia University, "Medical Research with Animals," http://cumc.columbia.edu/research/animal/standards.html

Craines Detroit Business, "Western Chic at the sixth-annual Cattle Baron's Ball," (September 30, 2008), http://www.crainsdetroit.com/article/20080930/GIVERS/809309985

Cruel Science, "Animal Use Statistics," http://www.cruelscience.ca/resources-stat.htm

CSPI Newsroom, "Americans and Europeans Want Tougher Action on Childhood Obesity and Diet-Related Disease," (April 2, 2008), http://www.cspinet.org/new/200804022.html

CSPI Newsroom, "Consumer Groups in 20 Countries Urge Coke, Pepsi to Limit Soft Drink Marketing to Children," (January 3, 2008), http://www.cspinet.org/new/200801031.html

Daily News Central, "US Turning Blind Eye to Rx Drug-Abuse Epidemic," http://health.dailynewscentral.com/content/view/1232/0

Daily Post (Liverpool, England), Daily Post Comment, "Junk Food Ad Ban Is a Drop in the Ocean," (November 15, 2004). http://www.highbeam.com/Search.aspx?q=Daily+Post+Comment+%e2%80%9cJunk+Food+Ad+Ban+Is+a+Drop+in+the+Ocean%e2%80%9d+

Davis, Carole and Etta Saltos, "Dietary Recommendations and How They Have Changed Over Time," *USDA publication,* AIB-750, USDA/ERS, http://www.ers.usda.gov/publications/aib750/aib750b.pdf

Davis, Devra, *The Secret History of the War on Cancer,* (New York: Basic Books, 2007).

Demark-Wahnefried, Wendy, Thomas J. Polascik, Stephen L. George, Boyd R. Switzer, John F. Madden, Mack T. Ruffin, IV, Denise C. Snyder, Kouros Owzar, Vera Hars, David M. Albala, Philip J. Walther, Cary N. Robertson, Judd W. Moul,

Barbara K. Dunn, Dean Brenner, Lori Minasian, Philip Stella and Robin T. Vollmer, "Flaxseed Supplementation (Not Dietary Fat Restriction) Reduces Prostate Cancer Proliferation Rates in Men Presurgery," *Cancer Epidemiology Biomarkers & Prevention*, 17, 3577-3587, (December 1, 2008), doi10.1158/1055-9965.EPI-08-0008, http://cebp.aacrjournals.org/cgi/content/abstract/ 17/12/3577

De Monaco, Herald J., M.S., "The New NCEP Guidelines and Current Patterns of Statin Prescribing," in *Drug Therapy Management*, Massachusetts General Hospital, Vol. XI, Issue 5, http://www2.massgeneral.org/pharmacy/Newsletters/2001/June%202001/New%20NCEP%20Guidelines%20and%20Current%20Patterns%20of%20Statin%20Prescribing.htm

Dennis, Leslie K., Linda G. Snetselaar, Brian J. Smith, Ron E. Stewart, and Michael E. C. Robbins, "Problems with the Assessment of Dietary Fat in Prostate Cancer Studies," *American Journal of Epidemiology*, (2004), 160(5):436-444; doi:10.1093/aje/kwh243, http://aje.oxfordjournals.org/cgi/content/full/160/5/436

Department of Health and Human Services, Center for Disease Control, "National Diabetes Fact Sheet 2007," http://www.cdc.gov/diabetes/pubs/pdf/ndfs_2007.pdf

Derson, Daniela, "Just Like South Africa," *New Voices, National Jewish Student Magazine*, (November 17, 2002), http://newvoices.org/features/just-like-south-africa.html

Diabetes Care, "A Low-Fat Vegan Diet Improves Glycemic Control and Cardiovascular Risk Factors in a Randomized Clinical Trial in Individuals With Type 2 Diabetes," (August 2006), Volume 29, No. 8, http://www.nealbarnard.org/pdfs/Diabetes-Care.pdf

Epstein, Dr. Samuel, interviewed by Amy Goodman, "Most Censored Story: Does the American Cancer Society Work to Prevent Cancer?" *Democracy Now, daily TV/radio news program*, (April 13, 2000), http://www.democracynow.org/

2000/4/13/most_censored_story_does_the_american

Epstein, Samuel S., *The Politics of Cancer Revisited*, (New York: East Ridge Press, 1998).

Esselstyn, Caldwell B., Jr., MD, *Prevent and Reverse Heart Disease*, (New York: Penguin Group, 2007), http://books.google.com/books?id=hihHaBiKKU8C&dq=Caldwell+Esselstyn,+B.+Jr.,+MD,+Prevent+and+Reverse+Heart+Disease&printsec=frontcover&source=bn&hl=en&ei=OrIxSsqTA4zyMpDhqYcK&sa=X&oi=book_result&ct=result&resnum=4

Eves, Howard W., *Mathematical Circles Adieu and Return to Mathematical Circles*, Mathematical Circles, Vol. III (Washington, D.C.: The Mathematical Association of America, Inc., 2003).

femail.com.au, "The Reverse Diabetes Diet," http://www.femail.com.au/the-reverse-diabetes-diet.htm

Food and Agriculture Organization of the United Nations, "Livestock's Long Shadow," Summary and Conclusions, (Rome 2007), http://www.fao.org/docrep/010/a0701e/a0701e00.HTM

Food & Water Europe, "A Factory Farm Force: US Multinational Smithfield Moves into Europe," (2008), see Scribd, http://www.scribd.com/doc/6303027/A-Factory-Farm-Force-US-Multinational-Smithfield-Moves-into-Europe*The Food Studies Institute*, http://www.foodstudies.org/Curriculum/LessonSummaries.htm

Forbes.com, "David R. Bethune," http://people.forbes.com/profile/david-r-bethune/14859

Forbes.com, "Essex Dental Benefits to Cover Zila's ViziLite Plus for Oral Cancer Screenings" (Nov. 4, 2008), http://www.forbes.com/businesswire/feeds/businesswire/2008/11/04/businesswire20081104005228r1.html

Framingham Study, "The Framingham Heart Beat," (Winter 2005), http://www.framinghamheartstudy.org/participants/new

sletters/winter2005.pdf

Freston, Kathy, "On Cancer and a Vegetarian Diet," *The Huffington Post,* (January 12, 2009), http://www.huffington post.com/kathy-freston/on-cancer-and-a-vegetaria_b_46661. html

Fried, Ellen and Michele Simon, "The Competitive Food Conundrum: Can Government Regulations Improve School Food?" *Duke Law Journal,* (2007), 56, no. 6, www.law. duke.edu/shell/cite.pl?56+Duke+L.+J.+1491+pdf

Friends of Narconnon, "History of Methamphetamine," http://www.friendsofnarconon.org/drug_education/drug_inf ormation/meth_%10_speed/history_ of_methamphetamine/

Frontline, "ADHD — An Update," http://www.pbs.org/wgbh/ pages/frontline/shows/medicating/etc/adhdupdate.html

Galland, Leo, "Four Patterns of Dysbiosis" in Comprehensive Digestive Stool Analysis Application Guide, *Genova Diagnostic,* http://www.genovadiagnostics.com/files/profile_ assets/referenced_materials/CDSA-AppGuide.pdf

Galland, Leo, *Power Healing,* (New York: Random House, 1997).

Gersh, Bernard J. M.D., ed., *Mayo Clinic Heart Book,* 2nd ed., (New York: William Morrow, 2000), pp. 190-196,

Garfalk, Connie, "Help, My Cat Loves Me," *Offbeat Cats,* http://www.offbeat-cats.com/feature_feelings_e.html

Giles, Jim and Meredith Wadman, "Grants Fall Victim to NIH Success," Nature (October 26, 2006), 443, 894-89, http://www. nature.com/nature/journal/v443/n7114/full/443894a.html

Giovannucci, E, "Dietary influences of 1,25 (OH)2 vitamin D in relation to prostate cancer: a hypothesis." *Cancer Causes and Control* 9 (1998): 567-582.

Gold, Mark, "The Global Benefits of Eating Less Meat," *Compassion in World Farming Trust,* (2004), 16, http://www.wellfedworld.org/PDF/CIWF%20Eat%20Less%20 Meat.pdf

goveg.com, "Cancer: Killing Animals is Killing Us," http://www.

goveg.com/cancer.asp

goveg.com, "Meat and Strokes," http://www.goveg.com/strokes-meat.asp

goveg.com, "PETA Undercover: Sacred and Federal Laws Violated at Iowa Slaughterhouse," http://www.goveg.com /feat/agriprocessors/

Green, Matthew, "Udder Confusion: Difficult Choices in the Dairy Aisle," *Edible East Bay*, (Spring 2008), http://www. edibleeastbay.com/content/pages/articles/spring08/udder.pdf

Gursche, Siegfried, "I have A," *Alive Academy*, (February 2003), # 244, http://www.alive.com/1252a4a2.php?subject_bread_ cramb=852

Halweil, Brian, "Meat Production Continues to Rise," *Worldwatch Institute*, (August 20, 2008), http://www.worldwatch.org/ node/5443

Hardinge, Mervyn G., "The Protein Myth: when too much of a good thing is a bad thing," *BNET*, http://findarticles.com/ p/articles/mi_m0826/is_n1_v6/ai_8174479

Harkin, Tom, *Iowa's Senator*, "It's time for better nutrition in our schools," *United States Senate*, http://harkin.senate.gov/pr /col.cfm?id=274213

Harvard School of Public Health, "Fats and Cholesterol: Out with the Bad, In with the Good," http://www.hsph.harvard. edu/nutritionsource/what-should-you-eat/fats-full-story/index.html

Harvard School of Public Health, "The Nutrition Source, Low-Fat Diet Not a Cure -All," http://www.hsph.harvard.edu /nutritionsource/nutrition-news/low-fat/*HealthCentral.com*, "About Dr. Dean," http://www.healthcentral.com/drdean/408/deana bout.html

Holguin, Jamie, "Statins' Side Effects Under Fire," *CBS Evening News*, (October 11, 2004), http://www.cbsnews.com/stories/ 2004 /10/11/eveningnews/main648685.shtml

Howard, B.V., L. Van Horn, J. Hsia et al., "Low-fat dietary

pattern and risk of cardiovascular disease: the Women's Health Initiative Randomized Controlled Dietary Modification Trial," *JAMA*, (2006), 295:6, 655-66, http://jama.ama-assn.org/cgi/content/full/295/6/655

Horton, Richard, *Health Wars: On the Global Front Lines of Modern Medicine*, (New York: The New York Review of Books, 2003).

The Huffington Post, "Low-Carb? Low-Fat? Study finds calories count more," (February 25, 2009), http://www.huffingtonpost.com/huff-wires/20090225/med-dueling-diets/

The Huffington Post, "T. Colin Campbell: Biography," *T. Colin Campbell Blog*, http://www.huffingtonpost.com/t-colin-camp bell/

Human Ecology Forum, "China study shows diet-disease connection," 22.n3 (Fall 1994): 9(1),
http://www.accessmylibrary.com/article-1G1-16642776/china-study-shows-diet.html

Humane Society of the United States, "Undercover Investigation Reveals Rampant Animal Cruelty at California Slaughter Plant — A Major Beef Supplier to America's School Lunch Program," (January 30, 2008), http://www.hsus.org/farm/news/ournews/undercover_investigation.html

Humane Society of the United States, "USDA Animal Welfare Act Enforcement Report," http://www.hsus.org/animals_in_research/animals_in_research_news/usda_report_on_animal_welfare.htm

Iaccobo, Karen and Michael Iaccobo, *Vegetarian America*, (Westport, CT.: Greenwood Publishing Group, Inc., 2004), http://books.google.com/books?id=0AiAz62C_jc C&printsec=copyright&dg=had+a+heart+attack+in+Framingham+in +35+years+in+anyone+who+had+a+cholesterol+under+150 #PPA210,M1

In Defense of Animals, "Help End Nicotine Experiments on Monkeys at OHSU," http://www.vivisectioninfo.org/campa igns/spindel/

In Defense of Animals, "IDA's Response to NIH Defense of Lisberger," http://www.vivisectioninfo.org/uscf/nihresponse.html

In Defense of Animals, "The Horrific Monkey Experiments of New York University," http://www.vivisectioninfo.org/nyu.html

In Defense of Animals, "The Truth About Vivisection," http://www.vivisectioninfo.org/lisberger.html

Integrity in Science, "American Cancer Society, Tied to Drug companies, von Eschenbach," *Center for Science in the Public Interest*, (March 3, 2006), http://www.cspinet.org/integrity/watch/200603241.html

International Vegetarian Union, "Ancient Greece and Rome: Socrates (470-399 BCE)," http://www.ivu.org/history/greece_rome/socrates.html

International Vegetarian Union, "Herodotus (484-425 B.C.)," http://www.ivu.org/history/greece_rome/herodotus.html

Jarvis, William T., Ph.D., *"The Physicians Committee for Responsible Medicine,"* National Council Against Health Fraud, http://www.ncahf.org/articles/o-r/pcrm.html

The Journal of Physical Education, Recreation & Dance, "Child Obesity-What Can Schools Do?" (2001), vol. 72, Issue: 2.

Katch, Frank L., "History Makers, Wilbur Olin Atwater (1844-1907)," http://www.sportsci.org/news/history/atwater/atwater.html

Kaiseredu.org, "U.S. Healthcare Costs: Background Brief," http://www.kaiseredu.org/topics_im.asp?imID=1&parentID=61&id=358#1b

Kassirer, Jerome P., *On the Take: How Medicine's Complicity with Big Business Can Endanger Your Health*, (New York: Oxford University Press, 2005), http://books.google.com/books?id=5jsiffLtnm8C&dq=Jerome+P.+Kassirer,+On+the+Take,+How+Medicine%E2%80%99s+Complicity+with+Big+Business+Can+Endanger+Your+Health&printsec=frontcover&source=bl&ots=NCo-gfZpj&sig=WJ4Mb79aF8z7XijQEvPkKSCwa7s&hl=

en&ei=d8UxStLtN-CLtgfVu5SwCQ&sa= X&oi= book_result& ct=result&resnum=3

Kestin et al., "Cardiovascular Disease Risk Factors in Free-Living Men: Comparison of Two Prudent Diets," *American Journal of Clinical Nutrition*, (1989) 50, 280, http:// interactive.zogby.com/fuse/messageview.cfm?catid=25&threa did=22066

Knight, Matthew, "Scientist: stem cells could end animal testing," (Dec. 22, 2008), Animals and Animal Rights in the Media Worldwide, http://animals-in-the-news.blogspot.com /2008/12/professor-christine-mummery-van-leids.html

Koplan, Jeffrey P., Catharyn T. Liverman, Vivica I. Kraak, Eds., *Preventing Childhood Obesity, Health in the Balance*, Institute of Medicine of the National Academies, (Washington, D.C.: The National Academies Press, 2005), http://www.nap.edu/ openbook.php?isbn=0309091969&page=1

Kover, Amy, "Wall Street Week: Unhip, Unabashed, Unbeaten Louis Rukeyser, Superstar," *Fortune*, (Aug. 3, 1998), http:// money.cnn.com/magazines/fortune/fortune_archive/1998/08/0 3/246302/index.htm

Kwiterovich, Peter O., Jr., M.D., *The Johns Hopkins Complete guide for Preventing and Reversing Heart Disease*, (Rocklin, California: Rima Publishing, 1993), Appendix B. Kushi, Mishio, *The Macrobiotic Approach to Cancer*, (New York: Avery, 1991), http://books.google.com/books?id=H_DSJn3DCeYC&pg =PA7&lpg=PA7&dq=Mishio+Kushi,+The+Macrobiotic+Appro ach+to+Cancer&source=bl&ots=DeoVWPMiau&sig=8o0emRn qzN7hXdCyUQkvDrpiKKo&hl=en&ei=dkp8StiyNJHONej0te UC&sa=X&oi=book_result&ct=result&resnum=1#v=onepage &q=&f=false

Lammers, Stephen E. and Allan Verhey, *On Moral Medicine: Theological Perspectives in Medical Ethics*, 2 ed. (Grand Rapids, MI: William B. Eerdmans Publishing, 1998), http://books. google.com/books?id=HStj9xiKx44C&pg=PA889&lpg=PA889

&dq=Men+who+have+practiced+tortures+on+animals+witho
ut+pity,+relating+them+without+shame&source=bl&ots=EM
mhH4DYwE&sig=X_BYsgnLbuyAhoBsZlh0IzRmJw4&hl=en
&ei=20w1SvnyO5qltgf99rW8CQ&sa=X&oi=book_result&ct=r
esult&resnum=6#PPA889,M1

Lappé, Francis Moore, *Diet for a Small Planet Revisited*, (New
York: Random House, Inc. 1982), http://books.google.com/
books?id=djAaUJlny0cC&pg=PA115&lpg=PA115&dq=Franci
s+Moore+Lapp%C3%A9,+Diet+for+a+Small+Planet+Revisite
d,&source=bl&ots=FsOcs5YR1V&sig=QtyF5uZM3Jv7XCHN
G3Hst8x1Qgo&hl=en&ei=Y7AxSur-M4-oM-iFgZcK&sa=
X&oi=book_result&ct=result&resnum=2

Layton, Lindsay, "Peanut Executive Takes The Fifth," *Washington
Post*, (February 12, 2009), http://www.washingtonpost.com/
wp-dyn/content/article/2009/ 02/11/AR2009021104174.html

Leckie, Stephen, "How Meat-Centered Eating Patterns Affect
Food Security and the Environment," *International
Development Research Center*, http://www.idrc.ca/en/ev-30610-
201-1-DO_TOPIC.html

Lee, Christopher, "Doctors, Legislators Resist Drugmakers'
Prying Eyes," *The Washington Post*, (May 22, 2007), see
http://www.washingtonpost.com/wpdyn/content/article/200
7/05/21/AR2007052101701.html

Lindeberg, Staffan, "Paleolithic diet ('stone age' diet),"
Scandinavian Journal of Food & Nutrition, (June 2005), 49 (2):
75-7, http://www.foodandnutritionresearch.net/index.php/
fnr/article/viewFile/1526/1394

Linn, Susan and Diane E. Levin, "Stop marketing 'yummy' food
to children," Commentary, *The Christian Science Monitor*,
(June 20, 2002). http://www.csmonitor.com/2002/0620/p09
s01-coop.htm

Lipsky, Martin S. MD, Marla Mendelson, MD, Stephen Havas,
MD, MPH, and Michael Miller, MD, *American Medical
Association Guide to Preventing and Treating Heart Disease*,

(Hoboken, New Jersey: John Wiley & Sons, Inc., 2008), http://books.google.com/books?id=4iSoMzkwStMC&print sec=frontcover&dq=American+Medical+Association+Guide+t o+Preventing+and+Treating+Heart+Disease&source=bl&ots= Wu7XOW5le&sig=yOOT2N6ljFl_R11wUOyWzfuLQD8&hl=e n&ei=KXxETKvYFsL6lwfCvIDjDQ&sa=X&oi=book_result&ct =result&resnum=2&ved=0CCEQ6AEwAQ#v=onepage&q&f=f alse

Lyman, Howard F. and Glen Merzer, *Mad Cowboy: Plain Truth from the Cattle Rancher Who Won't Eat Meat*, (New York: Touchstone, 1998).

Mahar, Maggie, "The Bad Science that Created the Cholesterol Con," (March 3, 2008), Alternet, http://www.alternet.org/ healthwellness/78554/the_bad_science_that_created_the_chol esterol_con/

Martin, Darlene, "NF97-315 Overview of the USDA School Meals Initiative for Healthy Children," Historical Materials from University of Nebraska - Lincoln Extension, (January 1997), http://digitalcommons.unl.edu/cgi/viewcontent.cgi?article= 1416&context=extensionhist

Mason, Stephen F., *A History of the Sciences*, (New York: Collier Books, 1977).

Matthews, Robert A.J., "Medical progress depends on animals, doesn't it," *Podium*, (2008), J R Soc Med, 101: 95-98. DOI 10.1258/jrsm.2007.070164, http://www.animalexperiments. info/assets/studies/Human%20relevance%20Contributions% 20to%20medical%20progress%20Matthews%202008%20JRS M.pdf

McDougall, John, Dr., "A Brief History of Protein: Passion, Social Bigotry, Rats, and Enlightenment," http://www.all-creatures.org/mfz/health-protein-jm.html

McDougall Newsletter, (February 2006), Vol 5, No. 2, http://www. drmcdougall.com/misc/2006nl/february/response.htm

McGee, Charles T., *Heart Frauds*, (Colorado Springs: Health Wise

Publications, 2001), http://books.google.com/books?id=4tr IQScMS_UC&dq=Charles+T.+McGee,+Heart+Frauds&printse c=frontcover&source=bn&hl=en&ei=R7QxStmIKJuetweCpO THCQ&sa=X&oi=book_result&ct=result&resnum=4

McLean, Rob, "Calcium and Osteoporosis," *Cyberparent*, http:// www.cyberparent.com/nutrition/osteoporosiscausemilk.htm

McNeil, Donald G., Jr., "Group Documents Cruelty to Turkeys," *The New York Times*, (November 18, 2008), http://www. nytimes.com/2008/11/19/dining/19peta.html?_r=1&scp=1&sq =Aviagen%20Turkey%20Plant&st=cse

Melton, Doug, interviewed by Charlie Rose in "Stem Cells with Dr. Doug Melton," *Charlie Rose Show*, http://www. charlierose.com/view/interview/10274

Merck Source, "For Your Heart's Sake Lower Your Cholesterol," http://www.mercksource.com/pp/us/cns/cns_healthink_tem plate.jspzQzpgzEzzSzppdocszSzuszSzcnszSzcontentzSzheal thinkzSzlowercholesterolzPzhtml

Moss, Ralph W., *The Cancer Industry* (New York: Paragon House, 1991).

Moss, Ralph W., *Cancer Therapy* (Brooklyn: Equinox Press, 2001).

Moynihan, Ray, "Disease-Mongers: How Doctors, Drug Companies, and Insurers Are Making You Feel Sick," Review, *BMJ* 2002;324(7342):923, http://ukpmc.ac.uk/ articlerender.cgi?artid=477342

Moynihan, Ray and Alan Cassels, *Selling Sickness: How the World's Biggest Pharmaceutical Companies are Turning us All Into Patients*, (New York: Nation Books, 2006), http://books. google.com/books?id=fftKR4y2NMIC&dq=Ray+Moynihan+a nd+Alan+Cassels,+Selling+Sickness:+How+the+World%E2%8 0%99s+Biggest+Pharmaceutical+Companies+are&printsec=fr ontcover&source=bl&ots=4yKwHKtMch&sig=DYvqecWKTd 120JpENJAfHfCEcgA&hl=en&ei=x8QxSpqpHY7KtgeG-ZG4CQ&sa=X&oi=book_result&ct=result&resnum=2

Mukerjee, Madhusree, "Trends in Animal Research," *Scientific*

American Magazine, (February 1997).

My Fox Detroit, "2008 American Cancer Society Cattle Barron's Ball," WJBK Web Team, (Sept. 7, 2008), http://www.myfoxdetroit.com/myfox/pages/InsideFox/Detail?contentId=7377482&version=2&locale=EN-US&layoutCode=TSTY&pageId=5.7.1

Nationmaster.com, "Health Statistics: Life expectancy at birth, Total population by country, 2008," http://www.nationmaster.com/graph/hea_lif_exp_at_bir_tot_pop-life-expectancy-birth-total-population&date=2008

The National Cancer Institute, "Breast Cancer Prevention, Estrogen (Endogenous)," http://www.cancer.gov/cancertopics/pdq/prevention/breast/Patient/page3#Keypoint5

National Cancer Institute, "The National Cancer Institute: More Than 70 Years of Excellence in Cancer Research," http://www.cancer.gov/aboutnci/excellence-in-research

National Center for Health Statistics http://www.cdc.gov/nchs/products/pubs/pubd/hestats/overweight/overwght_adult_03.htm

National Cholesterol Education Program, "High Blood Cholesterol, What You Need to Know," http://www.nhlbi.nih.gov/health/public/heart/chol/wyntk.htm#numbers

National Dairy Council, "Educators Journey Into Nutrition Education," Nutrition Explorations, (March 2009), http://www.nutritionexplorations.com/educators/lessons/chef-combo/chef-combo.asp?tab=1

National Institutes of Health, "Women's Health Trial, Feasibility Study in Minority Populations," http://clinicaltrials.gov/ct2/show/NCT00000481

National Institutes of Health, National Heart, Lung, and Blood Institute, "Dash Eating Plan: Your Guide to Lowering Your Blood Pressure with Dash," http://www.nhlbi.nih.gov/health/public/heart/hbp/dash/new_dash.pdf

National Research Council, National Academy of Sciences, "Diet, Nutrition, and Cancer," (1982), http://www.nutritioncancer.

com/history.html

Natural News.com, "JAMA refuses to exclude authors who hide financial ties to drug companies," (Aug. 6, 2006), http://www. naturalnews.com/019914.html

Nestle, Marion, *Food Politics: How the Food Industry Influences Nutrition and Health*, (University of California Press, 2003), http://books.google.com/books?id=yD_RCqOE5goC& dq=Marion+Nestle,+Food+Politics:+How+the+Food+Industry +Influences+Nutrition+and+Health&printsec=frontcover&so urce=bn&hl=en&ei=wasxSrjFCIHcM7GpwPsJ&sa=X&oi=boo k_result&ct=result&resnum=4

Nichols, Bradford L., Jr. and Peter J. Reeds, "History of Nutrition: History and Current Status of *Research in Human Energy Metabolism*," (USDA Symposium, Baylor College of Medicine and Texas Children's Hospital, Houston, TX), *American Institute of Nutrition*, (*Journal of Nutrition*, (April 1991), 121: 1889-1890), http://jn.nutrition.org/cgi/reprint/121/ 11/1889.pdf

NIH News, "Heart-Healthy, Reduced-Calorie Diets Promote Long-term Weight Loss," (February 25, 2009), *U.S. Department of Health and Human Services*, http://public.nhlbi. nih.gov/newsroom/home/GetPressRelease.aspx?id=2624

North Carolina Associates for Biomedical Research, "How Many and What Kinds of Animals are Used in Biomedical Research," http//www.ncabr.org/biomzed/FAQ_animal/faq_animal_13. html

NutritionCancer.com, "History of the Link Between Nutrition and Cancer," http://www.nutritioncancer.com/history.html

Oceans Alert, "PCB Information," http://www.oceansalert .org/pcbinfo.htm

Office of Technology Assessment, Congress of the United States, "Unconventional Cancer Treatments," (1990), http://www. nutritioncancer.com/history.html

Oregon Health and Science University, "Eliot Spindel," http://www.

ohsu.edu/xd/research/centers-institutes/onprc/scientific-discovery/scientists/eliot-spindel.cfm

Ornish, Dean, M.D., Dr. *Dean Ornish's Program for Reversing Heart Disease*, (New York: Ballantine Books, 1991).

Ornish, Dean, M.D., *Eat More, Weigh Less*, (New York: Harper Perennial, 1994).

Payer, Lynn, *Disease-Mongers: How Doctors, Drug Companies, and Insurers Are Making You Feel Sick*, (New York: Wiley & Sons, 1992).

Patterson, Charles, *Eternal Treblinka: Our Treatment of Animals and the Holocaust*, (New York: Lantern Books, 2002).

PBS interview of Dr. John Young, "Animal Testing Ethics," *Religious & Ethics Newsweekly*, (August 15, 2008), Episode no. 1150, http://www.pbs.org/wnet/religionandethics/week1150 /cover.html

Pearson, Thomas A., "The Prevention Of Cardiovascular Disease: Have We Really Made Progress?" (2007), *Health Affairs*, 26, no. 1, 49-60, http://content.healthaffairs .org/cgi/content/full/26/1/49

Pelto, Gretel H. and Pertti J. Pelto, *The Human Adventure: An Introduction to Anthropology* (New York: Macmillan Publishing Co., 1976).

PETA, "Undercover Investigations: Thousands of Chickens Tortured by KFC Supplier," http://www.kentuckyfriedcruelty .com/u-pilgrimspride.asp

PETA Media Center, "Animal Experiments: Overview, Funding and Accountability," http://www.peta.org/mc/factsheet_ display.asp?ID=126

PETATV.com, "Undercover Investigation Reveals Hormel Supplier's Abuse of Mother Pigs and Piglets," http:// getactive.peta.org/campaign/iowa_pigfarm_abuse2. See video, http://www.petatv.com/tvpopup/video.asp?video= iowa_sow_farm_investigation_9-08_web_edit_peta&Player= wm

Peta2 Free For All, "Take Charge: Stop School Slaughter," http://www.peta2.com/takecharge/t-stoptheslaughter.asp

Piccolo, Cynthia M., "Timeline: Ibn al-Nafis, c. 1210-1288," *Medhunters*, http://www.medhunters.com/articles/timeline IbnAlNafis.html

Physicians Committee for Responsible Medicine, "Good Medicine, Illegal Experiments: Physicians File Lawsuit Against USCF for Violating Animal Welfare Law," (Autumn, 2007), Volume XVI, Number 4, http://www.pcrm.org/magazine/gm07au umn/illegal_experiments.html

Physicians Committee for Responsible Medicine, "March of Dimes-Funded Animal Experiments: An Overview," reviewed by Peggy Carlson, M.D., and Kristie Stoick, M.P.H., http:// www.pcrm.org/resch/charities/mod_overview.html

Physicians Committee for Responsible Medicine, "PCRM Sues Glickman and Shalala, "Dietary Guidelines for 2000, the Politics of Food: A Brief History of the U.S. Dietary Guidelines," http://www.pcrm.org/news/lawsuit_history. html

Poetwilll.org, "Running for Their Lives," http://www.poetwill. org /billman_dogs.htm

Prentice, RL, B. Caan, RT Chlebowski, et al., "Low-fat dietary pattern and risk of invasive breast cancer: the Women's Health Initiative Randomized Controlled Dietary Modification Trial," *JAMA*, 2006; 295:629-42.

Preston, Julia, "Meatpacker Is Fined Nearly $10 Million," *The New York Times*, (October 29, 2008), http://www.nytimes.com /2008/10/30/us/30fine.html

Prevention Magazine, "Take This Letter To Your Doctor," (Reader Service Report), (November 1996).

Proctor , Robert N., *Cancer Wars: How Politics Shapes What We know & Don't Know*, (New York: Basic Books, 1995).

The Products, Tools & Info that you need to choose Health over Disease, "The Hoxsey Formula," https://www.illnessisoptional.com/cms/index2.php?option=com_content&do_pdf=1 &id=104

Quillin, Patrick, PhD, RD, CNS and R. Michael Williams, MD, PhD (co-editors), "Adjuvant Nutrition in Cancer Treatment," (1993), *Research Foundation, Arlington Heights, IL,* http:// www.nutritioncancer.com/history.html

Rae, Helen, "Healthy Start to the War on Junk Foods: in Association with the NHS. A North East MP Is Keen to See an End to Junk Food Advertising," Report, *Evening Chronicle,* Newcastle, England, (May 19, 2008), http://www.entre-preneur.com/tradejournals/article/179162632.html

Raysahelian.com, "Alpha Linolenic Acid, ALA," http://www. raysahelian.com/linolenic.html

Reuters, "Humane Society Says Video Shows Abused Livestock," (May 7, 2008), http://www.reuters.com/article/domestic News/idUSN0716185920080507

Rifkin, Jeremy, "Our Fellow Creatures Have Feelings — So We Should Give Them Rights Too," *Common Dreams.Org,* (August 16, 2006), http://www.commondreams.org/views03/0816-05. htm

Rifkin, Jeremy, "The World's Problem on a Plate, 2002," *News Center, CommonDreams.org* Originally published in The Guardian of London, http://www.commondreams.org/views 02/0517-03.htm

Robertson, Laurel, Carol Flinders, Brian Ruppenthal, *The New Laurel's Kitchen, A Handbook for Vegetarian Cookery & Nutrition,* 2nd ed., (Berkeley, CA: Ten Speed Press, 1986), http://books. google.com/books?id=TsChEsPHL5cC&pg=PA407&lpg=PA40 7&dq=Laurel+Robertson+et+al,+The+New+Laurel%E2%80%9 9s+Kitchen:+A+Handbook+for+Vegetarian+Cookery+%26+Nu trition&source=bl&ots=yPaYQ8GbCb&sig=SX3MEQajgpIN_o mACcf_Ir3X9CQ&hl=en&ei=oK8xSqyyOYSoM4Sr5Z4K&sa= X&oi=book_result&ct=result&resnum=5

Robbins, John, *Reclaiming Our Health,* (Tiburon, CA: HJ Kramer,

Inc., 1996).

Roysten, Angela, *Proteins for a Healthy Body*, (Chicago: Heinemann Library, 2003).

Rush PR News, "Meet Dog 3017 - Ohio State University's Latest Lab Casualty," (April 22, 2009), http://www.rushprnews.com/2009/04/22/meet-dog-3017-ohio-state-universitys-latest-lab-casualty/

Sachiko, T. St. Jeor, RD PhD; Barbara V. Howard, PhD; T. Elaine Prewitt, RD DrPH; Vicki Bovee, RD MS; Terry Bazzarre, PhD; Robert H. Eckel, MD; "Dietary Protein and Weight Reduction," *The American Heart Association*," http://circ.ahajournals.org/cgi/content/full/104/15/1869?ijkey=02c8fa98ff287d30167717c3ee0f126da3311fa5

Schlosser, Eric, *Fast Food Nation*, (New York: Houghton Mifflin, 2001).

Schweitzer, Albert, *Reverence for Life*, trans., Reginald H. Fuller (New York: Harper & Row 1969).

Scientific American, "Feds Agree to Toxicity Tests That Cut Animal Testing," http://www.scientificamerican.com/article.cfm?id=feds-agree-to-toxicity-test&page=2

Sea Shepherd Conservation Society, "United States Senate Condemns the Canadian Seal Slaughter," (May 11, 2009), http://www.seashepherd.org/news-and-media/news-090511-1.html

Senior Journal.com, "Cancer to Replace Heart Disease as Leading Killer in World by 2010, Says International Study," Health and Medicine for Senior Citizens, http://seniorjournal.com/NEWS/Health/2008/20081209-CancerToReplaceHeart.htm

Severson, Kim, "National Briefing/Education; Trying Anew To Rein In School Foods," *The New York Times*, (December 18, 2007), http://query.nytimes.com/gst/fullpage.html?res=9C07E6DD1F3AF93BA25751C1A9619C8B63

Simplot, "Feedlots," http://www.simplot.com/land/cattle_feeding/feedlots.cfm

Sourcewatch Encyclopedia, "Animal Testing," http://www.source watch.org/index.php?title=Animal_testing#Government_fun ded_vivisection

Sourcewatch Encyclopedia, "Ten Worst Laboratories," http://www. sourcewatch.org/index.php?title=Ten_Worst_Laboratories

Sheldrake, Rupert, *The Rebirth of Nature: The Greening of Science and God*, (Rochester, VT: Park Street Press, 1994).

Smith, J. Clinton, M.D., M.P.H., *Understanding Childhood Obesity*, (Jackson, MS: University Press of Mississippi, 1999).

Snowdon, "Animal Product Consumption and Mortality... in Seventh-Day Adventists," *American Journal of Clinical Nutrition*, (1988), 48, 739, http://interactive.zogby.com/fuse /messageview.cfm?catid=25&threadid=22066

Sourcewatch Encyclopedia, "Animal Testing," http://www. source-watch.org/index.php?title=Animal_testing#Government_fun ded_vivisection

Sourcewatch Encyclopedia, "Ten Worst Laboratories."

Spacedoc.net, "Statin Drugs Side Effects," *Duane Graveline website*, http://www.spacedoc.net/index.php

Stamfordplus.com, "Stamford Hospital Unveils the New Center for Integrative Medicine and Wellness," http://www.pmri .org/publications/stamford_plus_article.pdf

Stauble, Ann, "Cats and NEAVS don't fancy this Cat Fancy Article," *New England Anti-Vivisection Society*, (June 29, 2001), http://www.neavs.org/programs/avoiceforanimals/lte_catfan cy_06292001.ht

Stein, Rob, "Diet, Exercise, and Reduced Stress Slow Prostate Cancer, Study Shows," Washington Post, (August 11, 2005), http://www.washingtonpost.com/wp-dyn/content/article/ 2005/08/10/AR2005081001882.html

Stobbe, Mike, "Cancer to be Top Killer by 2010, WHO says," *newsvine.com* http://www.newsvine.com/_news/2008/12/09/ 2194410-cancer-to-be-worlds-top-killer-by-2010-who-says

Stobbe, Mike, "Smoking ban leads to major drop in heart

attacks," *newsvine.com* http://www.newsvine.com/_news/2008/12/31/2262215-smoking

Stop Animal Exploitation Now (S.A.E.N.), "Animal Experimentation in the United States,", http://www.all-creatures.org/saen/fact-anex-2007.html

Stop Animal Exploitation Now (S.A.E.N.), "Government Grants Promoting Cruelty to Animals, University of Minnesota, Minneapolis, MN, Marilyn E. Carroll, Primate Testing, 2005 - 2007," http://www.all-creatures.org/saen/res-fr-mn-umgrant-carroll-2005.html

Story, Mary and Simone French, "Food Advertising and Marketing Directed at Children and Adolescents in the U.S.," *International Journal of Behavioral Nutrition and Physical Activity,* (2004), **1**:3doi:10.1186/1479-5868-1-3, http://www.ijbnpa.org/content/1/1/3

Surfwax Health News, "Zila sees revenue leap, continued loss as operations refocus," (Oct. 16, 2007), http://news.surfwax.com/health/archives/Oral_Cancer.html

Survive Treatments for Cancer, "Did Dr. Gerson Have a Cancer Cure - 4," http://www.asunburst.com/Dr-Gersons-Cancer Cure-4.html

Sustainweb.org., "Children's food campaigners complain about ads for 'manly' burgers," Children's food campaign, news, http://www.sustainweb.org/news.php?id=165

Takrouri, Mohamad S. M., MB. ChB. FFARCS, "Medical aspects of Ala al-Din Abu'l-Hasan Ali Ibn Abi'l-Haram al-Qurashi (Ibn al-Nafis)'s contributions to science," http://www.angelfire.com/md/Takrouri/Ibn_alNafis.htm

Tangley, Laura, "Animal Emotions," *U.S. News and World Report,* (October 22, 2000), http://www.usnews.com/usnews/culture/articles/001030/archive_010364_3.htm

Text of H.R. 1363, "Child Nutrition Promotion and School Lunch Protection Act of 2007," http://www.opencongress.org/bill/110-h1363/text

Thomas, Paul R. and Robert Earl, *Opportunities in the Nutrition and Food Sciences: Research Challenges and the Next Generation of Investigators*, (Washington, D.C.: National Academy Press, 1994), http://books.nap.edu/openbook.php?record_ id=2133& page=R1

Tom Harkin, Iowa's Senator, "It's Time For Better Nutrition In Our Schools," (May 14, 2007), http://harkin.senate.gov/pr/col.cfm? id=274213

Tietz, Jeff, "Boss Hog," *Rolling Stone*, (December 14, 2006), http://www.rollingstone.com/politics/story/12840743/porks_ dirty_secret_the_nations_top_hog_producer_is_also_one_ of_americas_worst_polluters

Tuller, David, "Seeking a Fuller Picture of Statins," *The New York Times*, (July 20, 2004), http://www.nytimes.com/2004/07/20/ health/seeking-a-fuller-picture-of-statins.html?sec=health &&fta=y

University of California San Francisco, "UCSF Institutional Animal Care and Use Committee," http://www.iacuc.ucsf.edu/

University of Michigan Health System, "Calcium and Vitamin D," http://www.med.umich.edu/1libr/guides/calcium.htm

UniSci, "Lower Cholesterol Reading Can Mask Heart Attack Risk," (March 2001), http://www.unisci.com/stories/20011/ 0321013.htm

USDA Agricultural Research Service, "ARS Timeline: Founding American Nutrition Science," http://www.ars.usda.gov/is/ timeline/nutrition.htm

USDA website, "Nutrition and Your Health: Dietary Guidelines, Choose a diet that is low in fats, saturated fats, and cholesterol," http://www.nal.usda.gov/fnic/dga/dguide95.html

U.S. National Libraries of Medicine, NIH, "The Reports of the Surgeon General: The 1964 Report on Smoking and Health," http://profiles.nlm.nih.gov/NN/Views/Exhibit/narrative/smo king.html

Veracity, Dani, "Is the American Cancer Center more interested in cancer profit than cancer prevention?" (July 31, 2005), http://www.naturalnews.com/010244.html

VegWeb.com, "Forced Molting in Laying Hens," Association of Veterinarians for Animal Rights, http://vegweb.com/index.php?topic=12178.0

Ward & Lopez-Carrillo, "Dietary Factors and the Risk of Gastric Cancer in Mexico City," *American Journal of Epidemiology*, (1999), 149, 925, http://interactive.zogby.com/fuse/message view.cfm?catid=25&threadid=22066

Wasserman, Harvey , "Ethics into Action: Henry Spira and the Animal Rights Movement," *The Nation*, (October 19, 1998).

WebMD Health, "Sudden Death in 12 Kids on ADHD Drug Adderall," http://www.webmd.com/add-adhd/news/20050210/sudden-death-in-12-kids-on-adhd-drug-adderall-news

WebMD, "What is Atherosclerosis?" http://www.webmd.com/heart-disease/what-is-atherosclerosis

Weil, Andrew, *Eating Well for Optimal Health*, (New York: Random House, 2001).

Wellness Forum, http://www.wellnessforum.com/

Winston, Robert and Lori Oliwenstein, *Superhuman* (New York: Dorling Kindersly, 2000).

Winters, Lynn, "Our Judaic-Christian Heritage," Albert Schweitzer, http://www.entheology.org/library/winters/

Wolinsky, Howard, "Disease Mongering and Drug Marketing," *EMBO* (European Molecular Biology Organization), (July 6(7) 2002), Report 612-614; doi: 10.1038/sj.embor.7400476. http://www.pubmedcentral.nih.gov/articlerender.fcgi?artid=1369125

World Health Organization, The Lancet: The Lancet's Series on Maternal and Child Undernutrition, Executive Summary, http://www.who.int/nutrition/topics/Lancetseries_Executive Summary.pdf

World Health Organization, "Launch of the Chronic Disease Report," (2006), http://www.oxha.org/knowledge/publica-

tions/mauritius-launch-of-the-who-chronic-disease-report.
pdf

World Health Organization,"Undernutrition is the underlying cause of death for at least 30% of all children under age five," *Fact File,* http://www.who.int/features/factfiles/global_burden/facts/en/index9.html

Yarri, Dana, *The Ethics of Animal Experimentation: A Critical Analysis and Constructive Christian Proposal,* (Oxford University Press, 2005).

Yeager, Selene, Jennifer Haigh, Sari Harrar, Selene Y. Craig, *Complete Book of Alternative Nutrition,* (Emmaus, PA,: Rodale Press, 1997).

Young, John, interviewed by Saul Gonzalez on PBS with Tim O'Brien, anchor, "Animal Testing Ethics," *Religious & Ethics Newsweekly,* (August 15, 2008), Episode no. 1150, contains interview transcription and video, http://www.pbs.org/wnet/religionandethics/week1150/cover.html

Zamir, Tzachi, *Ethics and the Beast,* (Princeton University Press, 2007), http://books.google.com/books?id=3oEKodnhg48C&dq=Tzachi+Zamir,+Ethics+and+the+Beast&printsec=frontcover&source=bn&hl=en&ei=2LwxSovNN56qtgePz_yqCQ&sa=X&oi=book_result&ct=result&resnum=4.

Index

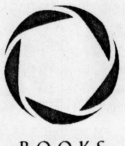

BOOKS

O is a symbol of the world, of oneness and unity. In different cultures it also means the "eye," symbolizing knowledge and insight. We aim to publish books that are accessible, constructive and that challenge accepted opinion, both that of academia and the "moral majority."

Our books are available in all good English language bookstores worldwide. If you don't see the book on the shelves ask the bookstore to order it for you, quoting the ISBN number and title. Alternatively you can order online (all major online retail sites carry our titles) or contact the distributor in the relevant country, listed on the copyright page.

See our website www.o-books.net for a full list of over 500 titles, growing by 100 a year.

And tune in to myspiritradio.com for our book review radio show, hosted by June-Elleni Laine, where you can listen to the authors discussing their books.

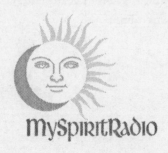

MySpiritRadio